Cerebrovascular disease

Prevention, diagnosis and treatment are the watchwords in stroke research, for basic neuroscientists and clinicians alike. This book, from the 22nd Princeton Conference on Cerebrovascular Disease, contains contributions from outstanding investigators on current topics in stroke research.

The contents cover the current status and future directions of stroke pathophysiology, diagnosis and treatment, with special emphasis on the molecular and cellular mechanisms of ischemic cell death and repair, and clinical issues including imaging, risk factors, and therapeutic strategies in stroke.

Available in print and online, this survey of the basic and clinical science of stroke is an essential resource for all involved in advancing knowledge of cerebrovascular disease.

Pak H. Chan is Professor of Neurosurgery, Neurology and Neurological Sciences at Stanford University. He holds a Javits Neuroscience Investigator Award from the National Institutes of Health, is President of the National Neurotrauma Society and is currently an editorial board member for *Stroke, Journal of Neuroscience, Journal of Cerebral Blood Flow & Metabolism* and *Journal of Neurotrauma*.

Cerebrovascular Disease

22nd Princeton Conference

Edited by

Pak H. Chan, Ph.D.

Professor of Neurosurgery, Neurology & Neurological Sciences
Faculty, Program in Neurosciences
Director, Neurosurgical Laboratories
Stanford University School of Medicine

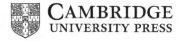

CAMBRIDGE
UNIVERSITY PRESS

CAMBRIDGE UNIVERSITY PRESS
Cambridge, New York, Melbourne, Madrid, Cape Town, Singapore,
São Paulo, Delhi, Dubai, Tokyo, Mexico City

Cambridge University Press
The Edinburgh Building, Cambridge CB2 8RU, UK

Published in the United States of America by Cambridge University Press, New York

www.cambridge.org
Information on this title: www.cambridge.org/9780521187534

First published 2002
First paperback edition 2010

A catalogue record for this publication is available from the British Library

Library of Congress Cataloguing in Publication data

Cerebrovascular disease : 22nd Princeton Conference / edited by Pak H. Chan.
p.   cm.
The 22nd Princeton Conference on Cerebrovascular Disease held in Redwood City,
California, March 20–12, 2000.
Includes bibliographical references and index.
ISBN 0 521 80254 7 (hardback)
1. Cerebrovascular disease – Pathophysiology – Congresses. 2. Cerebrovascular
disease – Treatment – Congresses. 1. Chan, Pak H. 11. Princeton Conference on
Cerebrovascular Disease (22nd : 2000 Redwood City, Calif.)
[DNLM: 1. Cerebrovascular Accident – physiopathology – Congresses. 2. Cell
Death – Congresses. 3. Cerebrovascular Accident – diagnosis – Congresses. 4.
Cerebrovascular Accident – therapy – Congresses. WL 355 C413435 2002]
RC388.5 .C3995 2002
616.1–dc21   2001025936

ISBN 978-0-521-80254-3 Hardback
ISBN 978-0-521-18753-4 Paperback

Additional resources for this publication at www.cambridge.org/9780521187534

Contents

The plate section is between pp.138 and 139 (and is also available for download from www.cambridge.org/9780521187534).

Contributors

Koji Abe
Department of Neurology
Okayama University Medical School
2-5-1 Shikatacho
Okayama 700-8558
Japan

Stuart M. Allan
School of Biological Sciences
1.124 Stopford Building
University of Manchester
Oxford Road
Manchester M13 9PT
England
UK

Susan Alexander
Department of Neurology
University of New Mexico
Albuquerque, NM 87131
USA

Minoru Asahi
Neuroprotection Research Laboratory
Harvard Medical School
MGH East 149-2322
Charlestown, MA 02129
USA

Joseph S. Beckman
Department of Anesthesiology, THT 958
University of Alabama at Birmingham
1530 Third Avenue South
Birmingham, AL 35294-0006
USA

A. Lorris Betz
Moran Eye Center, 5th Floor
50 North Medical Drive
Salt Lake City, UT 84132-0001
USA

Andrew W. Bollen
Department of Pathology
University of California
Box 0102
San Francisco, CA 94143-0102
USA

Dale Bredesen
The Buck Center for Research in Aging
PO Box 638
Novato, CA 94948
USA

Ross Bullock
Division of Neurosurgery
Medical College of Virginia
PO Box 980631
Richmond, VA 23298-0631
USA

Susana Castro-Obregon
The Buck Center for Research in Aging
PO Box 638
Novato, CA 94948
USA

Pak H. Chan
Department of Neurosurgery
Stanford University School of Medicine
1201 Welch Road
MSLS #P304
Stanford, CA 94305-5487
USA

Dennis W. Choi
Center for the Study of Nervous System
    Injury and Department of Neurology
Washington University School of Medicine
660 South Euclid Avenue, Campus Box 8111
St. Louis, MO 63105
USA

John Crow
Department of Anesthesiology, THT 958
University of Alabama at Birmingham
1530 Third Avenue South
Birmingham, AL 35294-0006
USA

Ted M. Dawson
Department of Neurology
Johns Hopkins University School of
    Medicine
600 North Wolfe Street, Carnegie 2-214
Baltimore, MD 21287
USA

Valina L. Dawson
Department of Neurology
Johns Hopkins University School of Medicine
600 North Wolfe Street, Carnegie 2-214
Baltimore, MD 21287
USA

Ian deBelle
The Buck Center for Research in Aging
PO Box 638
Novato, CA 94948
USA

Gabriel del Rio
The Buck Center for Research in Aging
PO Box 638
Novato, CA 94948
USA

Gregory J. del Zoppo
Department of Molecular and Experimental
    Medicine
The Scripps Research Institute
10550 North Torrey Pines Road, MEM 132
La Jolla, CA 92037
USA

Deborah Dewar
Wellcome Surgical Institute and Hugh
    Fraser Neuroscience Laboratories
University of Glasgow
Garscube Estate, Bearsden Road
Glasgow, G61 1QH
Scotland
UK

Rick M. Dijkhuizen
Neuroprotection Research Laboratory
Harvard Medical School
MGH East 149-2322
Charlestown, MA 02129
USA

Alvaro G. Estévez
Department of Physiology
McCallum Building
MCLM 850
University of Alabama at Birmingham
Birmingham, AL 35294-0005
USA

Edward Y. Estrada
Department of Neurology
University of New Mexico
Albuquerque, NM 87131
USA

Itaf Fakhry
Department of Internal Medicine–Clinical
    Pharmacology,
Medical College of Virginia
Virginia Commonwealth University
Box 980160
Richmond, VA 23298
USA

Frank M. Faraci
Department of Internal Medicine
University of Iowa
200 Hawkins Drive, E329-2 GH
Iowa City, IA 52242-1081
USA

Giora Z. Feuerstein
DuPont Pharmaceuticals Company
Experimental Station E400/3257
Rt. 141 & Henry Clay Roads
Wilmington, DE 19880-0400
USA

Ferda Filiz
Departments of Medicine and Physiology
Cardiovascular Research Institute
University of California
Box 0130
San Francisco, CA 94143-0130
USA

Miki Fujimura
Stanford University School of Medicine
1201 Welch Road
MSLS #P304
Stanford, CA 94305-5487
USA

Irene Ginis
Stroke Branch, NINDS, NIH
36 Convent Drive, MSC 4128
Building 36/Room 4A03
Bethesda, MD 20892-4128
USA

Mark P. Goldberg
Department of Neurology, Campus Box
    8111
Washington University School of Medicine
660 South Euclid Avenue
St. Louis, MO 63110
USA

Mark Grostette
Department of Neurology
University of New Mexico
Albuquerque, NM 87131
USA

James Grotta
University of Texas-Houston Medical School
6431 Fannin Street, MSB 7.044
Houston, TX 77030
USA

Robert I. Grundy
School of Biological Sciences
1.124 Stopford Building
University of Manchester
Oxford Road
Manchester M13 9PT
England
UK

Vladimir Hachinski
Department of Clinical Neurological
    Sciences
The University of Western Ontario
339 Windermere Road
London, Ontario
Canada N6A 5A5

John M. Hallenbeck
Stroke Branch, NINDS, NIH
36 Convent Drive, MSC 4128
Building 36/Room 4A03
Bethesda, MD 20892-4128
USA

Takayuki Hara
Max-Planck-Institute for Neurological
    Research
Department of Experimental Neurology
Gleueler Strasse 50
D-50931 Cologne
Germany

M. Josh Hasbani
Department of Neurology, Campus Box 8111
Washington University School of Medicine
660 South Euclid Avenue
St. Louis, MO 63110
USA

Ryuji Hata
Max-Planck-Institute for Neurological
    Research
Department of Experimental Neurology
Gleueler Strasse 50
D-50931 Cologne
Germany

Takeshi Hayashi
Department of Neurology
Okayama University Medical School,
2-5-1 Shikatacho
Okayama 700-8558
Japan

Donald D. Heistad
Department of Internal Medicine
University of Iowa
200 Hawkins Drive, E315-GH
Iowa City, IA 52242-1081
USA

Konstantin-Alexander Hossmann
Max-Planck-Institute for Neurological
    Research
Department of Experimental Neurology
Gleueler Strasse 50
D-50931 Cologne
Germany

Costantino Iadecola
Center for Clinical and Molecular
    Neurobiology
Department of Neurology
University of Minnesota
Box 295 UMHC
420 Delaware Street SE
Minneapolis, MN 55455
USA

Olav Jansen
Neuroradiology
University of Kiel
Weimarer Str. 8
D-24106 Kiel
Germany

Barbro B. Johansson
Division for Experimental Brain Research
Wallenberg Neuroscience Center
University Hospital
S-221 85 Lund
Sweden

Ahmad Khaldi
Division of Neurosurgery
Medical College of Virginia
PO Box 980631
Richmond, VA 23298-0631
USA

Chelsea Kidwell
UCLA Stroke Center
710 Westwood Plaza
Los Angeles, CA 90095
USA

Hisashi Kitagawa
Second Institute of New Drug Research
Otsuka Pharmaceutical Co., Ltd.
463-10 Kagasuno
Kawauchi-cho Tokushima 771-0192
Japan

Jari Koistinaho
A.I. Virtanen Institute
University of Kuopio
PO Box 1627
FIN-70211, Kuopio
Finland

Katalin Komajti
Wellcome Surgical Institute and Hugh
    Fraser Neuroscience Laboratories
University of Glasgow
Garscube Estate
Bearsden Road
Glasgow G61 1QH
Scotland
UK

Richard P. Kraig
Department of Neurology, MC2030
University of Chicago
5841 South Maryland Avenue
Chicago, IL 60637
USA

Philip E. Kunkler
Department of Neurology
University of Chicago
SBRI J209, MC 2030
Chicago, IL 60637
USA

Kennedy R. Lees
University Department of Medicine &
    Therapeutics
Western Infirmary
Glasgow G11 6NT
Scotland
UK

Jane H.-C. Lin
Department of Cell Biology and Anatomy
New York Medical College
Valhalla, NY 10595
USA

Stuart A. Lipton
The Burnham Institute
Center for Neuroscience and Aging
10901 North Torrey Pines Road
La Jolla, CA 92037
USA

Jialing Liu
Department of Neurological Surgery (112C)
Department of Veterans Affairs Medical
    Center
4150 Clement Street
San Francisco, CA 94121
USA

Jie Liu
Stroke Branch, NINDS, NIH
36 Convent Drive, MSC 4128
Building 36/Room 4A03
Bethesda, MD 20892-4128
USA

Eng H. Lo
Neuroprotection Research Laboratory
Harvard Medical School
MGH East 149-2322
Charlestown, MA 02129
USA

Tonghui Ma
Department of Medicine and Physiology
Cardiovascular Research Institute
University of California, Box 0130
San Francisco, CA 94143-0130
USA

Geoffrey T. Manley
Department of Neurological Surgery
University of California
505 Parnassus Avenue, Box 0112
San Francisco, CA 94143-0112
USA

Michael P. Marks
Stanford University Medical Center
300 Pasteur Drive
Stanford, California 94305-5105
USA

James McCulloch
Wellcome Surgical Institute and Hugh
　Fraser Neuroscience Laboratories
University of Glasgow
Garscube Estate
Bearsden Road
Glasgow G61 1QH
Scotland
UK

José G. Merino
Department of Clinical Neurological
　Sciences
The University of Western Ontario
339 Windermere Road
London, Ontario
Canada N6A 5A5

Michael A. Moskowitz
Massachusetts General Hospital
149 13th Street Room 6403
Charlestown, MA 02129
USA

Toshiaki Nagafuji
Shionogi & Co.
1–8 Disho-machi 3-chome
Chuo-ku
Osaka 541
Japan

Maiken Nedergaard
Department of Cell Biology and Anatomy
New York Medical College
Valhalla, NY 10595
USA

Nobuo Noshita
Stanford University School of Medicine
1201 Welch Road
MSLS #P304
Stanford, CA 94305-5487
USA

Kook In Park
Department of Pediatrics and Pharmacology
Yonsei University College of Medicine
Seoul
Korea

Lisa C. Parker
School of Biological Sciences
1.124 Stopford Building
University of Manchester
Oxford Road
Manchester M13 9PT
England
UK

Elaine E. Peters
DuPont Pharmaceuticals Company
Experimental Station E400/3257
Rt. 141 & Henry Clay Roads
Wilmington, DE 19880-0400
USA

Nikolaus Plesnila
Stroke and Neurovascular Regulation
   Laboratory
Massachusetts General Hospital
Harvard Medical School
Charlestown, MA 01129
USA

Michael Reinert
Division of Neurosurgery
Medical College of Virginia
PO Box 980631
Richmond, VA 23298-0631
USA

Bruce R. Rosen
NMR Center
Massachusetts General Hospital
Harvard Medical School
55 Fruit Street
Boston, MA 02114
USA

Gary A. Rosenberg
Department of Neurology
University of New Mexico
Albuquerque, NM 87131
USA

Nancy J. Rothwell
School of Biological Sciences
1.124 Stopford Building
University of Manchester
Oxford Road
Manchester M133 9PT
England
UK

Jeffrey L. Saver
UCLA Stroke Center
710 Westwood Plaza
Los Angeles, CA 90095
USA

Peter D. Schellinger
Department of Neurology
University of Heidelberg Medical School
Heidelberg
Germany

Frank R. Sharp
Department of Neurology
University of Cincinnati
2624 Clifton Avenue
Cincinnati, OH 45221
USA

Domenic A. Sica
Department of Clinical Pharmacology
Medical College of Virginia
Virginia Commonwealth University
Box 980160
Richmond, VA 23298
USA

Roger P. Simon
R.S. Dow Center for Neurobiology
Legacy Research
1225 Northeast 2nd Avenue
Portland, OR 97232
USA

Evan Y. Snyder
Children's Hospital, Boston
Harvard Medical School
300 Longwood Avenue
248 Enders Building
Boston, MA 02115
USA

Maria Spatz
Stroke Branch, NINDS, NIH
36 Convent Drive, MSC 4128
Building 36/Room 4A03
Bethesda, MD 20892-4128
USA

Sabina Sperandio
The Buck Center for Research in Aging
PO Box 638
Novato, CA 94948
USA

Philip E. Stieg
Brigham and Women's Hospital
Div of Neurosurgery
75 Francis Street PBBH-BALC 2
Boston, MA 02115
USA

Selva Baltan Tekkök
Department of Neurology, Campus Box
   8111
Washington University School of Medicine
660 South Euclid Avenue
St. Louis, MO 63110
USA

Suzanne Underhill
Department of Neurology, Campus Box 8111
Washington University School of Medicine
660 South Euclid Avenue
St. Louis, MO 63110
USA

*Valerio Valeriani
Wellcome Surgical Institute
and Hugh Fraser Neuroscience Laboratories
University of Glasgow
Garscube Estate
Bearsden Road
Glasgow G61 1QH
Scotland
UK

Alan S. Verkman
Departments of Medicine and Physiology
University of California
Box 0521
San Francisco, CA 94143-0521
USA

Xiaoying Wang
Neuroprotection Research Laboratory
Harvard Medical School
MGH East 149-2322
Charlestown, MA 02129
USA

Xinkang Wang
DuPont Pharmaceuticals Company
Experimental Station E400/3257
Rt. 141 & Henry Clay Roads
Wilmington, DE 19880-0400
USA

Steven Warach
NIH, NINDS
Section on Stroke Diagnostics &
   Therapeutics
10 Center Drive, Room 3B10A
MSC 1247
Bethesda, MD 20892-1247
USA

Philip R. Weinstein
Department of Neurological Surgery
University of California
Box 0112
San Francisco, CA 94143-0112
USA

* Permanent Address:
Experimental Research Department
2nd Institute of Physiology
1082 Budapest
Hungary

Guo-Yuan Yang
Department of Surgery, Section of
   Neurosurgery
University of Michigan
Room 5550 Kresge I
Ann Arbor, MI 48109-0532
USA

Alois Zauner
Division of Neurosurgery
Medical College of Virginia
PO Box 980631
Richmond, VA 23298-0631
USA

Justin A. Zivin
Department of Neurosciences
University of California
9500 Gilman Drive
La Jolla, CA 92093-0624
USA

Preface

The 22nd Princeton Conference on Cerebrovascular Disease, held in Redwood City, California, 10–12 March 2000, was hosted by the Stanford University School of Medicine, with administrative support provided by the Neurosurgical Laboratories, Department of Neurosurgery. The Conference focused on the current status and future directions of stroke pathophysiology, diagnosis and treatment, with special emphasis on the cellular and molecular mechanisms of ischemic cell death and repair, and clinical aspects of imaging, risk factors and therapeutic strategies in stroke. This 2 day conference was exciting and productive, with a consensus that the goals that were set forth for this meeting had been accomplished, and perhaps far exceeded expectations. First, the meeting provided a unique forum for promoting collaborative interaction in stroke research among the attendees. Second, many of the speakers presented state-of-the-art and up-to-date information, and the vigorous interactive discussions among the participants made this conference a successful and memorable one.

The first three topics in this monograph are directed toward the cellular and molecular mechanisms of ischemic cell death. Zinc and caspases, which are emerging as important mediators involved in ischemic cell death, have been fully elaborated in the two special invited lectures. Other important mediators including oxygen radicals, NMDA receptors and genes involved in ischemic tolerance are discussed. Two major concepts, parapoptosis and ischemic white matter injury in culture, are introduced.

One major area that distinguishes this meeting from other stroke conferences is that late-breaking news in stroke research was presented, and appears in this book in Part IV. These hot topics include the gap junction between astrocytes, the aquaporin-4 water channel, tetracycline neuroprotection and spreading depression.

Postischemic pathophysiological events are discussed in Parts V and VI. Hemorrhage and inflammation are two major areas of focus. New concepts in the role of thrombolytic tissue plasminogen activator and cytokines in postischemic pathophysiology and injury have evolved from these presentations.

Parts VII and VIII focus on the preclinical utility of gene transfer in stroke, and neural stem cell transplantation and its involvement in neural plasticity after cere-bral ischemia. These studies present up-to-date and unique therapeutic strategies and potentials employing gene transfer and stem cells in clinical stroke.

Diffusion/perfusion magnetic resonance imaging in clinical stroke dominate the discussions in Part IX. New and innovative approaches using these imaging tech-niques in addressing acute ischemic stroke, transient ischemic attack and early recanalization in acute ischemic stroke have been vigorously discussed and debated.

Finally, a particular section (Part X) is devoted to risk factors, clinical trials and new therapeutic horizons. This section presents a unique perspective for consider-ing vascular factors and white matter as the new neuroprotection targets in stroke clinical trials.

The enthusiasm and excitement reflected in the presentations and the vigorous interactive discussions among the participants reflect the success of the conference. This momentum is likely to continue. Tremendous advances in both basic and clin-ical sciences were demonstrated during the 2 day meeting. It is our hope that these advances, as communicated through this volume, will provide an impetus for stroke researchers to maintain and exceed these excitements in advancing our knowledge in both the basic and clinical sciences of stroke.

P. H. Chan

Acknowledgments

The success of the 22nd Princeton Conference on Cerebrovascular Disease was very dependent on the contributions and cooperation of many individuals including those who gave generously of their time as part of the Organizing Committee (Gregory W. Albers, M.D., Rona G. Giffard, M.D., Ph.D., Michael E. Moseley, Ph.D., Robert M. Sapolsky, Ph.D., Frank R. Sharp, M.D., Gary K. Steinberg, M.D., Ph.D., Raymond A. Swanson, M.D., Midori A. Yenari, M.D. and Philip R. Weinstein, M.D.) and the Scientific Advisory Committee (Nicolas Bazan, M.D., Ph.D., Dennis W. Choi, M.D., Ph.D., Michael Chopp, Ph.D., Marc Fisher, M.D., Myron D. Ginsberg, M.D., Philip Gorelick, M.D., M.P.H., Chung Y. Hsu, M.D., Ph.D., John R. Marler, M.D., Michael A. Moskowitz, M.D., James T. Robertson, M.D., Bo K. Siesjö, M.D., Ph.D., Bryce Weir, M.D. and Justin A. Zivin, M.D., Ph.D.). Ms. Aileen Beals and Ms. Cheryl Christensen are greatly appreciated for their outstanding contribution of coordinating the Conference. As in the past, the Princeton Conference received generous support from the National Institute of Neurological Disorders and Stroke and from our colleagues in the pharmaceutical industry. A list of these contributors can be found below. Special thanks to our colleagues at the NINDS who provided encouragement and support: Gerald D. Fischbach, M.D., the past Director, Michael D. Walker, M.D., past Director of the Stroke and Trauma Division, John R. Marler, M.D., Associate Director of Clinical Trials and Thomas P. Jacobs, Ph.D., Program Director. The significant fundraising efforts of many colleagues are acknowledged, in particular, Marc Fisher, M.D., and Justin A. Zivin, M.D., Ph.D. Finally, the untiring effort of Ms. Cheryl Christensen, who also served as the assistant editor of this monograph, is appreciated.

Major contributors

Janssen Pharmaceuticals Inc.
Parke-Davis Pharmaceutical Research
American Heart Association

Abbott Laboratories

AstraZeneca

Boehringer Ingelheim Pharmaceuticals

Bristol-Myers Squibb Company

DuPont Pharmaceuticals Company

Hoffmann La Roche Inc.

Knoll Pharmaceutical Company

Amgen Inc.

Genentech, Inc.

Guilford Pharmaceuticals Inc.

ICOS Corporation

La Jolla Pharmaceutical Company

Lilly Research Laboratories

SmithKline Beecham Pharmaceuticals

Part I

Special lectures

Moderator: Richard J. Traystman

Zinc toxicity in the ischemic brain

Dennis W. Choi

Center for the Study of Nervous System Injury and Department of Neurology, Washington University School of Medicine, St. Louis, MO

Growing evidence indicates that the brain's heightened vulnerability to ischemia, in large part, reflects a propensity for its intrinsic cell–cell and intracellular signaling mechanisms, normally responsible for information processing, to turn lethal under ischemic conditions. The most extensively studied example of such a signaling mechanism is that mediated by the excitatory neurotransmitter glutamate. In health, glutamate mediates most fast excitatory neurotransmission, but, under ischemic conditions, glutamate floods out from both neurons and astrocytes, building up in the extracellular space and becoming a killer that facilitates excess calcium entry into neurons, contributing to their demise.

Two Princeton Conferences ago, that is in Memphis in 1996, I presented then emerging evidence from my laboratory supporting the idea that another neurotransmitter released from excitatory nerve terminals might become a killer in the ischemic brain: the metal zinc. Besides the "transmitter killer" parallel to glutamate, I noted that there was also a parallel between zinc and calcium, in that both were divalent cation metals mediating ischemic neuronal death via excess influx across the plasma membrane [1].

A substantial body of evidence suggests that zinc is a neurotransmitter/neuromodulator [reviewed by refs. 2–4], although this possibility has had, to date, a rather low profile within the scientific community. The central nervous system contains a pool of relatively free zinc, separate from the zinc tightly bound to metalloenzymes and transcription factors in all cells. This free central nervous system zinc is concentrated in vesicles within central nerve terminals throughout the telencephalon, largely colocalized (albeit in distinct vesicles) with transmitter glutamate. Consistent with a neurotransmitter role, it is released upon membrane depolarization in a calcium-dependent fashion and then taken back up.

Little is currently known about the functional significance of the zinc neurotransmitter system, probably reflecting a paucity of directed studies. An experience reported a quarter of a century ago in the neurology literature suggests that acute zinc depletion through oral chelation can produce profound reversible changes in mentation [5]. Certainly, there are many candidates for relevant target actions of synaptically released zinc at the micromolar concentrations that it may well reach [6], as these zinc concentrations can modify the behavior of many important membrane proteins including transmitter receptors, channels and transporters. Of particular relevance, given its systematic colocalization with glutamate, extracellular zinc reduces N-methyl-D-aspartate (NMDA) receptor activation by both a voltage-independent reduction of channel opening frequency, and a voltage-dependent channel block [7]. Modulation of zinc release, therefore, may provide a mechanism for modifying the relative proportion of NMDA vs. α-amino-3-hydroxy-5-methyl-4-isoxazole propionic acid (AMPA) or kainate receptors activated by glutamate. It can also enter postsynaptic neurons (see below), whereupon it may modify signaling, metabolism or gene transcription in a lasting fashion. We have recently found evidence that brief exposure to non-toxic levels of extracellular zinc can activate mitogen-activated protein (MAP) kinase and Src family kinase signaling in neurons, the latter leading to phosphorylation of the NMDA receptor subunits (NR2A and NR2B) and consequent enhancement of NMDA receptor activity [8]. Thus normal zinc actions on the NMDA receptor may be biphasic: an initial direct inhibition followed by more lasting kinase-mediated upregulation.

After transient global ischemia, chelatable Zn^{2+} translocates from nerve terminals into cell bodies of vulnerable neurons, not just in the hippocampus, but also in the cortex, striatum, amygdala and thalamus [9]. This translocation precedes neuronal degeneration, and its interruption by the intracerebroventricular injection of a chelator, ethylenediaminetetra-acetic acid saturated with equimolar Ca^{2+} (CaEDTA), reduces subsequent neuronal death. Exposure to the high micromolar concentrations of zinc likely to occur in brain extracellular space after synchronous cellular depolarization is sufficient to kill cultured neurons, especially if the neurons are depolarized, a state that facilitates toxic entry of zinc across the plasma membrane through several routes. Most prominent among these depolarization-facilitated entry routes are L-type voltage-gated calcium channels, but we now have evidence for participation of N-type voltage-gated calcium channels, agonist-gated calcium channels (especially calcium-permeable AMPA receptors when present, for example, on GABAergic neurons (GABA is γ-aminobutyric acid)) and exchanger-mediated transport (exchanged for sodium, presumably via the sodium–calcium exchanger) [10]. Lower levels of toxic zinc exposure induce apoptosis sensitive to deletion of the bax gene or inhibition of caspases; higher levels induce explosive necrosis associated with fulminant cell swelling [11,12].

Using mag-fura-5 initially, and later using the lower affinity, albeit non-ratiometric, indicator dye Newport Green, my colleagues and I have estimated levels of intracellular free zinc attained in neurons subjected to toxic levels of extracellular zinc, and found them to be on the order of 200 to 300 nM [13]. This is a tremendous concentration of free zinc, many orders of magnitude above the affinity of intracellular binding sites on metallothioneins and other metalloproteins. It is plausible that many metabolic disturbances might result from such extreme elevations in zinc availability within the intracellular milieu, but an especially consequential disturbance may be caused by a reduction in glycolysis, secondary to inhibition of glyceraldehyde 3-phosphate dehydrogenase (GAPDH) [14]. Rather than occurring by direct interaction with zinc, this inhibition appears to reflect depletion of oxidized nicotinamide-adenine dinucleotide (NAD$^+$) by some catabolic process sensitive to inhibition by benzamide. Administration of benzamide, niacinamide or pyruvate increases NAD$^+$ levels, restoring GAPDH function and neuronal ATP levels, and attenuating zinc-induced death. Interestingly, the neuroprotective effects of niacinamide and benzamide in brain ischemia have already been established by studies motivated by considering the ability of these substances to enhance ATP synthesis [15] or inhibit poly(ADP-ribose) polymerase activity [16].

In addition to the contribution of zinc toxicity to selective neuronal loss after transient global ischemia, recent observations from our laboratory spearheaded by Jin-Moo Lee have suggested that it may contribute to the development of cerebral infarction after mild transient focal ischemia. Adult male Long–Evans rats subjected to middle cerebral artery occlusion for 30 minutes followed by reperfusion, developed delayed cerebral infarction reaching completion 3 days after the insult. One day after the insult, many degenerating cerebral neurons exhibited increased intracellular zinc, some labeling with an antibody against activated caspase-3. Intracerebroventricular administration of CaEDTA 15 minutes prior to ischemia attenuated subsequent zinc translocation into the cortical neurons, and reduced infarct volume measured 3 days after ischemia. Although the protective effect of CaEDTA at this end-point was substantial (about 70% infarct reduction), it was lost when insult severity was increased from 30 to 60 minutes of arterial occlusion, or when infarct volume was measured 14 days after ischemia. These observations suggest that toxic zinc translocation may accelerate the development of cerebral infarction after mild transient focal ischemia. Our preliminary studies have not demonstrated any protective effects of intracerebroventricular CaEDTA in more traditional models of focal ischemia, using longer periods of reversible ischemia or permanent ischemia, in which infarction develops more rapidly (complete within a matter of hours after insult).

Why might zinc contribute more prominently to neuronal loss after global ischemia than after focal ischemia? Further studies will be needed to answer this important question, but as a working hypothesis, I am inclined to consider that two related factors are especially influential. First, it is clear from the work of many laboratories that NMDA receptor-triggered, calcium-mediated excitotoxicity is a larger component of focal ischemic injury than global ischemic injury. My colleagues and I have called this form of excitotoxicity "rapidly triggered" to emphasize how quickly it can occur; in cortical neuronal cell cultures, 3 to 5 minutes of sustained NMDA receptor activation is sufficient to destroy most neurons [17]. In contrast, AMPA receptor-triggered, calcium-mediated excitotoxicity, a larger component of global ischemic injury, typically occurs more slowly, requiring hours of sustained receptor activation to induce lethal injury in the same cell cultures. Thus one could imagine that zinc-mediated injury might have more opportunity to lead to cell death after global ischemia; whereas after focal ischemia, more fulminant NMDA receptor-triggered, calcium-mediated injury might supervene and render zinc-mediated injury largely invisible to therapeutic interference.

Second, and probably in part responsible for the first factor (the greater involvement of NMDA receptors in focal ischemic injury as compared with global ischemic injury), extracellular pH in brain tissue does not fall as much in the penumbra of focal ischemia as it does in global ischemia, where it may reach values in mid to upper 6s. Not only does this extracellular acidity selectively downregulate NMDA receptor activation and NMDA receptor-mediated injury [18–20], but it appears to shift L-type voltage-gated calcium channels toward a zinc-preferring mode. In recent experiments using whole cell clamp physiology to measure currents through high voltage-activated calcium channels on cultured cortical neurons, we confirmed earlier studies that indicated that lowering the pH to 6.4 reduced calcium currents through these channels, but we were surprised to see that the same pH manipulation markedly enhanced the zinc current through presumably the same channels [21].

The implication of zinc in the pathogenesis of neuronal loss after ischemic insults raises consideration of several novel therapeutic strategies. In broad categories, these would include:

1 Reduction of presynaptic zinc stores. For example, through acute reduction of dietary zinc intake, coupled with oral chelation, as a prophylactic measure before high-risk surgery or other anticipated ischemic stress.
2 Reduction of zinc release. Can this be accomplished independent of altering glutamate release?
3 Extracellular chelation.
4 Block of postsynaptic entry routes, such as voltage-gated calcium channels, calcium-permeable AMPA receptors or the sodium–calcium exchanger. Weak neuroprotective effects of dihydropyridines and other L-type voltage-gated calcium channel blockers have been observed in previous studies with both experimental models and human patients. Could these suggestions of benefit reflect the reduction of zinc toxicity in addition to the intended reduction of calcium overload? To attain higher levels of neuroprotection, it may be necessary to concurrently block multiple pathways of zinc entry.
5 Enhancement of zinc buffering, sequestration or export via plasma membrane transporters.

6 Elevation of intracellular NAD^+ or ATP levels.

7 Blockade of zinc-induced apoptosis.

The most logical clinical setting to begin testing anti-zinc strategies for neuro-protective effect would be that of hospitalized patients resuscitated after cardiac arrest. No effective neuroprotective treatments are currently available for global ischemia in humans, and the natural history of cerebral degeneration has a well-defined relationship to arrest duration. Patients sustaining longer periods of global ischemia at a normal body temperature prior to effective restoration of cerebral blood flow inevitably develop serious neurological morbidity due to delayed selected neuronal death. These patients could be treated immediately with all the resources of the inpatient setting, and ethical risk/benefit considerations would justify relatively aggressive experimental approaches. Other settings where toxic zinc translocation has been identified in animal models and hence, where anti-zinc approaches might be of clinical value, would include head trauma or sustained seizures [22–24].

Lastly, I will speculate that anti-zinc approaches could find a place in the treatment of stroke, in settings where the ischemic insult is limited. Even if these approaches cannot by themselves prevent infarction from ultimately occurring, perhaps they might be useful in buying time, increasing the temporal therapeutic window for other approaches.

REFERENCES

1 Choi DW & Koh JY (1998) Zinc and brain injury. *Annual Review of Neuroscience*, 21, 347–75.

2 Frederickson CJ (1989) Neurobiology of zinc and zinc-containing neurons. *International Review of Neurobiology*, 31, 145–238.

3 Harrison NL & Gibbons SJ (1994) Zn^{2+}: an endogenous modulator of ligand- and voltage-gated ion channels. *Neuropharmacology*, 33, 935–52.

4 Smart TG, Xie X & Krishek BJ (1994) Modulation of inhibitory and excitatory amino acid receptor ion channels by zinc. *Progress in Neurobiology*, 42, 393–441.

5 Henkin RI, Patten BM, Re PK & Bronzert DA (1975) A syndrome of acute zinc loss. Cerebellar dysfunction, mental changes, anorexia, and taste and smell dysfunction. *Archives of Neurology*, 32, 745–51.

6 Assaf SY & Chung SH (1984) Release of endogenous Zn^{2+} from brain tissue during activity. *Nature*, 308, 734–6.

7 Christine CW & Choi DW (1990) Effect of zinc on NMDA receptor-mediated channel currents in cortical neurons. *Journal of Neuroscience*, 10, 108–16.

8 Manzerra P, Behrens MM, Heidinger V, Ichinose T, Yu SP & Choi DW (2000) Zinc exposure results in the activation of Src kinase and the phosphorylation of NMDA receptor subunits (NR2A/2B). *Society for Neuroscience Abstract*, 26, 2145.

9 Koh JY, Suh SW, Gwag BJ, He YY, Hsu CY & Choi DW (1996) The role of zinc in selective neuronal death after transient global cerebral ischemia. *Science,* **272,** 1013–16.

10 Sensi SL, Canzoniero LM, Yu SP, Ying HS, Koh JY, Kerchner GA & Choi DW (1997) Measurement of intracellular free zinc in living cortical neurons: routes of entry. *Journal of Neuroscience,* **17,** 9554–64.

11 Manev H, Kharlamov E, Uz T, Mason RP & Cagnoli CM (1997) Characterization of zinc-induced neuronal death in primary cultures of rat cerebellar granule cells. *Experimental Neurology,* **146,** 171–8.

12 Lobner D, Canzoniero LMT, Manzerra P, Gottron F, Ying H, Knudson M, Tian M, Dugan LL, Kerchner GA, Sheline CT, Korsmeyer SJ & Choi DW (2000) Zinc-induced neuronal death in cortical neurons. *Cellular & Molecular Biology,* **46,** 797–806.

13 Canzoniero LMT, Turetsky DM & Choi DW (1999) Measurement of intracellular free zinc concentrations accompanying zinc-induced neuronal death. *Journal of Neuroscience,* **19 RC31,** 1–6.

14 Sheline CT, Behrens MM & Choi DW (2000) Zinc-induced cortical neuronal death: contribution of energy failure attributable to loss of NAD^+ and inhibition of glycolysis. *Journal of Neuroscience,* **20,** 3139–46.

15 Ayoub IA, Lee EJ, Ogilvy CS, Beal MF & Maynard KI (1999) Nicotinamide reduces infarction up to two hours after the onset of permanent focal cerebral ischemia in Wistar rats. *Neuroscience Letters,* **259,** 21–4.

16 Eliasson MJL, Sampei K, Mandir AS, Hurn PD, Traystman RJ, Bao J, Pieper A, Wang Z-Q, Dawson TM, Snyder SH & Dawson VL (1997) Poly(ADP-ribose) polymerase gene disruption renders mice resistant to cerebral ischemia. *Nature Medicine,* **3,** 1089–95.

17 Choi DW (1992) Excitotoxic cell death. *Journal of Neurobiology,* **23,** 1261–76.

18 Tang CM, Dichter M & Morad M (1990) Modulation of the *N*-methyl-D-aspartate channel by extracellular H^+. *Proceedings of the National Academy of Sciences, USA,* **87,** 6445–9.

19 Giffard RG, Monyer H, Christine CW & Choi DW (1990) Acidosis reduces NMDA receptor activation, glutamate neurotoxicity, and oxygen-glucose deprivation neuronal injury in cortical cultures. *Brain Research,* **506,** 339–42.

20 Tombaugh GC & Sapolsky RM (1990) Mild acidosis protects hippocampal neurons from injury induced by oxygen and glucose deprivation. *Brain Research,* **506,** 343–5.

21 Kerchner GA, Canzoniero LMT, Yu SP, Ling C & Choi DW (2000) Zn^{2+} current is mediated by voltage-gated Ca^{2+} channels and enhanced by extracellular acidity in mouse cortical neurones. *Journal of Physiology,* **528,** 39–52.

22 Sloviter RS (1985) A selective loss of hippocampal mossy fiber Timm stain accompanies granule cell seizure activity induced by perforant path stimulation. *Brain Research,* **330,** 150–3.

23 Suh SW, Koh JY & Choi DW (1996) Extracellular zinc mediates selective neuronal death in hippocampus and amygdala following kainate-induced seizure. *Society for Neuroscience Abstract,* **22,** 2101.

24 Suh SW, Chen JW, Motamedi M, Bell B, Listiak K, Pons NF, Danscher G & Frederickson CJ (2000) Evidence that synaptically-released zinc contributes to neuronal injury after traumatic brain injury. *Brain Research,* **852,** 268–73.

Central nervous system ischemia: diversity among the caspases

Nikolaus Plesnila[1] & Michael A. Moskowitz[2]

[1,2] Stroke and Neurovascular Regulation Laboratory, Massachusetts General Hospital, Boston, MA

Introduction

Ischemic neurons die acutely by osmotically driven rupture of cellular and subcellular membranes by a process called necrosis, but may also die in a delayed manner, dependent on the activation of a family of cysteine proteases named caspases. Caspases are synthesized as inactive proenzymes containing three subunits, an N-terminal prodomain, a large (~20 kDa) and a small subunit (~10 kDa), which form heterotetromers on cleavage and activation. Family members show a near absolute specificity for cleavage at the N-terminal of aspartate residues. At least 14 caspases have been identified to date, designated 1 to 14. Caspases -1, -2, -3, -7, -8 and -9 are constitutively expressed in the brain. In the spinal cord, caspases -2, -3 and -8 are constitutively expressed. Caspases -1, -4 and -5 (caspase-1 family members) promote cytokine maturation and mediate inflammation whereas caspases -2, -3, -6, -7, -8 and -9 (caspase-3 family members) promote apoptotic cell death. On activation, caspase-11, which is found only in mice, promotes both cytokine maturation and apoptosis.

In this review, we will briefly summarize the evidence implicating caspases in cerebral and spinal cord ischemia. Caspase-driven cell death may have important therapeutic implications for ischemia as well as for other acute and chronic central nervous system (CNS) conditions in which cell death is prominent.

Global ischemia

Early evidence for the involvement of caspases in global ischemia came from two studies showing upregulation of caspase-1 mRNA by reverse transcriptase–polymerase chain reaction [1] and in situ hybridization [2] beginning 24 hours after forebrain ischemia in the gerbil (see also Table 2.1). The protein was found at 48 hours [1]. Upregulation of caspase-3 mRNA (in situ hybridization) plus a

Table 2.1. Literature overview on caspases in ischemic brain injury

Global ischemia

Reference	Ischemia (min)	Caspase	Species	Model	Finding
8	5	Caspase-3	Gerbil	BCAO	−
2	5 or 10	Caspase-1	Gerbil	BCAO	+
1	7	Caspase-1	Gerbil	BCAO	+
9	10	Caspase-9	Dog	Cardiac arrest	+
3	10	Caspase-3	Rat	Cardiac arrest	+
53	12	Caspase-3	Rat	4VO	+
4	15	Caspase-3	Rat	4VO	+
6	15	Caspase-3	Rat	4VO	+
7	15	Caspase-3	Rat	BCAO/hypotension	+
5	30	Caspase-3	Rat	4VO	+

Focal ischemia (MCAO)

Reference	Ischemia	Caspase	Species	Model	Finding
18	Permanent	Caspase-1	Mouse (KO)	Filament	+
20	Permanent	Caspase-3	Rat	Filament	+
54	Permanent	Caspase-3	Mouse	Distal	+
26	Permanent	Caspases -3, -8	Rat	Distal	+
19	Permanent	Caspase-11	Mouse	Filament	+
17	3 hours	Caspase-1	Mouse	Filament	+
21	2 hours	Caspase-3	Mouse	Filament	+
22	30 min	Caspase-3	Mouse	Filament	+

Notes:
BCAO, bilateral carotid artery occlusion; 4VO, four-vessel occlusion; MCAO, middle cerebral artery occlusion; KO, knockout.
Source: From ref. 53.

two-fold increase in DEVD (Asp-Glu-Val-Asp) cleaving activity was identified at 24 hours in rat CA1 hippocampal neurons after 10 minutes of cardiac arrest [3]. These findings were confirmed [4–7], along with additional evidence for increased caspase-3 protein and enzyme activity within the hippocampus after global ischemia. One report, however, failed to show active caspase-3 after global ischemia in the gerbil by immunohistochemistry, although the constitutive proform was widely expressed in the CA1 hippocampus [8]. More recently, caspase-9 release from mitochondria was documented by electron microscopy and fluorescence microscopy after canine cardiac arrest [9]. In vitro, caspase-9 forms a complex (apoptosome) with apoptosis activating factor-1, cytochrome c and deoxy-adenosine triphosphate, thereby promoting downstream caspase cleavage and activation. Because cytochrome c release was detected in hippocampal neurons up to 2 hours after a global ischemic insult [10–12], formation of a mitochondrial death complex might play a role in delayed neuronal death after global ischemia.

The importance of caspases and cell death in global ischemia was further established by pharmacological evidence showing enhanced resistance to ischemic injury after caspase inhibition (Table 2.2). Himi et al. [13] injected into the gerbil hippocampus an irreversible pancaspase inhibitor, benzyloxycarbonyl-Asp-CH$_2$-dichlorobenzene (zD), and achieved near-complete rescue of CA1 neurons after 8 days. Performance on memory tests was better and cleavage of a caspase-3 substrate, poly(ADP-ribose) polymerase, was inhibited. Several other groups confirmed these findings [4,6,14]. For example, Chen et al. [4] and Gillardon et al. [6] showed that cell death was decreased by 30% to 85% in the CA1 region after inhibition of caspase-3. However, Li and colleagues [15] injected zVAD.FMK or zDEVD.FMK, both as a pre- and post-treatment, but did not find protection, possibly because a 10-fold lower dose (2×200 ng vs. 3×1.5 μg) was used in their global ischemia model compared with the previous studies.

Focal ischemia

Early evidence for the significance of caspases in focal ischemia came from a preliminary study using repeated administration of a pancaspase inhibitor, z-VAD, before and after permanent focal ischemia in the rat. Twenty-four hours later, a 50% reduction of total infarct volume was observed [16] (Table 2.2). Hara et al. [17] confirmed these findings in models of transient focal ischemia (2 hours) in mice and rats and showed 25% protection 24 hours after zDEVD.FMK injection, a more selective caspase inhibitor without inhibition of interleukin-1β formation. The same group demonstrated the importance of caspase-1 by showing neuroprotection (45% decrease of infarct volume) using transgenic mice expressing a dominant negative inhibitor of caspase-1 [17]. A similar infarct reduction (-50%) was also found in caspase-1-deficient animals [18]. However, these data might be difficult to interpret because caspase-1 null mice do not express caspase-11 [19], which is also cleaved and activated during cerebral ischemia and seems to be an upstream modulator of caspase-1 (see below).

Caspase-3 has been implicated in focal ischemic brain damage as evidenced by increased rat caspase-3 mRNA 1 hour after the induction of permanent ischemia [20]. Upregulation of murine caspase-3 protein in neurons plus increased enzyme activity in homogenates was shown by Namura et al. [21] and Fink et al. [22], respectively, after severe and mild focal ischemia. After a more severe reversible ischemia (2 hours of occlusion), caspase-3 was maximally active shortly after

Table 2.2. Literature overview on caspase inhibitors in cerebral ischemia

Global ischemia

Reference	Ischemia (min)	Species	Model	Inhibitor and dosage	Protection
13	5	Gerbil	BCAO	zD (1 μmol) intrahippocampal (CA1); 0, 12 + 24 hours	+
14	10	Rat	BCAO/hypotension	zVAD (200 μg) icv; 60 min	+
15	10	Rat	4VO	zVAD (200 ng)/DEVD (200 ng) icv; −15 min, 10 min	−
4	15	Rat	4VO	zDEVD (1.5 μg) icv; −30 min, 2 + 24 hours	+
6	15	Rat	4VO	zDEVD icv; cont. 0 to 24 hours (50 pmol/hour)	+

Focal ischemia (MCAO)

Reference	Ischemia	Species	Model	Inhibitor and dosage	Protection
22	30 min	Mouse	Filament	zDEVD (480 ng) icv; −10 min, or 6 or 9 hours	+
23	30 min	Mouse	Filament	zVAD (120 ng)/DEVD (480 ng) icv; −10 min, or 3 or 6 hours	+
15	90 min	Rat	Distal	zVAD (200 ng)/DEVD (200 ng) icv; −30 min, 30 min, 60 min, 2 hours	+
17	2 hours	Rat	Filament	zVAD (160 ng) icv; −15 min, 2 hours, 10 min	+
17	2 hours	Mouse	Filament	zVAD (80 ng)/DEVD (240 ng)/YVAD (400 ng) icv; −15 min, 2 hours	+
16	Permanent	Rat	Distal	zVAD (1 pmol) icv; −30 min, 15 min, 2, 4, 6 + 8 hours	+
24	Permanent	Rat	Distal	zVAD icv; −30 min (120 ng), cont. for 24 hours (40 ng/hour)	+

Notes:

BCAO, bilateral carotid artery occlusion; icv, intracerebroventricular; 4VO, four-vessel occlusion; MCAO, middle cerebral artery occlusion.

Source: From ref. 54.

reperfusion, whereas after mild ischemia (30 minutes) the enzyme was maximally active only after 12 hours. Consistent with these results and in line with prior findings [23], the infarct volume decreased by 60% at 3 days when zDEVD was administered up to 9 hours after mild ischemia. Accordingly, severe injury is less responsive to a delayed application of caspase inhibitors [15,17,24].

In addition to caspase-1 and -3, caspases -7, -8 and -11 and cytochrome c, a coactivator of caspase-9, have been implicated in ischemic brain injury [19,25,26]. Caspase 11, for example, is upregulated and cleaved at least 12 hours after permanent ischemia. Caspase-11 null mice exhibit a 75% reduction in terminal deoxynucleotidyl transferase-mediated uridine 5′-triphosphate-biotin nick end labeling (TUNEL)-positive cells and a decrease in caspase-3 cleavage within the ischemic cortex [19]. Velier et al. [26] showed that caspase-8 was cleaved in the ischemic cortex beginning 6 hours after permanent middle cerebral artery occlusion. Because caspase-8 processing is at times coupled to tumor necrosis factor-like receptor activation (e.g., Fas-R, tumor necrosis factor-R), cell surface receptors may promote ischemic neuronal cell death [27].

Recently we showed constitutive caspase-7 mRNA and protein expression in the mouse brain. After 2 hours of distal middle cerebral artery occlusion and 24 hours of reperfusion, caspase-7 mRNA is upregulated and the proform decreased, suggesting increased caspase-7 turnover (Y. Wu, personal communication, 2000).

Not all caspases participate in ischemic cell death, at least as reflected in tested models. For example, caspase-2 protein levels are unchanged after 2 hours of reversible cerebral ischemia in the mouse, and mice deficient in caspase-2 are not protected from ischemic brain damage [28].

Neonatal hypoxic–ischemic brain injury

In rodent models, neuronal cell death develops after a delay of 6 to 12 hours and is paralleled by activation of downstream caspases, as shown by DEVD cleaving activity [29], and the appearance of active caspase-3 [30] and actin cleavage fragment [31]. Caspase-1-deficient neonatal mice are more resistant to 70 minutes but not to 120 minutes of ischemia–hypoxia [32], possibly reflecting a role for caspases in milder forms of cerebral ischemia. Finally, pancaspase inhibitors (BAF) reduced injured brain tissue by >50% even when given systemically 3 hours after insult [29].

Spinal cord ischemia

Caspases -2, -3 and -8 are constitutively expressed in the spinal cord [33,34] and motor neurons can be protected from programmed cell death during development by caspase inhibitors [35,36].

The ischemic spinal cord of rabbits and rats shows a large number of TUNEL-positive neurons and apoptotic cell morphology beginning 12 to 24 hours after reperfusion [37,38]. In a similar model in the rat, motor neurons also die selectively, but with an even greater delay of more than 2 days; moreover, more than 50% of motor neurons show DNA fragmentation [39]. Cleavage of caspases -1, -2 and -3 develops as early as 8 hours after reperfusion. In a novel mouse spinal cord ischemia model [40], procaspase-8 was upregulated 3 hours after reperfusion, as shown by immunohistochemistry and in situ hybridization. Active caspase-8 (p18) was detected by immunoblot and immunohistochemistry some time between 3 and 18 hours and increased 1 day after reperfusion. A high proportion of TUNEL-positive motor neurons showed double staining for active caspase-3 and -8 and the anatomical distribution of those markers was overlapping. The peak of active caspase-8-positive neurons preceded that of caspase-3-positive neurons, indicating that caspase-8 activation might precede that of caspase-3 [34]. It remains unclear how the caspase cascade is triggered after spinal cord ischemia, although recent evidence implicates cell surface receptors as a potential source. Cell surface receptors promote cell death, for example the Fas (Apo1/CD95) cell death receptor [41], and have been implicated in focal brain ischemia [42] or during programmed cell death of motor neurons in the spinal cord [43].

In the immune system, Fas receptor (FasR) and Fas ligand (FasL) are involved in elimination of mature T cells, infected cells or tumor cells. FasL triggers cell death by trimerizing FasR at the cell surface. Under these conditions, the cytoplasmic domain of FasR binds the adapter protein FasR-associated death domain [44]. FasR-associated death domain in turn binds procaspase-8, which can thereby self-activate [45]. Cleavage of downstream substrates by caspase-8 rapidly triggers death in cells expressing FasR [46]. FasL can also activate FasR in an autocrine manner: T lymphocytes committed to die upregulate FasL and FasR and thus support their own death [47,48].

In the normal spinal cord FasL mRNA was identified by Southern blot analysis [43,49], while FasR expression was observed in neurons and microvessels by immunohistochemistry [34]. After spinal cord ischemia in adult rabbits, FasR immunoreactivity was selectively increased in spinal motor neurons 8 hours to 1 day after reperfusion and preceded typical ladders of oligonucleosomal DNA fragments by 24 hours [50]. Similar results were obtained in a newly developed mouse spinal cord ischemia model [34]. The latter work provided the first suggestive evidence that FasR upregulation is actually leading to caspase activation and is therefore linked to subsequent cell death. A complex containing Fas and procaspase-8 in ischemic spinal cord was found by immunoprecipitation. Hence, spinal cord ischemia appears to augment the death inducing signaling complex thereby first activating caspase-8 and, later, caspase-3 (see above).

Conclusion

There is already sufficient evidence to implicate caspases in ischemic pathophysiology and to suggest targeting one or more family members for treatment of acute CNS injury. Together, the data suggest that caspases are constitutively expressed in the adult nervous system and become activated after brain and spinal cord ischemia. The onset and extent of cleavage depends to some degree on the magnitude and duration of insult, with evidence favoring a greater role for caspase-mediated cell death during brief and mild or moderate ischemic injury. The mechanisms appear to be distinct from necrotic cell death mediated by excitotoxicity, and there is in vivo and in vitro evidence to suggest synergistic effects that may have important implications for combination therapy [51,52]. The two mechanisms of cell death are, however, not mutually exclusive. The use of caspase inhibitors for human stroke and spinal cord ischemia will depend on the successful development of drugs that cross the blood–brain barrier and penetrate CNS cells at sufficient levels to achieve enzyme inhibition. The expression and activation of other caspases (e.g., caspase-8 and caspase-7) suggest the advantages of developing pancaspase inhibitors.

Acknowledgments

The current work was supported by the National Institutes of Health (NS10828 and NS374141–02, M.A.M.) and the Deutsche Forschungsgemeinschaft (Pl 249/5–1, N.P.).

REFERENCES

1 Bhat RV, DiRocco R, Marcy VR, Flood DG, Zhu Y, Dobrzanski P, Siman R, Scott R, Contreras PC & Miller M (1996) Increased expression of IL-1β converting enzyme in hippocampus after ischemia: selective localization in microglia. *Journal of Neuroscience*, **16**, 4146–54.
2 Honkaniemi J, Massa SM, Breckinridge M & Sharp FR (1996) Global ischemia induces apoptosis-associated genes in hippocampus. *Molecular Brain Research*, **42**, 79–88.
3 Gillardon F, Bottiger B, Schmitz B, Zimmermann M & Hossmann K-A (1997) Activation of CPP-32 protease in hippocampal neurons following ischemia and epilepsy. *Molecular Brain Research*, **50**, 16–22.
4 Chen J, Nagayama T, Jin K, Stetler RA, Zhu RL, Graham SH & Simon RP (1998) Induction of caspase-3-like protease may mediate delayed neuronal death in the hippocampus after transient cerebral ischemia. *Journal of Neuroscience*, **18**, 4914–28.

5 Ni B, Wu X, Su Y, Stephenson D, Smalstig EB, Clemens J & Paul SM (1998) Transient global forebrain ischemia induces a prolonged expression of the caspase-3 mRNA in rat hippocampal CA1 pyramidal neurons. *Journal of Cerebral Blood Flow & Metabolism*, **18**, 248–56.

6 Gillardon F, Kiprianova I, Sandkuhler J, Hossmann K-A & Spranger M (1999) Inhibition of caspases prevents cell death of hippocampal CA1 neurons, but not impairment of hippocampal long-term potentiation following global ischemia. *Neuroscience*, **93**, 1219–22.

7 Ouyang YB, Tan Y, Comb M, Liu CL, Martone ME, Siesjö BK & Hu BR (1999) Survival- and death-promoting events after transient cerebral ischemia: phosphorylation of Akt, release of cytochrome *c* and activation of caspase-like proteases. *Journal of Cerebral Blood Flow & Metabolism*, **19**, 1126–35.

8 Nakatsuka H, Ohta S, Tanaka J, Toku K, Kumon Y, Maeda N, Sakanaka M & Sakaki S (2000) Histochemical cytochrome *c* oxidase activity and caspase-3 in gerbil hippocampal CA1 neurons after transient forebrain ischemia. *Neuroscience Letters*, **285**, 127–30.

9 Krajewski S, Krajewska M, Ellerby LM, Welsh K, Xie Z, Deveraux QL, Salvesen GS, Bredesen DE, Rosenthal RE, Fiskum G & Reed JC (1999) Release of caspase-9 from mitochondria during neuronal apoptosis and cerebral ischemia. *Proceedings of the National Academy of Sciences, USA*, **96**, 5752–7.

10 Antonawich FJ (1999) Translocation of cytochrome *c* following transient global ischemia in the gerbil. *Neuroscience Letters*, **274**, 123–6.

11 Nakatsuka H, Ohta S, Tanaka J, Toku K, Kumon Y, Maeda N, Sakanaka M & Sakaki S (1999) Release of cytochrome *c* from mitochondria to cytosol in gerbil hippocampal CA1 neurons after transient forebrain ischemia. *Brain Research*, **849**, 216–19.

12 Sugawara T, Fujimura M, Morita-Fujimura Y, Kawase M & Chan PH (1999) Mitochondrial release of cytochrome *c* corresponds to the selective vulnerability of hippocampal CA1 neurons in rats after transient global cerebral ischemia. *Journal of Neuroscience*, **19 RC39**, 1–6.

13 Himi T, Ishizaki Y & Murota S (1998) A caspase inhibitor blocks ischaemia-induced delayed neuronal death in the gerbil. *European Journal of Neuroscience*, **10**, 777–81.

14 Rami A, Agarwal R, Botez G & Winckler J (2000) μ-Calpain activation, DNA fragmentation, and synergistic effects of caspase and calpain inhibitors in protecting hippocampal neurons from ischemic damage. *Brain Research*, **866**, 299–312.

15 Li H, Colbourne F, Sun P, Zhao Z, Buchan AM & Iadecola C (2000) Caspase inhibitors reduce neuronal injury after focal but not global cerebral ischemia in rats. *Stroke*, **31**, 176–82.

16 Loddick SA, MacKenzie A & Rothwell NJ (1996) An ICE inhibitor, z-VAD-DCB attenuates ischaemic brain damage in the rat. *Neuroreport*, **7**, 1465–8.

17 Hara H, Fink K, Endres M, Friedlander RM, Gagliardini V, Yuan J & Moskowitz MA (1997) Attenuation of transient focal cerebral ischemic injury in transgenic mice expressing a mutant ICE inhibitory protein. *Journal of Cerebral Blood Flow & Metabolism*, **17**, 370–5.

18 Schielke GP, Yang GY, Shivers BD & Betz AL (1998) Reduced ischemic brain injury in interleukin-1β converting enzyme-deficient mice. *Journal of Cerebral Blood Flow & Metabolism*, **18**, 180–5.

19 Kang SJ, Wang S, Hara H, Peterson EP, Namura S, Amin-Hanjani S, Huang Z, Srinivasan A, Tomaselli KJ, Thornberry NA, Moskowitz MA & Yuan J (2000) Dual role of caspase-11 in

mediating activation of caspase-1 and caspase-3 under pathological conditions. *Journal of Cell Biology*, **149**, 613–22.

20 Asahi M, Hoshimaru M, Uemura Y, Tokime T, Kojima M, Ohtsuka T, Matsuura N, Aoki T, Shibahara K & Kikuchi H (1997) Expression of interleukin-1β converting enzyme gene family and bcl-2 gene family in the rat brain following permanent occlusion of the middle cerebral artery. *Journal of Cerebral Blood Flow & Metabolism*, **17**, 11–18.

21 Namura S, Zhu J, Fink K, Endres M, Srinivasan A, Tomaselli KJ, Yuan J & Moskowitz MA (1998) Activation and cleavage of caspase-3 in apoptosis induced by experimental cerebral ischemia. *Journal of Neuroscience*, **18**, 3659–68.

22 Fink K, Zhu J, Namura S, Shimizu-Sasamata M, Endres M, Ma J, Dalkara T, Yuan J & Moskowitz MA (1998) Prolonged therapeutic window for ischemic brain damage caused by delayed caspase activation. *Journal of Cerebral Blood Flow & Metabolism*, **18**, 1071–6.

23 Endres M, Namura S, Shimizu-Sasamata M, Waeber C, Zhang L, Gomez-Isla T, Hyman BT & Moskowitz MA (1998) Attenuation of delayed neuronal death after mild focal ischemia in mice by inhibition of the caspase family. *Journal of Cerebral Blood Flow & Metabolism*, **18**, 238–47.

24 Wiessner C, Sauer D, Alaimo D & Allegrini PR (2000) Protective effect of a caspase inhibitor in models for cerebral ischemia in vitro and in vivo. *Cellular & Molecular Biology*, **46**, 53–62.

25 Fujimura M, Morita-Fujimura Y, Murakami K, Kawase M & Chan PH (1998) Cytosolic redistribution of cytochrome *c* after transient focal cerebral ischemia in rats. *Journal of Cerebral Blood Flow & Metabolism*, **18**, 1239–47.

26 Velier JJ, Ellison JA, Kikly KK, Spera PA, Barone FC & Feuerstein GZ (1999) Caspase-8 and caspase-3 are expressed by different populations of cortical neurons undergoing delayed cell death after focal stroke in the rat. *Journal of Neuroscience*, **19**, 5932–41.

27 Harrison DC, Roberts J, Campbell CA, Crook B, Davis R, Deen K, Meakin J, Michalovich D, Price J, Stammers M & Maycox PR (2000) TR3 death receptor expression in the normal and ischaemic brain. *Neuroscience*, **96**, 147–60.

28 Bergeron L, Perez GI, Macdonald G, Shi L, Sun Y, Jurisicova A, Varmuza S, Latham KE, Flaws JA, Salter JC, Hara H, Moskowitz MA, Li E, Greenberg A, Tilly JL & Yuan J (1998) Defects in regulation of apoptosis in caspase-2-deficient mice. *Genes & Development*, **12**, 1304–14.

29 Cheng Y, Deshmukh M, D'Costa A, Demaro JA, Gidday JM, Shah A, Sun Y, Jacquin MF, Johnson EM & Holtzman DM (1998) Caspase inhibitor affords neuroprotection with delayed administration in a rat model of neonatal hypoxic-ischemic brain injury. *Journal of Clinical Investigation*, **101**, 1992–9.

30 Han BH, D'Costa A, Back SA, Parsadanian M, Patel S, Shah AR, Gidday JM, Srinivasan A, Deshmukh M & Holtzman DM (2000) BDNF blocks caspase-3 activation in neonatal hypoxia-ischemia. *Neurobiology of Disease*, **7**, 38–53.

31 Pulera MR, Adams LM, Liu H, Santos DG, Nishimura RN, Yang F, Cole GM & Wasterlain CG (1998) Apoptosis in a neonatal rat model of cerebral hypoxia-ischemia. *Stroke*, **29**, 2622–30.

32 Liu XH, Kwon D, Schielke GP, Yang GY, Silverstein FS & Barks JD (1999) Mice deficient in interleukin-1 converting enzyme are resistant to neonatal hypoxic–ischemic brain damage. *Journal of Cerebral Blood Flow & Metabolism*, **19**, 1099–108.

33 Hayashi T, Sakurai M, Abe K, Sadahiro M, Tabayashi K & Itoyama Y (1998) Apoptosis of motor neurons with induction of caspases in the spinal cord after ischemia. *Stroke*, **29**, 1007–12.

34 Matsushita K, Wu Y, Qiu J, Lang-Lazdunski L, Hirt L, Waeber C, Hyman BT, Yuan J & Moskowitz MA (2000) Fas receptor and neuronal cell death after spinal cord ischemia. *Journal of Neuroscience*, **20**, 6879–87.

35 Milligan CE, Prevette D, Yaginuma H, Homma S, Cardwell C, Fritz LC, Tomaselli KJ, Oppenheim RW & Schwartz LM (1995) Peptide inhibitors of the ICE protease family arrest programmed cell death of motoneurons in vivo and in vitro. *Neuron*, **15**, 385–93.

36 Li L, Prevette D, Oppenheim RW & Milligan CE (1998) Involvement of specific caspases in motoneuron cell death in vivo and in vitro following trophic factor deprivation. *Molecular & Cellular Neurosciences*, **12**, 157–67.

37 Kato H, Kanellopoulos GK, Matsuo S, Wu YJ, Jacquin MF, Hsu CY, Kouchoukos NT & Choi DW (1997) Neuronal apoptosis and necrosis following spinal cord ischemia in the rat. *Experimental Neurology*, **148**, 464–74.

38 Mackey ME, Wu Y, Hu R, DeMaro JA, Jacquin MF, Kanellopoulos GK, Hsu CY & Kouchoukos NT (1997) Cell death suggestive of apoptosis after spinal cord ischemia in rabbits. *Stroke*, **28**, 2012–7.

39 Sakurai M, Aoki M, Abe K, Sadahiro M & Tabayashi K (1997) Selective motor neuron death and heat shock protein induction after spinal cord ischemia in rabbits. *Journal of Thoracic & Cardiovascular Surgery*, **113**, 159–64.

40 Lang-Lazdunski L, Matsushita K, Hirt L, Waeber C, Vonsattel JP, Moskowitz MA & Dietrich WD (2000) Spinal cord ischemia. Development of a model in the mouse. *Stroke*, **31**, 208–13.

41 Nagata S & Golstein P (1995) The Fas death factor. *Science*, **267**, 1449–56.

42 Martin-Villalba A, Herr I, Jeremias I, Hahne M, Brandt R, Vogel J, Schenkel J, Herdegen T & Debatin KM (1999) CD95 ligand (Fas-L/APO-1L) and tumor necrosis factor-related apoptosis-inducing ligand mediate ischemia-induced apoptosis in neurons. *Journal of Neuroscience*, **19**, 3809–17.

43 Raoul C, Henderson CE & Pettmann B (1999) Programmed cell death of embryonic motoneurons triggered through the Fas death receptor. *Journal of Cell Biology*, **147**, 1049–62.

44 Chinnaiyan AM, O'Rourke K, Tewari M & Dixit VM (1995) FADD, a novel death domain-containing protein, interacts with the death domain of Fas and initiates apoptosis. *Cell*, **81**, 505–12.

45 Muzio M, Chinnaiyan AM, Kischkel FC, O'Rourke K, Shevchenko A, Ni J, Scaffidi C, Bretz JD, Zhang M, Gentz R, Mann M, Krammer PH, Peter ME & Dixit VM (1996) FLICE, a novel FADD-homologous ICE/CED-3-like protease, is recruited to the CD95 (Fas/APO-1) death-inducing signaling complex. *Cell*, **85**, 817–27.

46 Scaffidi C, Fulda S, Srinivasan A, Friesen C, Li F, Tomaselli KJ, Debatin KM, Krammer PH & Peter ME (1998) Two CD95 (APO-1/Fas) signaling pathways. *EMBO Journal*, **17**, 1675–87.

47 Brunner T, Mogil RJ, LaFace D, Yoo NJ, Mahboubi A, Echeverri F, Martin SJ, Force WR, Lynch DH, Ware CF & Green DR (1995) Cell-autonomous Fas (CD95)/Fas-ligand interaction mediates activation-induced apoptosis in T-cell hybridomas. *Nature*, **373**, 441–4.

48 Dhein J, Walczak H, Baumler C, Debatin KM & Krammer PH (1995) Autocrine T-cell suicide mediated by APO-1/(Fas/CD95). *Nature*, **373**, 438–41.

49 French LE & Tschopp J (1996) Constitutive Fas ligand expression in several non-lymphoid mouse tissues: implications for immune-protection and cell turnover. *Behring Institute Mitteilungen*, **97**, 156–60.

50 Sakurai M, Hayashi T, Abe K, Sadahiro M & Tabayashi K (1998) Delayed selective motor neuron death and fas antigen induction after spinal cord ischemia in rabbits. *Brain Research*, **797**, 23–8.

51 Schulz JB, Weller M, Matthews RT, Heneka MT, Groscurth P, Martinou JC, Lommatzsch J, von Coelln R, Wullner U, Loschmann PA, Beal MF, Dichgans J & Klockgether T (1998) Extended therapeutic window for caspase inhibition and synergy with MK-801 in the treatment of cerebral histotoxic hypoxia. *Cell Death & Differentiation*, **5**, 847–57.

52 Ma J, Endres M & Moskowitz MA (1998) Synergistic effects of caspase inhibitors and MK-801 in brain injury after transient focal cerebral ischaemia in mice. *British Journal of Pharmacology*, **124**, 756–62.

53 Xu D, Bureau Y, McIntyre DC, Nicholson DW, Liston P, Zhu Y, Fong WG, Crocker SJ, Korneluk RG & Robertson GS (1999) Attenuation of ischemia-induced cellular and behavioral deficits by X chromosome-linked inhibitor of apoptosis protein overexpression in the rat hippocampus. *Journal of Neuroscience*, **19**, 5026–33.

54 Guegan C & Sola B (2000) Early and sequential recruitment of apoptotic effectors after focal permanent ischemia in mice. *Brain Research*, **856**, 93–100.

Part II

Oxidative stress

Co-Chairs: Raymond A. Swanson & Bo K. Siesjö

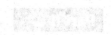

Peroxynitrite and injury to the vasculature and central nervous system in stroke and neurodegeneration

Joseph S. Beckman,[1] John Crow[2] & Alvaro G. Estévez[3]

[1] Departments of Anesthesiology, Biochemistry, and Neurobiology, University of Alabama at Birmingham, Birmingham, AL
[2] Departments of Anesthesiology and Pharmacology, University of Alabama at Birmingham, Birmingham, AL
[3] Departments of Pharmacology and Physiology, University of Alabama at Birmingham, Birmingham, AL

Introduction

Oxidative stress is a widely recognized but poorly understood component in stroke and neurodegeneration. Antioxidant enzymes as well as a variety of low molecular weight antioxidants can be remarkably protective in animal models in stroke, trauma and neurodegenerative diseases [1–5]. However, the targets and even the nature of the reactive species themselves have so far been poorly delineated. The extraordinary reactivity of some oxidants such as the hydroxyl radical has masked the search for specific targets of oxidative damage in vivo. Growing evidence indicates that oxygen radicals can produce remarkably specific actions far upstream in signaling cascades that can initiate apoptosis in neurodegeneration [6]. In addition, oxygen radicals exert an important role in promoting thrombosis and permeability increases in the vasculature that can greatly complicate the final outcome from stroke [7]. In this chapter, we will review how oxidative stress resulting from the interactions of superoxide with nitric oxide could be involved in damage both to the cerebral vasculature and to neurons in stroke.

Oxygen toxicity and superoxide

A strong case can be made for molecular oxygen in the air we breathe being the most dangerous toxin and carcinogen in the environment [8]. From a thermodynamic point of view, molecular oxygen is capable of oxidizing any biological molecule [9] and routinely does so as the terminal electron acceptor in normal metabolism. However, the rates of such reactions occurring spontaneously with oxygen are quite slow, which allows us to exist in an atmosphere containing 20%

oxygen. Molecular oxygen has a most unusual bonding arrangement, with two unpaired electrons occupying separate orbitals. In essence, this small molecule preferentially exists as two free radicals rather than having all of the electrons paired. Consequently, oxygen can accept only one electron sequentially from biological molecules at a time. This prevents oxygen from rapidly oxidizing most biological materials because they have filled orbitals containing two electrons of opposite spin and giving up only one electron is energetically highly unfavorable.

However, oxygen can be reduced by a variety of enzymes in the body, including reduced nicotinamide adenine dinucleotide phosphate (NADPH) oxidases and xanthine oxidase, to produce free radicals. The addition of one electron to molecular oxygen produces superoxide anion. Superoxide was named by Linus Pauling [10], who predicted that it would be an exceptionally strong oxidant, capable of grabbing a second electron to form hydrogen peroxide. However, superoxide at neutral pH is not a strong oxidant because it is negatively charged. Since oxidation would require withdrawing an electron from another molecule, the overall reaction would be quite slow because the reaction involves transferring a negative charge to a small molecule that is already negatively charged (Figure 3.1). While not a general oxidizing agent, superoxide is quite reactive with iron–sulfur centers commonly found in mitochondria, which are positively charged and contain electron-rich sulfurs as ligands [9]. The positive charge attracts and then neutralizes the negatively charged superoxide anion, which then oxidizes adjacent sulfurs. This is known to inactivate a variety of enzymes including aconitase and amino acid dehydratases [11–13].

From the viewpoint of patients recovering from stroke, oxidative stress is generally bad because it amplifies tissue injury. However, there has also been strong evolutionary pressure for cells to produce oxygen radicals as antimicrobial defenses. Because these molecules are generally reactive, they are produced by a variety of inflammatory cells including neutrophils and macrophages to injure or kill invading microorganisms and parasites. These inflammatory cells contain highly active NADPH oxidases that donate electrons from NADPH univalently to reduce oxygen to superoxide. Activation of these complexes in the vicinity of invading microorganisms can produce a substantial flux of superoxide and hydrogen peroxide [14]. Neutrophils also contain the enzyme myeloperoxidase, which uses hydrogen peroxide plus chloride to produce hypochlorous acid, the principal ingredient in Clorox bleach. More recently, it has been recognized that macrophages [15–19] and even neutrophils can produce nitric oxide [20]. Nitric oxide itself is not toxic, but adds a whole new layer of secondary reactive species that can be generated within these inflammatory cells. Even more surprising, expression of NADPH oxidases is not restricted to inflammatory cells but is also found in endothelium and neurons [21,22]. Because of the great importance in surviving

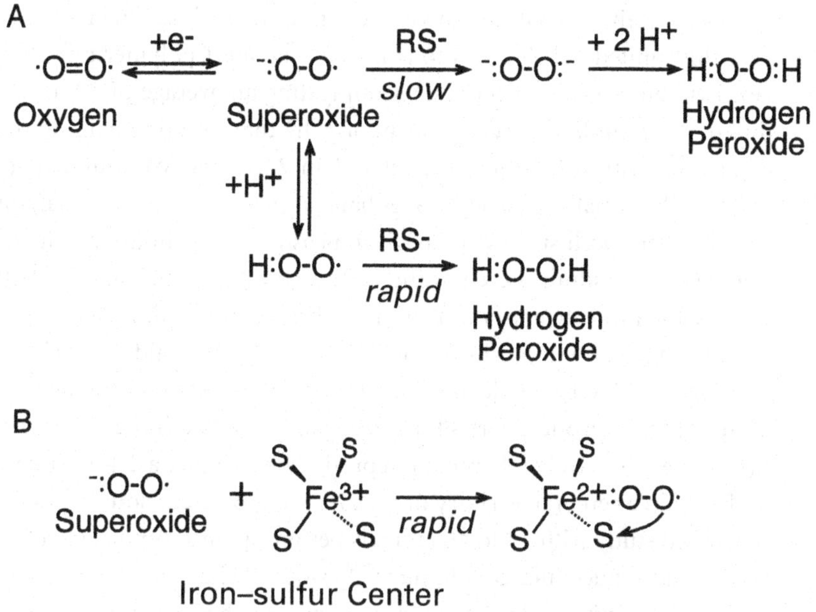

A

$$\cdot O{=}O\cdot \underset{}{\overset{+e^-}{\rightleftharpoons}} \;\; \overset{..}{\cdot}O{-}O\cdot \;\; \underset{slow}{\overset{RS{-}}{\longrightarrow}} \;\; \overset{..}{\cdot}O{-}O{:}^{-} \;\; \overset{+2\,H^+}{\longrightarrow} H{:}O{-}O{:}H$$

Oxygen   Superoxide   Hydrogen
                                                                Peroxide

$+H^+$

$$H{:}O{-}O\cdot \;\; \underset{rapid}{\overset{RS{-}}{\longrightarrow}} \;\; H{:}O{-}O{:}H$$

Hydrogen
Peroxide

B

$$\overset{..}{\cdot}O{-}O\cdot \;\; + \;\; \overset{S}{\underset{S}{\diagdown}}Fe^{3+}\overset{S}{\underset{S}{\diagup}} \;\; \underset{rapid}{\longrightarrow} \;\; \overset{S}{\underset{S}{\diagdown}}Fe^{2+}{:}O{-}O\cdot\overset{S}{\underset{S}{\diagup}}$$

Superoxide

Iron–sulfur Center

Figure 3.1   (A) The reactivity of superoxide is surprisingly limited. Transferring an electron to a
negatively charged superoxide is slow because the intermediate has two negative charges.
Consequently, superoxide is slow to oxidize biological materials, including ionized
sulfhydryls (RS⁻). These are among the groups most susceptible to autooxidation.
(B) However, positively charged metals such as the iron in iron–sulfur proteins can react
rapidly with superoxide. Once the electrical charge of superoxide is neutralized, the
superoxide-Fe adduct can rapidly attach the sulfur.

infection and the huge selective pressures imposed by infectious diseases during
early childhood, it is not surprising that the body produces large amounts of oxidants as antimicrobial defenses at the expense of suffering greater collateral
damage in neurological disease, occurring well past the age of reproduction. There
is growing recognition that inflammation plays a major role in neurodegeneration
as well [23].

Superoxide and stroke

Oxygen radicals can clearly amplify the injury produced by cerebral ischemia. My
own interest in this field began by using the antioxidant enzyme superoxide dismutase (SOD) as a therapeutic agent to treat stroke. SOD was first identified in 1969
by McCord and Fridovich [24] and by the 1980s was being produced in large
amounts by biotech companies as a possible therapeutic agent for intestinal and
myocardial ischemia. A problem with the use of SOD was its rapid clearance by the

kidneys, limiting its half-life in vivo to 6 minutes or less. One method to circumvent this limited half-life was to conjugate the inert polymer polyethylene glycol (PEG) to amino groups on SOD. Conjugating an average of 10 to 12 PEGs produced a high molecular weight form of SOD that would remain detectable in the circulation with a half-life of greater than 24 hours. We found that PEG-SOD would substantially protect Mongolian gerbils subjected to bilateral common carotid artery occlusion [25]. Survival measured at 24 hours was increased when PEG-SOD was administered at the end of carotid occlusion. PEG-SOD was also remarkably protective in a model of cerebral ischemia developed by Chung Hsu [26]. In this highly reproducible model of stroke, the middle cerebral artery was occluded distal to the circle of Willis and then blood flow was reduced by clamping both common carotid arteries for a fixed period of 90 minutes. This was one of the first models that could reliably and reproducibly produce a defined infarct confined to the middle cerebral territory of rats. In a randomized, double-blinded placebo-controlled study with 38 to 40 animals per group, intravenous injections of PEG-SOD could reduce infarct volume by 35% [27]. The placebo control consisted of PEG-SOD inactivated by treatment with alkaline hydrogen peroxide to selectively damage one of the histidine ligands to copper in the active site. In a subsequent study, Hsu showed that the dosage of PEG-SOD was extremely important and that a three-fold higher concentration of PEG-SOD could make edema even worse rather than providing protection [28]. This loss of protection could not be attributed to toxicity of the PEG-SOD itself and remained largely unexplained. Pharmaceutical companies began to test PEG-SOD as a possible therapeutic reagent for treating traumatic brain injuries. A phase II trial showed some efficacy at the same dosage of PEG-SOD as we used in our initial trials [29]. However, expanded phase III trials subsequently found little or no protective effect of PEG-SOD [30].

The failure of phase III trials with PEG-SOD points to our limited and even naïve understanding of the role of free radicals in traumatic brain injury and cerebral ischemia. For example, PEG-SOD was injected directly into the circulation and it is too large to readily cross the blood–brain barrier except at sites of injury [31,32]. This suggests that PEG-SOD may be active at the level of the vasculature rather than directly affecting neuronal survival. A second gap in our knowledge is the target of superoxide that is responsible in increased injury. A third difficulty is to explain how high doses of SOD are less protective and possibly even increase brain edema. The last point has become particularly important to understand, since mutations to SOD have since been discovered to cause selective degeneration of motor neurons in amyotrophic lateral sclerosis (ALS). To better understand these issues, it is necessary to consider the normal functions of SOD in greater depth.

SOD and the scavenging of superoxide

There are three isozymes of SOD found in vivo. We will concentrate here only on the cytosolic form of the enzyme, which is a dimer containing 153 amino acid residues and in which each subunit contains one atom of copper (Cu) and one atom of zinc (Zn). The enzyme is particularly abundant in cells and constitutes 0.5% by weight of liver and brain. In the spinal cord we have estimated the concentration of SOD may be as high as 0.7% of total cell protein. The enzyme is distributed throughout the cytosol and is found in peroxisomes as well as in the nucleus. Mitochondria contain a distinct 24 kDa isozyme of SOD that contains manganese. We will not consider this enzyme further in this chapter, although it also has a major role in our understanding of oxidative stress in neurodegeneration [33]. Because CuZnSOD is a relatively small protein and constitutes a large fraction of total cell protein, its concentration in vivo is surprisingly high, estimated to be roughly 10 μM [34]. The concentration of oxygen is roughly 200 μM in the bloodstream and in the range of 30 μM or below in neurons. Given the high concentrations of SOD and limited solubility of oxygen, the concentration of superoxide has to be incredibly small in vivo.

The catalytic mechanism of scavenging of superoxide by CuZnSOD is remarkably simple (Figure 3.2A). Copper normally exists in its oxidized or cupric state (Cu^{2+}). Superoxide is attracted to the active site of SOD containing the copper, and an electron is rapidly transferred from superoxide to copper. This generates oxygen and leaves copper in its cuprous or Cu^{1+} state. When a second superoxide encounters the enzyme, the electron is transferred from the Cu^{1+} to the superoxide to produce hydrogen peroxide and regenerates the SOD enzyme in the cupric state. Both steps of the reaction occur quite rapidly, making SOD the fastest enzyme known. However, the mechanism is subtler, with the structural zinc atom playing an important role in the second half of the dismutation cycle. A bridging histidine spans the copper and the zinc in SOD, which is a unique structure that has not been identified in any other protein to date. In the oxidized state, the copper is bound to a total of four histidines including the bridging histidine ligand to zinc. However, copper becomes reduced, the bridging ligand bound to the zinc detaches and the copper remains coordinated to only three histidine residues (Figure 3.2B). The bridging histidine still bound to the zinc atom becomes protonated and the high positive charge density on the zinc atom makes this proton a strong Lewis acid. This helps facilitate the second half of the reaction, where an electron needs to be transferred onto the negatively charged superoxide. The proton can be transferred to the negatively charged superoxide to form its conjugate acid, HOO$^{\cdot}$. This intermediate is a powerful oxidant and will rapidly oxidize Cu^{1+} to regenerate Cu^{2+} SOD into the native state while producing hydrogen peroxide (the additional proton is

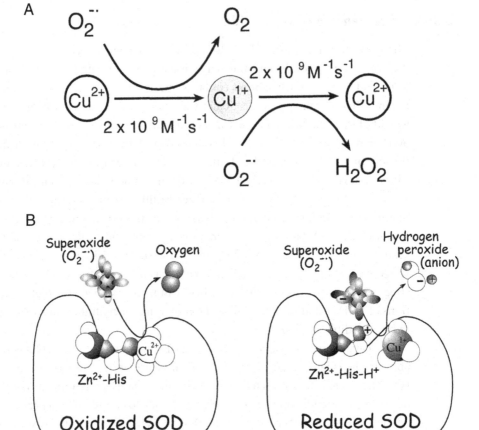

Figure 3.2   (A) At a simple level, the catalytic mechanism of SOD can be viewed simply as an alternating reduction and reoxidation of the copper atom in the active site. (B) However, the zinc atom plays an important role in neutralizing the negative charge and protonate superoxide, which then rapidly removes the electron stored on the copper atom. Loss of this zinc from SOD makes this protein far more toxic.

provided by the solvent). Consequently, the zinc atom plays an important role in promoting the rapid oxidation of Cu^{1+} in the formation of hydrogen peroxide. The loss of zinc greatly changes the properties of SOD and makes it toxic to neurons.

The high concentrations of SOD present in cells and its near diffusion-limited reaction with superoxide raises questions about what can be the biological targets of superoxide in vivo. Such targets must be both abundant and react rapidly with superoxide to have a chance of competing with SOD. One of the few such types of chemical moieties are iron–sulfur centers found in electron transport enzymes. The positive charge of the iron helps to attract and neutralize the negative charge on superoxide, while the electron-rich sulfur groups provide a substrate that can be easily oxidized once superoxide interacts with the iron atom. One example is the citric acid cycle enzyme aconitase, which is slowly inactivated by superoxide in vivo [11,35].

Nitric oxide and peroxynitrite

However, a major target for the reaction with superoxide became apparent with the discovery of nitric oxide as a biological molecule [36]. Nitric oxide was originally described as the endothelium-derived relaxing factor. It can be produced by any of three different isozymes through the oxidation of a guanidino nitrogen. Nitric oxide has been shown to activate guanylate cyclase to promote the vasorelaxation of blood vessels [37,38]. It is also a major modulator of neuronal transmission and is produced in much greater concentrations throughout the central nervous system [39–41]. While nitric oxide was originally described as highly reactive and toxic, further studies showed that nitric oxide itself was relatively inert with most biological molecules [42,43]. Its toxicity was derived from the formation of secondary reactive species. At the low concentrations of nitric oxide produced for single transduction, the molecule is rapidly removed by diffusing into blood vessels where it reacts with hemoglobin to form met-hemoglobin plus nitrate, or to a lesser extent nitrosyl(Fe^{2+})hemoglobin complexes.

Because both nitric oxide and superoxide have unpaired electrons, they react at near diffusion-limited rates to form peroxynitrite anion. The diffusion-limited limit implies that essentially every collision between nitric oxide and superoxide results in the formation of peroxynitrite. Because small molecules can diffuse much more rapidly than large proteins, the reaction of nitric oxide is several times faster with superoxide than the scavenging of superoxide by SOD. This allows nitric oxide to outcompete SOD for superoxide under physiological conditions. The high intracellular concentrations of SOD, estimated to be as high as 10 μM [34], greatly reduce the formation of peroxynitrite in vitro. However, the formation of peroxynitrite can still occur in the presence of SOD and is even more favorable than a simple competitive analysis of the relative rate constants would indicate. This point is essential for understanding how SOD participates in ALS.

Peroxynitrite is a far stronger oxidant and much more toxic than either nitric oxide or superoxide acting separately. One can consider peroxynitrite to be a binary weapon assembled from two less reactive intermediates. Peroxynitrite anion is remarkably stable. We have kept crystals of peroxynitrite for as long as 10 years with little decomposition. Peroxynitrite anion has a pK_a of 6.8, allowing a substantial fraction to be protonated at neutral pH. The resulting peroxynitrous acid is far more reactive, with 30% decomposing to form hydroxyl radical and nitrogen dioxide ($\cdot NO_2$) [14,44]. In addition, peroxynitrite can react with metal ions bound

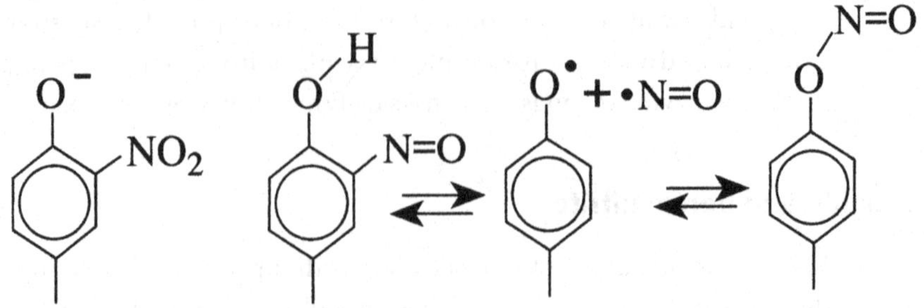

3-Nitrotyrosine   *C*-Nitrosotyrosine   Tyrosine radical   *O*-Nitrosotyrosine

Figure 3.3   Structure of nitrotyrosine vs. nitrosotyrosine and tyrosine radical plus nitric oxide. Nitrosotyrosine is relatively unstable whereas nitrotyrosine is effectively a permanent modification. The NO group on nitrosotyrosine can move between the oxygen and 3′-carbon of the phenyl group.

to proteins as well as carbon dioxide that catalyzes the addition of nitro (NO_2) groups to nitrate biological molecules. The most common targets include tyrosine, tryptophan and guanine.

Tyrosine nitration

The ability of peroxynitrite to nitrate biological molecules has been an important factor for establishing a role for peroxynitrite in many pathological processes. It is important to distinguish between nitration, nitrosation and nitrosylation (Figure 3.3). Nitration is the addition of an NO_2 group to tyrosine or other chemical moieties. In a biological system, molecules with aromatic rings are more susceptible to nitration than most other biological molecules. These form stable chemical adducts that are generally removed by degradation of the macromolecule and secretion in urine. Nitrosation is the addition of a nitroso (NO) group, which occurs most commonly on thiols but also is well known on hydroxyl groups and amines. Thiol nitrosation is generally a rapidly reversible process and tends to be rather short lived in biological systems, where an excess of thiols will reduce S-nitroso groups back to thiols. Nitrosotyrosine can be formed by the addition of the NO to tyrosine radicals, which is readily reversible [45].

Because the nitro group is a stable chemical modification that dramatically changes the chemical properties of tyrosine, it can have long lasting effects upon protein function. The nitro group is a large, bulky addition that is strongly electron withdrawing. This decreases the pK_a of the phenol hydroxy group on tyrosine from 10 to approximately 7.5. At neutral pH, approximately 50% of nitrotyrosine is negatively charged. In the negatively charged form, nitrotyrosine is visibly yellow. We initially discovered tyrosine nitration by peroxynitrite by observing that proteins became yellow after exposure to peroxynitrite. This was particularly dramatic with bovine CuZnSOD. Bovine SOD contains a single tyrosine far removed from its active site. However, we discovered that at high concentrations bovine SOD catalyzed the nitration of this tyrosine, turning the normally blue-green SOD into a yellow enzyme that remained fully active. A careful kinetic analysis showed that one bovine SOD molecule was forming a complex with peroxynitrite that catalyzed the nitration of a tyrosine on a completely separate SOD molecule. In a mixture of proteins, SOD will catalyze the nitration of many other proteins before it will catalyze nitration of itself [46]. Curiously, many of the proteins most susceptible to nitration in such a complex biological mixture appear to be subunits of structural proteins including neurofilaments and actin [47]. The ability of SOD to catalyze tyrosine nitration by peroxynitrite led us to propose in 1993 that catalysis of tyrosine nitration may be the gain of function accounting for the dominant phenotype of mutations to SOD in ALS [48].

Because antibodies to phosphotyrosine have been extremely useful, we undertook the development of antibodies to recognize nitrotyrosine [49,50]. Multiple polyclonal and monoclonal antibodies were successfully generated and are now commercially available from several sources. These antibodies work particularly well for immunohistochemistry. We first described tyrosine nitration occurring in human atherosclerosis, pulmonary lesions resulting from adult respiratory distress syndrome and myocarditis [49,51–53]. The literature has rapidly grown to include over 600 publications showing tyrosine nitration is present in a wide range of diseases [54]. Tyrosine nitration is reported to occur in ALS, Alzheimer's disease, Huntington's disease, multiple sclerosis and bacterial meningitis. Specific antibodies raised to nitrated α-synuclein have been shown to colocalize with Lewy bodies in Parkinson's disease and related syndromes [55]. Tyrosine nitration also occurs in stroke [56], although nitration is not particularly dramatic compared with inflammatory diseases. Curiously, endothelium in blood vessels in both stroke and traumatic brain injury appears to be the most susceptible cell type to tyrosine nitration.

An important contribution by the use of nitrotyrosine antibodies has been to show that substantial amounts of reactive nitrogen species can be produced in human diseases. In the early 1990s, strong criticisms were expressed that human monocytes and other human cells did not produce significant amounts of nitric oxide and therefore nitric oxide was not playing a major role in human disease [57–59]. The identification of nitrotyrosine immunohistochemically colocalized with active inflammatory processes provided dramatic confirmation that reactive nitrogen species were being produced in substantial quantities in a wide range of disease processes. It turns out that induction of the inducible nitric oxide synthase in humans is regulated by mechanisms quite different from that found in rats and mice. Only recently have some of the complexities of the regulation of nitric oxide synthesis in humans been partially unraveled [60,61].

Specificity of the nitrotyrosine antibodies can be confirmed by blocking the nitrotyrosine antibodies with small peptides containing nitrotyrosine. A second important control is to treat tissue sections or Western blot membranes with the potent reducing agent dithionite. Dithionite will rapidly reduce nitrotyrosine to aminotyrosine, which is not recognized by the antibody. Immunoreactivity is lost after the treatment. The immunoreactivity can be largely restored by reacting a dithionite-treated sample with hydrogen peroxide plus copper, which reoxidizes a substantial portion of aminotyrosine back to nitrotyrosine. The presence of nitrotyrosine in these tissue sections can be confirmed by hydrolyzing proteins followed by high performance liquid chromatography analysis of the individual amino acids. In some human samples, the amount of nitrotyrosine can exceed 1% of total tyrosines present in proteins isolated from diseased tissues [62]. While there have been a number of controversies over possible artifactual formation of nitrotyrosine during tissue hydrolysis, we have found that these artifacts are relatively easy to control and minimize. Multiple methods have confirmed high levels of nitrotyrosine in essentially all tissues. In addition, for some proteins in tissue samples, acid hydrolysis can destroy a substantial amount of nitrotyrosine during sample preparation. With appropriate cautions followed during sample preparation, tyrosine nitration is a useful marker for the formation of peroxynitrite and possibly other oxidants derived from nitric oxide in biological samples.

Although controversial, we believe that tyrosine nitration is an excellent marker of peroxynitrite formation in vivo. The production of nitric oxide itself does not result in tyrosine nitration and can substantially inhibit nitration in vitro. Substantial criticisms have been raised recently about other mechanisms of tyrosine nitration occurring in vivo. Two major culprits that might result in tyrosine nitration include $\cdot NO_2$ and nitrylchloride, which can be formed by the reaction of hypochlorous acid with nitrite [63,64]. Within an acute inflammatory lesion, multiple mechanisms undoubtedly could contribute to tyrosine nitration occurring at once. We have found that while $\cdot NO_2$ and nitrylchloride can nitrate free tyrosine in simple phosphate buffers, these oxidants barely nitrate proteins in complex biological mixtures because they are simply too reactive with other biological targets to nitrate tyrosine. In contrast, peroxynitrite is quite efficient at modifying specific tyrosines in certain proteins in cells [65]. In biological systems, not all tyrosine nitration necessarily results from peroxynitrite, but strong evidence indicates that peroxynitrite is likely to play a major role in tyrosine nitration. Wherever tyrosine nitration occurs in tissues, peroxynitrite is a major contributor even though other nitration mechanisms could also be operative.

Tyrosine nitration of selected proteins is difficult to identify by simple Western blotting using nitrotyrosine antibodies. However, immunoprecipation with nitrotyrosine antibodies to enrich nitrated proteins has resulted in approximately 20 different proteins that are nitrated in vivo being identified [54]. The first protein to be identified as nitrated is manganese (Mn) SOD [66], which is the major enzymatic defense against superoxide in mitochondria. Peroxynitrite itself rapidly inactivates MnSOD and results in the selective nitration of three different tyrosines of six in the protein [67]. Tyrosine 34 near the active site of MnSOD has been shown to be selectively nitrated by peroxynitrite [68]. However, mutation of this tyrosine to phenylalanine did not prevent the inactivation of MnSOD by peroxynitrite [69]. Still, nitration of MnSOD and the loss of its enzymatic activity is commonly observed in many different disease processes and strongly correlated with the production of nitric oxide.

Nitration of prostacyclin synthase

Ming Zou and Volker Ullrich have identified prostacyclin synthase as being remarkably susceptible to nitration and inactivation by peroxynitrite [70–72]. This enzyme converts the product prostaglandin (PG) H_2, produced by cyclooxygenase, into thromboxane. Submicromolar concentrations of peroxynitrite added to endothelium result in almost complete inactivation of this critical enzyme for maintaining antithrombotic activities of endothelium. Liberation of arachidonic acid by phospholipases can result in the formation of prostacyclin through two steps (Figure 3.4). The first step involves activation of cyclooxygenase to oxidize arachidonate to PGH_2. This enzyme contains an iron that must be converted to a higher oxidation state to oxidize arachidonate. To fully activate the enzyme, biochemists have found that a small amount of peroxide must be added to the enzyme to initiate the chemical reactions. The biological source of this peroxide tone in vivo has remained quite mysterious. Marnett et al. [73] showed that peroxynitrous acid, the protonated form of peroxynitrite, is an efficient activator of cyclooxygenase in vitro. More recently, they provided evidence that the formation of peroxynitrite in vivo is critical to the full activation of cyclooxygenase. On the other hand, peroxynitrite can rapidly inactivate prostacyclin synthase, which would take the product of cyclooxygenase and turn it into the vasodilating and anti-thrombogenic agent prostacyclin. Consequently, sustained production of peroxynitrite could completely inactivate prostacyclin synthase activity in seconds, while leading to the rapid formation of PGH_2. Curiously, PGH_2 is almost as effective at activating thromboxane receptors as thromboxane itself. Therefore, the build up of PGH_2 due to inactivation of prostacyclin synthase will produce the same vasoconstricting effects even in the absence of thromboxane synthase.

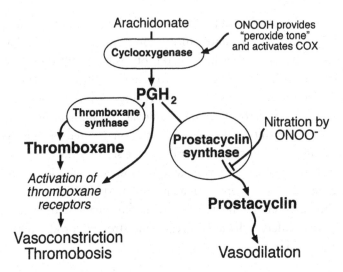

Figure 3.4   Dual actions of peroxynitrite on prostaglandin (PG) biosynthesis. Peroxynitrite can activate cyclooxygenase by providing the peroxide tone needed to put the iron in a highly oxidized state. This maximally stimulates the formation of PGH_2, which is a precursor for prostacyclin, thromboxane and PGE_2. However, prostacyclin synthase is also rapidly inactivated and nitrated by peroxynitrite, which results in the accumulation of PGH_2. PGH_2 has many of the same actions as thromboxane and will rapidly promote platelet aggregation and vasoconstriction. Thus inactivation of prostacyclin synthase alone is sufficient to cause the physiological actions of thromboxane even in tissues lacking thromboxane synthase.

Consequently, endothelium maintains an anti-thrombotic and vasodilating state through the combined production of nitric oxide and prostacyclin. However, inflammatory stimuli can activate superoxide production by endothelium [21,74], thereby forcing endogenous nitric oxide production to be rapidly converted to peroxynitrite. Peroxynitrite will increase the peroxide tone that can fully activate cyclooxygenase to oxidize more arachidonate to PGH_2, while shutting down the synthesis of prostacyclin through irreversible inactivation of prostacyclin synthase. The accumulating PGH_2 can act as thromboxane. In this manner, endothelium in a blood vessel can become strongly prothrombotic and constricted in a matter of seconds. While this would have negative effects in stroke and myocardial ischemia, it is an important adaptive response to limit trauma-induced bleeding and the spread of infectious agents.

Zou and Ullrich [70–72] have demonstrated nitration of prostacyclin synthase in atherosclerosis and have shown that exogenous PEG-SOD can prevent nitration of prostacyclin synthase in endothelium treated with pro-inflammatory stimuli. Given the propensity of endothelium to become positive for nitrotyrosine after cerebral ischemia, we suggest that nitration of prostacyclin synthase might be an important target of peroxynitrite in vivo. Protection of the endothelium may be a major contributing factor to explain how PEG-SOD was protective in our middle cerebral artery model of stroke [27].

Nitration of structural proteins

The other major target for nitration appears to be disassembled subunits of structural proteins. Structural proteins are the most abundant proteins expressed in cells. For instance, actin comprises about 8% of total brain protein, while neurofilaments are the predominant protein expressed in motor neurons. Structural proteins depend upon making many hydrophobic contacts between subunits to form stable macromolecular structures. Tyrosine tends to be particularly abundant in such proteins, occurring in 3% to 5% of total amino acids in a number of structural proteins. The hydroxyl group on tyrosine can hydrogen-bond to water, allowing it to be relatively hydrophilic but also stable within hydrophobic environments. When structural proteins are disassembled, many of these tyrosines become exposed to the solvent that greatly increases their susceptibility to nitration. We found that neurofilament-L, the smallest member of the neurofilament triplet family, was particularly susceptible to nitration at tyrosines located in the coiled coil domain [47].

Nitration of structural proteins can have major functional consequences. When nitrated neurofilaments are mixed with normal neurofilament protein, they greatly disrupt the assembly into functional neurofilament protein. Structural proteins are major targets for attack by peroxynitrite and other reactive nitrogen species because they are abundant, contain tyrosines that are susceptible to nitration, and nitration may have profound affects upon their ability to assemble into functional proteins. Tyrosine nitration adds a bulky hydrophilic group and introduces a negative charge to an amino acid residue that must normally fit tightly with the surface of other interacting subunits. Therefore, nitration has the capability of disrupting the assembly of macromolecular structures. Only a few tyrosines on a minority of subunits need to be modified to profoundly disrupt the assembly of functional, structural elements. In addition, nitrated neurofilaments can be found in the spinal cord of ALS patients as well as in patients suffering from a variety of other neurological diseases [75–77]. With the limited data available, one cannot say whether tyrosine nitration of neurofilament-L is more abundant in patients suffering from ALS versus other diseases [75].

SOD and motor neuron degeneration in ALS

ALS is characterized by the development of a progressive spastic paralysis resulting from the relentless death of lower and upper motor neurons. It is estimated that the adult spinal cord contains fewer than 1 millon to 2 million motor neurons. The loss of innervation by motor neurons leads to muscle degeneration, resulting in progressive paralysis. Motor neurons are the only means for the nervous system to activate muscles and thereby translate thought into action. Their complete loss eliminates the ability to communicate with the outside world.

In a landmark paper appearing in 1993, an international collaboration led by Siddique and Brown identified mutations to CuZnSOD as causing ALS in about 20% of familial patients [78]. Familial patients account for only about 10% of all patients suffering from this disease, so SOD mutations occur in only 2% to 3% of all ALS patients. No other defects in antioxidant defenses have been consistently identified in ALS. Of the ALS patients carrying SOD mutations, over 70 different mutations have been identified to the SOD protein [79]. The vast majority of these mutations are missense point mutations occurring in all five exons of this small protein. The SOD mutations are dominant, suggesting that they somehow confer a gain of function [79]. Overexpression of certain SOD mutations in transgenic mice results in the mice developing progressive paralysis [80]. In contrast, knocking out the endogenous mouse SOD gene does not result in the development of motor neuron disease [81], although motor neurons in these mice are more susceptible to injury.

To better characterize what the toxic gain of function might be for these mutations to SOD, we expressed a variety of the mutants in bacteria and purified the protein. Expression of the mutants was experimentally difficult to achieve because they have a much greater tendency to form inclusion bodies that could not be refolded into active SOD protein. However, small amounts of the protein could be expressed and purified. Working carefully to incorporate one zinc atom and one copper atom per subunit, we found that a range of the SOD proteins folded to give perfectly normal, functionally active CuZnSODs [82]. These SOD proteins scavenged superoxide at the same rate as the wild-type enzyme and also catalyzed tyrosine nitration by peroxynitrite of neurofilament proteins to the same extent as the wild-type enzyme [47]. While we could demonstrate no gain of function for the fully metal-containing form of the enzyme, it became clear that much of the SOD protein lacking zinc had been discarded during the purification procedures. This led us to the idea that the ALS mutants may have diminished affinity for zinc [82,83]. Similar conclusions were reached by Valentine's group [84].

The ALS-associated SOD mutations occur at sites that structurally weaken the β-barrel that forms the predominant backbone of the SOD protein [85,86]. Because zinc is held about 7000-fold less tightly than copper by the SOD protein, structural defects are more likely to cause the loss of zinc relative to copper [82]. Experimentally, we were able to demonstrate that the ALS mutants do have slightly smaller affinities for zinc as compared with the wild-type protein, and that one can

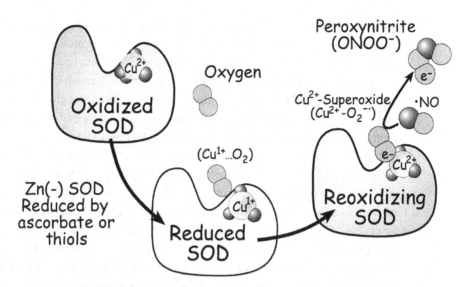

Figure 3.5   Zinc-deficient SOD is highly toxic to motor neurons because it can generate both superoxide and nitric oxide. The copper in zinc-deficient SOD rapidly oxidizes intracellular antioxidants such as ascorbate to become reduced. The reduced copper slowly reacts with oxygen and nitric oxide to form peroxynitrite, which is able to induce apoptosis in motor neurons.

roughly order zinc affinity of the SOD mutations with the rate of disease progression after diagnosis. There is no clear correlation with the age of onset.

The loss of zinc from SOD leads to a visibly distinct protein with different biochemical properties [87]. CuZnSOD is a blue-green protein, whereas zinc-deficient SOD is azure-blue. When ascorbate is added to the blue-colored zinc-deficient SOD, the protein quickly becomes colorless for a period of minutes until all the ascorbate is fully oxidized. The blue color gradually reappears as oxygen is reduced to superoxide. In the presence of a low concentration of nitric oxide, peroxynitrite can apparently be made by the reaction of nitric oxide with oxygen being reduced by the zinc-deficient SOD (Figure 3.5). In effect, zinc-deficient SOD can operate in reverse, stealing electrons from antioxidants present in the cell to reduce oxygen to superoxide, and can even catalyze the formation of peroxynitrite. Curiously, the addition of wild-type CuZnSOD does not slow the formation of peroxynitrite by zinc-deficient SOD. This is important because it shows how mutant SODs through the loss of zinc can confer a toxic gain of function involving oxidative stress, even in the presence of a large excess of wild-type CuZnSOD.

We have been able to show that a similar mechanism can operate within motor neurons in culture. To do this, we utilized a motor neuron system initially characterized by Alvaro Estévez during his Ph.D. work in Luis Barbeito's laboratory in

Uruguay. Motor neurons are one of the two neuronal cell cultures that can be grown in essentially pure culture without a mixture of neuronal types. When grown in the presence of any of several different trophic factors, motor neurons freshly isolated from embryonic day 15 spinal cords of rats will attach in cell culture plates and begin to spread neurites [88]. By day 3 an axon becomes clearly distinguished and by day 7 motor neurons take on what appears to be a mature phenotype of a motor neuron. If motor neurons are deprived of trophic factors under these culture conditions, they will still attach to plates and send out neurites for the first 12 to 24 hours. Then apoptosis occurs, with the vast majority of neurons dying within 3 days. Blockade of nitric oxide synthesis within these trophic factor-deprived motor neurons blocks the increase in apoptosis and keeps motor neurons alive for at least 6 days [88]. Generation of a constant flux of about 100 nM nitric oxide reversed the protection provided by nitric oxide synthase inhibitors to trophic factor-deprived motor neurons. However, this low flux of nitric oxide itself was not toxic to motor neurons cultured in the presence of trophic factors. Consequently, nitric oxide itself did not cause the death of the motor neurons. In addition, low molecular weight superoxide dismutase mimics, as well as liposomal delivery of CuZnSOD to motor neurons, were equally protective, blocking nitric oxide production [89]. As motor neurons were undergoing cell death, they became immunoreactive for nitrotyrosine. These results strongly indicate that trophic factor deprivation resulted in motor neurons producing peroxynitrite as an essential intermediate leading to apoptosis in these cells.

The results indicate that trophic factor deprivation somehow was activating a source of superoxide within motor neurons. So far, we have ruled out xanthine oxidase as a source of superoxide. More surprising was a recent discovery that nerve growth factor-deprived sympathetic neurons undergo cell suicide by turning on an NADPH oxidase [22]. This NADPH oxidase is normally found on the plasma membrane of inflammatory cells such as neutrophils and macrophages. However, strong evidence has been found that this oxidase can be expressed in neurons as well. At present, we do not know whether motor neurons express NADPH oxidase, but we are actively investigating this.

The ability to deliver SOD entrapped in liposomes enabled us to test the effects of metal status on the toxicity of SOD in vitro [89]. We expressed four different ALS mutants as well as wild-type SOD and prepared them to contain both copper plus zinc, as well as in the zinc-deficient state [87]. Delivery of wild-type CuZnSOD and any of the four ALS mutant SODs protected motor neurons from trophic factor deprivation equally well. These results indicate that the ALS mutant genes can yield fully active enzymes that are protective to motor neurons. However, the zinc-deficient SODs – whether ALS mutant or wild-type SOD – induce the death of motor neurons in the presence of trophic factor deprivation. This toxicity was blocked by inhibition of nitric oxide synthesis and was accompanied by the accumulation of tyrosine nitration. Copper chelators, such as bathocuproine, could fully protect against the toxicity of zinc-deficient SOD. John Crow (unpublished results) has separately shown that the copper from zinc-deficient SOD can be readily removed by bathocuproine in vitro. Further experiments showed that the apoSOD was not toxic to the motor neurons [87]. In addition, delivering copper citrate or copper bovine serum albumin at the same concentrations of the SOD protein was also not toxic to the motor neurons. These results indicate that copper in zinc-deficient SOD was increasing the death of motor neurons through the formation of peroxynitrite. Overall these results indicate that the loss of zinc from either wild-type or ALS mutant SOD is sufficient to cause the death of motor neurons. This suggests that mutations to SOD do not directly confer a gain of function on the protein but rather increase the susceptibility to the loss of zinc, and that the zinc-deficient SOD is responsible for the dominant gain of function. This provides an exciting connection whereby SOD may participate in sporadic ALS as well as in familial ALS.

Currently it is not possible to prove that zinc-deficient SOD is present in motor neurons. No one has been able to measure the amount of zinc bound to different proteins in vivo for any enzyme system. The problem is even more difficult with motor neurons, since they constitute less than 1% of the total cell volume in the spinal cord. Nevertheless, we are working to develop antibodies with phage display methodologies that bind selectively to zinc-deficient SOD to further test this hypothesis.

Concluding remarks

In experimental animals, administration of SOD as well as overexpression of the SOD protein can have profound protective effects in cerebral ischemia, trauma and in some models of neurodegeneration. Protection by PEG-SOD administered into the circulation suggests that the endothelium of the blood–brain barrier is an important target for oxidative stress in stroke. This is in part confirmed by the tendency to see increased nitration of the endothelium in stroke. Recent work by Ullrich's group strongly suggests that prostacyclin synthase is a major target of oxidative injury in these models. Nitration of prostacyclin synthase could have profound effects for understanding cerebral vasospasm that can result after trauma, stroke and subarachnoid hemorrhage.

In addition, nitrative and oxidative stresses directly affect the survival of neurons. The discovery of mutations to SOD causing ALS shows how surprisingly selective and subtle oxidative stress might be. Increasing the expression of CuZnSOD in neurons clearly shows that additional scavenging of superoxide can have protective effects. However, the loss of a zinc atom can turn this normally protective antioxidant protein into a potentially toxic form that appears to work in reverse to increase oxidative stress at the expense of lower molecular weight anti-oxidants. Recognition that specific targets of oxidative stress exist points the way toward identifying these targets, which will help to develop antioxidants as useful therapeutic strategies to attack cerebral injury.

REFERENCES

1 Beckman JS, Liu TH, Hogan EL, Lindsay SL, Freeman BA & Hsu CY (1988) Evidence for a role of oxygen radicals in cerebral ischemic injury. In *Cerebrovascular Diseases*, eds. MD Ginsberg & WD Dietrich, pp. 373–80. New York: Raven Press.

2 Chan PH (1996) Role of oxidants in ischemic brain damage. *Stroke*, **27**, 1124–9.

3 Chan PH, Kawase M, Murakami K, Chen SF, Li Y, Calagui B, Reola L, Carlson E & Epstein CJ (1998) Overexpression of SOD1 in transgenic rats protects vulnerable neurons against ischemic damage after global cerebral ischemia and reperfusion. *Journal of Neuroscience*, **18**, 8292–9.

4 Cao W, Carney JM, Duchon A, Floyd RA & Chevion M (1988) Oxygen free radical involve-ment in ischemia and reperfusion injury to brain. *Neuroscience Letters*, **88**, 233–8.

5 Matsumiya N, Koehler RC, Kirsch JR & Traystman RJ (1990) Superoxide dismutase reduces caudate infarct volume after transient focal ischemia. *15th International Joint Conference on Stroke and Cerebral Circulation*, **15**, 23 (Abstract).

6 Beckman JS, Estévez AG, Viera L, Spear N, Zhuang YX, Ye YZ & Crow JP (1998) Interactions between peroxynitrite and trophic support in apoptosis and cell survival. In *Pharmacology of Cerebral Ischemia*, ed. J Krieglstein, pp. 243–9. Marburg: MedPharm Scientific Publishers.

7 Kontos HA (1985) George E. Brown memorial lecture. Oxygen radicals in cerebral vascular injury. *Circulation Research*, **57**, 508–16.

8 Totter JR (1980) Spontaneous cancer and its possible relationship to oxygen metabolism. *Proceedings of the National Academy of Sciences, USA*, **77**, 1763–7.

9 Fridovich I (1986) Biological effects of the superoxide radical. *Archives of Biochemistry and Biophysics*, **247**, 1–11.

10 Pauling L (1979) The discovery of the superoxide radical. *Trends in Biochemical Sciences*, **4**, N270–N271.

11 Hausladen A & Fridovich I (1994) Superoxide and peroxynitrite inactivate aconitases, but nitric oxide does not. *Journal of Biological Chemistry*, **269**, 29405–8.

12 Benov L & Fridovich I (1999) Why superoxide imposes an aromatic amino acid auxotrophy on *Escherichia coli*. The transketolase connection. *Journal of Biological Chemistry*, **274**, 4202–6.

13 Gardner PR & Fridovich I (1991) Superoxide sensitivity of the *Escherichia coli* 6-phospho-gluconate dehydratase. *Journal of Biological Chemistry*, **266**, 1478–83.

14 Hurst JK & Lymar SV (1999) Cellularly generated inorganic oxidants as natural microbicidal agents. *Accounts of Chemical Research*, **32**, 520–8.

15 Drapier JC & Hibbs JB Jr (1988) Differentiation of murine macrophages to express nonspecific cytotoxicity for tumor cells results in L-arginine-dependent inhibition of mitochondrial iron–sulfur enzymes in the macrophage effector cells. *Journal of Immunology*, **140**, 2829–38.

16 Granger DL, Hibbs JB Jr, Perfect JR & Durack DT (1988) Specific amino acid (L-arginine) requirement for the microbiostatic activity of murine macrophages. *Journal of Clinical Investigation*, **81**, 1129–36.

17 Green SJ, Meltzer MS, Hibbs JB Jr & Nacy CA (1990) Activated macrophages destroy intracellular *Leishmania major* amastigotes by an L-arginine-dependent killing mechanism. *Journal of Immunology*, **144**, 278–83.

18 Hibbs JB Jr, Taintor RR & Vavrin Z (1987) Macrophage cytotoxicity: role for L-arginine deiminase and imino nitrogen oxidation to nitrite. *Science*, **235**, 473–6.

19 Hibbs JB Jr, Taintor RR, Vavrin Z & Rachlin EM (1988) Nitric oxide: a cytotoxic activated macrophage effector molecule. [erratum: *Biochemical and Biophysical Research Communications*, **158**, 624, 1989] *Biochemical and Biophysical Research Communications*, **157**, 87–94.

20 Evans TJ, Buttery LD, Carpenter A, Springall DR, Polak JM & Cohen J (1996) Cytokine-treated human neutrophils contain inducible nitric oxide synthase that produces nitration of ingested bacteria. *Proceedings of the National Academy of Sciences, USA*, **93**, 9553–8.

21 Pagano PJ, Griswold MC, Najibi S, Marklund SL & Cohen RA (1999) Resistance of endothelium-dependent relaxation to elevation of O_2^- levels in rabbit carotid artery. *American Journal of Physiology*, **277**, H2109–H2114.

22 Tammariello SP, Quinn MT & Estus S (2000) NADPH oxidase contributes directly to oxidative stress and apoptosis in nerve growth factor-deprived sympathetic neurons. *Journal of Neuroscience*, **20 RC53**, 1–5.

23 Floyd RA (1999) Neuroinflammatory processes are important in neurodegenerative diseases: an hypothesis to explain the increased formation of reactive oxygen and nitrogen species as major factors involved in neurodegenerative disease development. *Free Radical Biology & Medicine*, **26**, 1346–55.

24 McCord JM & Fridovich I (1969) Superoxide dismutase. An enzymic function for erythrocuprein (hemocuprein). *Journal of Biological Chemistry*, **244**, 6049–55.

25 Beckman JS, Campbell GA, Hannan J, Karfias CS & Freeman BA (1986) Involvement of superoxide and xanthine oxidase with death due to cerebral ischemia-induced seizures in gerbils. In *Superoxide and Superoxide Dismutase in Chemistry, Biology and Medicine*, ed. G Rotilio, pp. 602–7. Amsterdam: Elsevier Science.

26 Chen ST, Hsu CY, Hogan EL, Maricq H & Balentine JD (1986) A model of focal ischemic stroke in the rat: reproducible extensive cortical infarction. *Stroke*, **17**, 738–43.

27 Liu TH, Beckman JS, Freeman BA, Hogan EL & Hsu CY (1989) Polyethylene glycol-conjugated superoxide dismutase and catalase reduce ischemic brain injury. *American Journal of Physiology*, **256**, H589–H593.

28 He YY, Hsu CY, Ezrin AM & Miller MS (1993) Polyethylene glycol-conjugated superoxide dismutase in focal cerebral ischemia-reperfusion. *American Journal of Physiology*, **265**, H252–H256.

29 Muizelaar JP, Marmarou A, Young HF, Choi SC, Wolf A, Schneider RL & Kontos HA (1993) Improving the outcome of severe head injury with the oxygen radical scavenger polyethylene glycol-conjugated superoxide dismutase: a phase II trial. *Journal of Neurosurgery*, **78**, 375–82.

30 Young B, Runge JW, Waxman KS, Harrington T, Wilberger J, Muizelaar JP, Boddy A & Kupiec JW (1996) Effects of pegorgotein on neurologic outcome of patients with severe head injury. A multicenter, randomized controlled trial. *Journal of the American Medical Association*, **276**, 538–43.

31 Beckman JS, Minor RL Jr, White CW, Repine JE, Rosen GM & Freeman BA (1988) Superoxide dismutase and catalase conjugated to polyethylene glycol increases endothelial enzyme activity and oxidant resistance. *Journal of Biological Chemistry*, **263**, 6884–92.

32 Haun SE, Kirsch JR, Helfaer MA, Kubos KL & Traystman RJ (1991) Polyethylene glycol-conjugated superoxide dismutase fails to augment brain superoxide dismutase activity in piglets. *Stroke*, **22**, 655–9.

33 Gonzalez-Zulueta M, Ensz LM, Mukhina G, Lebovitz RM, Zwacka RM, Engelhardt JF, Oberley LW, Dawson VL & Dawson TM (1998) Manganese superoxide dismutase protects nNOS neurons from NMDA and nitric oxide-mediated neurotoxicity. *Journal of Neuroscience*, **18**, 2040–55.

34 Rae TD, Schmidt PJ, Pufahl RA, Culotta VC & O'Halloran TV (1999) Undetectable intracellular free copper: the requirement of a copper chaperone for superoxide dismutase. *Science*, **284**, 805–8.

35 Kennedy MC, Antholine WE & Beinert H (1997) An EPR investigation of the products of the reaction of cytosolic and mitochondrial aconitases with nitric oxide. *Journal of Biological Chemistry*, **272**, 20340–7.

36 Moncada S, Palmer RM & Higgs EA (1991) Nitric oxide: physiology, pathophysiology, and pharmacology. *Pharmacological Reviews*, **43**, 109–42.

37 Ignarro LJ, Adams JB, Horwitz PM & Wood KS (1986) Activation of soluble guanylate cyclase by NO-hemoproteins involves NO-heme exchange. Comparison of heme-containing and heme-deficient enzyme forms. *Journal of Biological Chemistry*, **261**, 4997–5002.

38 Ignarro LJ (1989) Heme-dependent activation of soluble guanylate cyclase by nitric oxide: regulation of enzyme activity by porphyrins and metalloporphyrins. *Seminars in Hematology*, **26**, 63–76.

39 Garthwaite J, Charles SL & Chess-Williams R (1988) Endothelium-derived relaxing factor release on activation of NMDA receptors suggests role as intercellular messenger in the brain. *Nature*, **336**, 385–8.

40 Garthwaite J (1991) Glutamate, nitric oxide and cell–cell signalling in the nervous system. *Trends in Neurosciences*, **14**, 60–7.

41 Garthwaite J & Boulton CL (1995) Nitric oxide signaling in the central nervous system. *Annual Review of Physiology*, **57**, 683–706.

42 Beckman JS (1996) The physiological and pathological chemistry of nitric oxide. In *Nitric Oxide: Principles and Actions*, ed. J Lancaster Jr, pp. 1–82. San Diego: Academic Press.

43 Beckman JS & Koppenol WH (1996) Nitric oxide, superoxide, and peroxynitrite: the good, the bad, and ugly. *American Journal of Physiology*, **271**, C1424–C1437.

44 Coddington JW, Hurst JK & Lymar SV (1999) Hydroxyl radical formation during peroxynitrous acid decomposition. *Journal of the American Chemical Society*, 121, 2438–43.

45 Goldstein S, Czapski G, Lind J & Merényi G (2000) Tyrosine nitration by simultaneous generation of $\cdot NO$ and O_2^- under physiological conditions. How the radicals do the job. *Journal of Biological Chemistry*, 275, 3031–6.

46 Beckman JS, Ischiropoulos H, Zhu L, van der Woerd M, Smith C, Chen J, Harrison J, Martin JC & Tsai M (1992) Kinetics of superoxide dismutase- and iron-catalyzed nitration of phenolics by peroxynitrite. *Archives of Biochemistry and Biophysics*, 298, 438–45.

47 Crow JP, Ye YZ, Strong M, Kirk M, Barnes S & Beckman JS (1997) Superoxide dismutase catalyzes nitration of tyrosines by peroxynitrite in the rod and head domains of neurofilament-L. *Journal of Neurochemistry*, 69, 1945–53.

48 Beckman JS, Carson M, Smith CD & Koppenol WH (1993) ALS, SOD and peroxynitrite. *Nature*, 364, 584 (Letter).

49 Beckman JS, Ye YZ, Anderson P, Chen J, Accavetti MA, Tarpey MM & White CR (1994) Extensive nitration of protein tyrosines in human atherosclerosis detected by immunohistochemistry. *Biological Chemistry Hoppe-Seyler*, 375, 81–8.

50 Ye YZ, Strong M, Huang Z-Q & Beckman JS (1996) Antibodies that recognize nitrotyrosine. In *Methods in Enzymology*, vol. 269, ed. L Packer, pp. 201–9. San Diego: Academic Press.

51 Haddad IY, Pataki G, Hu P, Galliani C, Beckman JS & Matalon S (1994) Quantitation of nitrotyrosine levels in lung sections of patients and animals with acute lung injury. *Journal of Clinical Investigation*, 94, 2407–13.

52 Kooy NW, Royall JA, Ye YZ, Kelly DR & Beckman JS (1995) Evidence for in vivo peroxynitrite production in human acute lung injury. *American Journal of Respiratory & Critical Care Medicine*, 151, 1250–4.

53 Kooy NW, Lewis SJ, Royall JA, Ye YZ, Kelly DR & Beckman JS (1997) Extensive tyrosine nitration in human myocardial inflammation: evidence for the presence of peroxynitrite. *Critical Care Medicine*, 25, 812–19.

54 Ischiropoulos H (1998) Biological tyrosine nitration: a pathophysiological function of nitric oxide and reactive oxygen species. *Archives of Biochemistry and Biophysics*, 356, 1–11.

55 Giasson BI, Duda JE, Murray I, Chen Q, Souza JM, Hurting HI, Ischiropoulos H, Trojanowski JQ & Lee M-Y (2001) Oxidative damage linked to neurodegeneration by selective alpha-synuclein nitration in synaclinopathy lesions. *Science*, 290, 985–9.

56 Xu J, He L, Ahmed S-H, Chen S-W, Goldberg MP, Beckman JS & Hsu CY (2000) Oxygen-glucose deprivation induces inducible nitric oxide synthase and nitrotyrosine expression in cerebral endothelial cells. *Stroke*, 31, 1744–51.

57 Cameron ML, Granger DL, Weinberg JB, Kozumbo WJ & Koren HS (1990) Human alveolar and peritoneal macrophages mediate fungistasis independently of L-arginine oxidation to nitrite or nitrate. *American Review of Respiratory Disease*, 142, 1313–19.

58 Padgett EL & Pruett SB (1992) Evaluation of nitrite production by human monocyte-derived macrophages. *Biochemical and Biophysical Research Communications*, 186, 775–81.

59 Albina JE (1995) On the expression of nitric oxide synthase by human macrophages. Why no NO? *Journal of Leukocyte Biology*, 58, 643–9.

60 Sherman MP, Loro ML, Wong VZ & Tashkin DP (1991) Cytokine- and *Pneumocystis carinii*-induced L-arginine oxidation by murine and human pulmonary alveolar macrophages. *Journal of Protozoology*, **38**, 234S–236S.

61 Weinberg JB (1998) Nitric oxide production and nitric oxide synthase type 2 expression by human mononuclear phagocytes: a review. *Molecular Medicine*, **4**, 557–91.

62 Banks BA, Ischiropoulos H, McClelland M, Ballard PL & Ballard RA (1998) Plasma 3-nitrotyrosine is elevated in premature infants who develop bronchopulmonary dysplasia. *Pediatrics*, **101**, 870–4.

63 van der Vliet A, Eiserich JP, O'Neill CA, Halliwell B & Cross CE (1995) Tyrosine modification by reactive nitrogen species: a closer look. *Archives of Biochemistry and Biophysics*, **319**, 341–9.

64 van der Vliet A, Eiserich JP, Halliwell B & Cross CE (1997) Formation of reactive nitrogen species during peroxidase-catalyzed oxidation of nitrite. A potential additional mechanism of nitric oxide-dependent toxicity. *Journal of Biological Chemistry*, **272**, 7617–25.

65 Souza JM, Daikhin E, Yudkoff M, Raman CS & Ischiropoulos H (1999) Factors determining the selectivity of protein tyrosine nitration. *Archives of Biochemistry and Biophysics*, **371**, 169–78.

66 MacMillan-Crow LA, Crow JP, Kerby JD, Beckman JS & Thompson JA (1996) Nitration and inactivation of manganese superoxide dismutase in chronic rejection of human renal allografts. *Proceedings of the National Academy of Sciences, USA*, **93**, 11853–8.

67 MacMillan-Crow LA, Crow JP & Thompson JA (1998) Peroxynitrite-mediated inactivation of manganese superoxide dismutase involves nitration and oxidation of critical tyrosine residues. *Biochemistry*, **37**, 1613–22.

68 Yamakura F (1997) Nitration of one tyrosine residue is responsible for inactivation of human mitochondrial Mn-superoxide dismutase by peroxynitrite. In *5th International Meeting on the Biology of Nitric Oxide*, eds. S Moncada, N Toda, H Maeda & EA Higgs, p. 34. Kyoto: Portland Press.

69 MacMillan-Crow LA & Thompson JA (1999) Tyrosine modifications and inactivation of active site manganese superoxide dismutase mutant (Y34F) by peroxynitrite. *Archives of Biochemistry and Biophysics*, **366**, 82–8.

70 Zou M-H & Ullrich V (1996) Peroxynitrite formed by simultaneous generation of nitric oxide and superoxide selectively inhibits bovine aortic prostacyclin synthase. *FEBS Letters*, **382**, 101–4.

71 Zou M, Martin C & Ullrich V (1997) Tyrosine nitration as a mechanism of selective inactivation of prostacyclin synthase by peroxynitrite. *Biological Chemistry*, **378**, 707–13.

72 Zou MH, Klein T, Pasquet JP & Ullrich V (1998) Interleukin 1β decreases prostacyclin synthase activity in rat mesangial cells via endogenous peroxynitrite formation. *Biochemical Journal*, **336**, 507–12.

73 Landino LM, Crews BC, Timmons MD, Morrow JD & Marnett LJ (1996) Peroxynitrite, the coupling product of nitric oxide and superoxide, activates prostaglandin biosynthesis. *Proceedings of the National Academy of Sciences, USA*, **93**, 15069–74.

74 Wolin MS, Burke-Wolin TM & Mohazzab-H KM (1999) Roles for NAD(P)H oxidases and reactive oxygen species in vascular oxygen sensing mechanisms. *Respiration Physiology*, **115**, 229–38.

75 Strong MJ, Sopper MM, Crow JP, Strong WL & Beckman JS (1998) Nitration of the low molecular weight neurofilament is equivalent in sporadic amyotrophic lateral sclerosis and control cervical spinal cord. *Biochemical and Biophysical Research Communications*, **248**, 157–64.

76 Chou SM, Wang HS & Taniguchi A (1996) Role of SOD-1 and nitric oxide/cyclic GMP cascade on neurofilament aggregation in ALS/MND. *Journal of the Neurological Sciences*, **139** Suppl, 16–26.

77 Chou SM, Wang HS & Komai K (1996) Colocalization of NOS and SOD1 in neurofilament accumulation within motor neurons of amyotrophic lateral sclerosis: an immunohistochemical study. *Journal of Chemical Neuroanatomy*, **10**, 249–58.

78 Rosen DR, Siddique T, Patterson D, Figlewicz DA, Sapp P, Hentati A, Donaldson D, Goto J, O'Regan JP, Deng H-X, Rahmani Z, Krizus A, McKenna-Yasek D, Cayabyab A, Gaston SM, Berger R, Tanszi RE, Halperin JJ, Herzfeldt B, Van den Bergh R, Hung W-Y, Bird T, Deng G, Mulder DW, Smyth C, Lang NG, Soriana E, Pericak-Vance MA, Haines J, Rouleau GA, Gusella JS, Horvitz HR & Brown RH Jr (1993) Mutations in Cu/Zn superoxide dismutase gene are associated with familial amyotrophic lateral sclerosis. [erratum: *Nature*, **364**, 362, 1993] *Nature*, **362**, 59–62.

79 Brown RH Jr (1996) Superoxide dismutase and familial amyotrophic lateral sclerosis: new insights into mechanisms and treatments. *Annals of Neurology*, **39**, 145–6.

80 Gurney ME, Pu H, Chiu AY, Dal Canto MC, Polchow CY, Alexander DD, Caliendo J, Hentati A, Kwon YW, Deng H-X, Chen W, Zhai P, Sufit RL & Siddique T (1994) Motor neuron degeneration in mice that express a human Cu,Zn superoxide dismutase mutation. [erratum: *Science*, **269**, 149, 1995] *Science*, **264**, 1772–5.

81 Reaume AG, Elliott JL, Hoffman EK, Kowall NW, Ferrante RJ, Siwek DF, Wilcox HM, Flood DG, Beal MF, Brown RH Jr, Scott RW & Snider WD (1996) Motor neurons in Cu/Zn superoxide dismutase-deficient mice develop normally but exhibit enhanced cell death after axonal injury. *Nature Genetics*, **13**, 43–7.

82 Crow JP, Sampson JB, Zhuang Y, Thompson JA & Beckman JS (1997) Decreased zinc affinity of amyotrophic lateral sclerosis-associated superoxide dismutase mutants leads to enhanced catalysis of tyrosine nitration by peroxynitrite. *Journal of Neurochemistry*, **69**, 1936–44.

83 Beckman JS (1996) Oxidative damage and tyrosine nitration from peroxynitrite. *Chemical Research in Toxicology*, **9**, 836–44.

84 Lyons TJ, Liu H, Goto JJ, Nersissian A, Roe JA, Graden JA, Café C, Ellerby LM, Bredesen DE, Gralla EB & Valentine JS (1996) Mutations in copper-zinc superoxide dismutase that cause amyotrophic lateral sclerosis alter the zinc binding site and the redox behavior of the protein. *Proceedings of the National Academy of Sciences, USA*, **93**, 12240–4.

85 Deng H-X, Hentati A, Tainer JA, Iqbal Z, Cayabyab A, Hung W-Y, Getzoff ED, Hu P, Herzfeldt B, Roos RP, Warner C, Deng G, Soriano E, Smyth C, Parge H, Ahmed A, Roses A, Hallewell R, Pericak-Vance M & Siddique T (1993) Amyotrophic lateral sclerosis and structural defects in Cu,Zn superoxide dismutase. *Science*, **261**, 1047–51.

86 Deng HX & Taylor R (1993) Superoxide dismutase dysfunction: a radical route to familial ALS. *Journal of National Institutes of Health Research*, **5**, 64–7.

87 Estévez AG, Crow JP, Sampson JB, Reiter C, Zhuang Y-X, Richardson GJ, Tarpey MM, Barbeito L & Beckman JS (1999) Induction of nitric oxide-dependent apoptosis in motor neurons by zinc-deficient superoxide dismutase. *Science*, **286**, 2498–500.

88 Estévez AG, Spear N, Manuel SM, Radi R, Henderson CE, Barbeito L & Beckman JS (1998) Nitric oxide and superoxide contribute to motor neuron apoptosis induced by trophic factor deprivation. *Journal of Neuroscience*, **18**, 923–31.

89 Estévez AG, Sampson JB, Zhuang Y-X, Spear N, Richardson GJ, Crow JP, Tarpey MM, Barbeito L & Beckman JS (2000) Liposome-delivered superoxide dismutase prevents nitric oxide-dependent motor neuron death induced by trophic factor withdrawal. *Free Radical Biology & Medicine*, **28**, 437–46.

4

Interaction between inducible nitric oxide and cyclooxygenase-2 in ischemic brain injury

Costantino Iadecola

Center for Clinical and Molecular Neurobiology, University of Minnesota, Minneapolis, MN

Introduction

Cerebral ischemic injury is the end product of a multitude of pathogenic factors acting in a coordinated fashion [1]. Thus ionic and chemical changes, initiated by ischemia-induced energy failure, lead to a wide variety of biochemical and genomic effects that ultimately result in tissue damage (Figure 4.1) (reviewed by ref. 2). These biochemical and molecular events are associated with marked cellular changes (reviewed by ref. 3). While neurons and glia develop swelling, circulating white cells adhere to cerebral endothelial cells and invade the brain parenchyma. Furthermore, astrocytes and microglia become activated, while macrophages accumulate in the injured areas [4]. Invasion of the brain tissue by blood-borne white cells and the activation of microglia contribute to the development of brain damage [1]. However, the mechanisms by which these inflammatory cells exert their deleterious effects are not well understood. Evidence accumulated over the past several years suggests that nitric oxide (NO) and cyclooxygenase (COX) products are involved in the mechanisms by which postischemic inflammation contributes to ischemic brain injury [1]. In this chapter, this evidence will be reviewed and discussed in the context of the interactions between NO produced by inducible nitric oxide synthase (iNOS) and COX-2.

Neuromodulatory and neurotoxic actions of nitric oxide

NO is a molecular mediator that is synthesized by the enzyme NOS from L-arginine [5]. Three isoforms of NOS have been described: neuronal NOS (nNOS), endothelial NOS (eNOS), and iNOS. eNOS is found mainly in endothelial cells, while nNOS is present in a selected group of neurons [6]. eNOS and nNOS are expressed

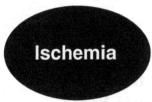

↓Oxidative Phosphorylation

Ionic and chemical changes
- ↓ pH, ATP
- ↑ Na+, Ca²+, glutamate
- ↑ Free radicals

Reprogramming gene expression
- Early genes, HSP
- Inflammation cascade
- Apoptosis

Activation of executioners
- Proteases, DNase
- Phospholipases
- Free radicals
- PARP

Cell Death

Figure 4.1   Summary of some of the mechanisms involved in ischemic brain injury. The reduction in oxidative phosphorylation produced by ischemia leads to ionic and chemical changes in the affected cells, which in turn lead to reprogramming of gene expression. Thus, immediate early genes, genes encoding for heat shock proteins (HSP), and genes for proteins involved in inflammation (cytokines, chemokines, adhesion molecules, iNOS, COX-2, etc.) and apoptosis (p53, Bax, Bad, Bcl-2, etc.) are expressed. These biochemical and molecular events lead to activation of "executioner" mechanisms that result in cell death. These include, for example, activation of proteases (calpain, caspases) DNase, phospholipases, and poly(ADP-ribose) polymerase (PARP). In addition, free radicals produce direct damage to cell membranes and proteins. The concerted action of these executioner mechanisms produces structural and functional changes leading to cell death.

constitutively and their activity is regulated by intracellular calcium [6]. Consequently, nNOS and eNOS produce "bursts" of NO during transient elevations in intracellular calcium. In contrast, iNOS is not normally present in most cells, but its expression is transcriptionally induced in pathological states, typically those associated with inflammation [7]. At variance with nNOS and eNOS, iNOS is not regulated by intracellular calcium and continuously synthesizes large amounts of NO [8]. Therefore, NO production by iNOS is thought to mediate some of the cytotoxic effects associated with inflammation [9].

NO and ischemic brain injury

There is substantial evidence that NO is involved in ischemic brain injury. The role of NO has been studied most extensively in rodent models of cerebral ischemia produced by occlusion of the middle cerebral artery (MCA). Depending upon the cellular compartment in which NO is generated, and on the stage of evolution of ischemic brain injury, this mediator can have either beneficial or deleterious effects (reviewed by refs. 10 and 11). Immediately after induction of ischemia the vasodilator effect of NO, produced mainly by eNOS, protects the brain by limiting the degree of flow reduction produced by the arterial occlusion [12]. However, after ischemia develops, NO, produced initially by nNOS and later by iNOS, contributes to the evolution of the brain injury [10]. The following section will focus on the role of iNOS.

iNOS and ischemic brain injury

Expression of iNOS occurs in the setting of the inflammatory reaction that involves the ischemic brain (reviewed by refs. 13 and 14). iNOS message, protein and enzymatic activity are expressed in the postischemic brain after permanent or transient MCA occlusion (MCAO) in rodents [15–18]. The expression peaks 12 to 48 hours after ischemia (Figure 4.2) and occurs in inflammatory cells that infiltrate the injured brain and in cerebral blood vessels. Recently, iNOS expression was studied in patients who died within 24 hours after a major stroke. iNOS immunoreactivity was found within neutrophils and vascular cells in the injured brains [19]. Interestingly, cells containing iNOS immunoreactivity were also positive for nitrotyrosine, a relatively specific marker of NO-derived peroxynitrite [20]. This finding indicates that iNOS is catalytically active in the postischemic human brain. The observation that iNOS is present in the human brain after stroke suggests that iNOS expression may be involved in the mechanisms of cerebral ischemia in humans as well.

The role of iNOS in ischemic stroke has been studied using relatively selective iNOS inhibitors such as aminoguanidine or 1400GW [21,22]. These drugs were administered beginning 12 to 24 hours after MCAO, because iNOS is expressed many hours after the induction of ischemia. It was found that iNOS inhibition reduced the infarct volume by 30% to 40% [18,21,22]. Importantly, the reduction in histological damage was associated with an improvement in neurological deficits

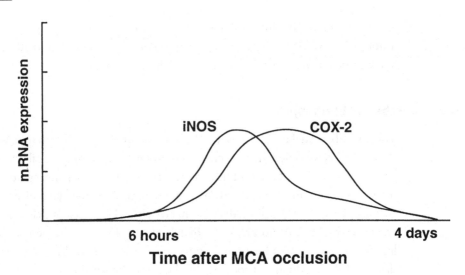

Figure 4.2   Time course of inducible nitric oxide synthase (iNOS) and cyclooxygenase-2 (COX-2) mRNA expression in brain following transient focal cerebral ischemia produced by occlusion of the rat middle cerebral artery (MCA) (data from ref. 35).

produced by the stroke [23]. Aminoguanidine did not influence cerebral blood flow, suggesting that the protection is not related to the preservation of postischemic blood flow [21]. These pharmacological data suggest that NO produced by iNOS contributes to the late stages of ischemic injury.

To provide non-pharmacological evidence of a role for iNOS in ischemic injury, mice lacking iNOS were used [24]. iNOS null mice did not express iNOS in the brain after MCAO [25]. It was found that iNOS null mice had smaller infarcts (−30%) and a better neurological outcome than wild-type littermates [25]. The reduction of infarct volume was more marked in homozygous rather than in heterozygous iNOS mice [26]. This observation is consistent with a gene-dosing effect of iNOS deletion. Because the reduction in cerebral blood flow produced by MCAO did not differ between iNOS null mice and controls, the protection could not result from cerebrovascular effects of iNOS deletion [25]. Furthermore, the reduction in infarct volume could not be attributed to effects on the cellular reaction that occurs after ischemia, because the degree of neutrophilic infiltration and astrocytic activation was comparable in iNOS null mice and controls [25]. Interestingly, the magnitude of protection resulting from deletion of the iNOS gene depends on the age of the mice. Thus the reduction in infarct volume is more marked at 1 or 2 months of age than at 6 months [27]. Although the precise mechanisms of the age dependence of the protection conferred by iNOS deletion remain to be defined, these observations suggest that age is an important variable in studies of neuroprotection in mice.

COX gene expression and inflammation

COX-2 is another gene that is expressed during inflammation. Cyclooxygenases are rate-limiting enzymes in the synthesis of prostaglandins and thromboxanes [28]. Two isoforms of COX have been described: COX-1 and COX-2. COX-1 is thought to play a role in platelet aggregation, gastric secretion and renal function, and is expressed in many cells [29]. COX-2 is constitutively expressed in excitatory neurons, wherein it is localized to dendritic spines [30,31]. In many organs, COX-2 expression is upregulated by a wide variety of stimuli, such as inflammatory mediators and mitogens [32]. In models of inflammation, COX-2 reaction products are believed to be destructive and to contribute to cytotoxicity [33]. The toxicity of COX-2 has been attributed to production of reactive oxygen species and toxic prostanoids [33].

COX-2 and cerebral ischemia

After cerebral ischemia, COX-2, mRNA and protein are upregulated, peaking 12 to 24 hours after ischemia [34–36] (Figure 4.2). COX-2 is expressed in neurons and vascular cells located at the border of the ischemic territory [35,36]. In neurons, COX-2 is expressed both in cells that exhibit ischemic changes, and in cells that are structurally normal [35]. Recently, COX-2 has also been found to be expressed in the human brain after ischemic stroke [37].

The role of COX-2 in the mechanisms of cerebral ischemia has not been completely elucidated. In a model of focal ischemia [35], initial data suggest that the relatively selective COX-2 inhibitor NS-398 reduces infarct volume by 20% to 30% [35]. Furthermore, COX-2 inhibition also reduced neuronal damage in a model of global cerebral ischemia [38]. The fact that delayed administration of NS-398 (6 hours after MCAO) reduces cerebral ischemic damage supports the notion that COX-2 is involved in the late stages of ischemic injury. However, evidence that NS-398 acts exclusively on COX-2 activity is lacking. NS-398, like other COX inhibitors, may also have effects on gene transcription, which may play a role in its protective effect [39,40].

Interaction between iNOS-derived NO and COX-2

Another line of evidence, suggestive of a pathogenic role for COX-2 in the mechanisms of cerebral ischemia, is provided by studies in which the interaction between NO produced by iNOS and COX-2 was investigated. iNOS and COX-2 are expressed with a similar time course and in cells that are close to each other, after cerebral ischemia [41] (Figure 4.2). The spatial and temporal proximity of iNOS

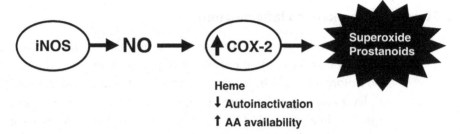

Figure 4.3   Model of interaction between iNOS-derived NO and COX-2. NO, or a derived species, possibly peroxynitrite, interacts with COX-2 and increases its catalytic activity. The mechanisms of the effects have not been elucidated, but they may include: (i) binding of NO to the heme group of COX-2 resulting in increased enzymatic activity; (ii) reduction of COX-2 autoinactivation; and (iii) increase in availability of arachidonic acid (AA), the substrate for COX-2 (see also ref. 44). For abbreviations see Figure 4.2.

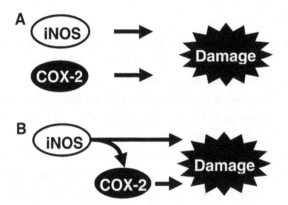

Figure 4.4   Potential pathogenic consequences of iNOS and COX-2 in the postischemic brain. iNOS-derived NO and COX-2 reaction products could contribute to ischemic injury by independent pathogenic mechanisms (possibility A). On the other hand, the deleterious effects of NO could be, in part, mediated through COX-2 reaction products (possibility B). For abbreviations, see Figure 4.2.

and COX-2 suggest that NO – or a derived species, possibly peroxynitrite – could activate COX-2 and enhance the toxic output of the enzyme (see refs. 42–44) (Figure 4.3). This possibility is supported by studies demonstrating that selective inhibition of iNOS reduces COX-2 reaction products in the postischemic brain [41]. Furthermore, COX-2 reaction products are reduced in iNOS null mice, which do not produce iNOS-derived NO after ischemia [41]. These data, collectively, suggest that NO produced by iNOS may "drive" COX-2 activity in the postischemic brain and increase COX-2 reaction products. Recent experimental evidence supports this hypothesis. If iNOS-derived NO and COX-2 reaction products contribute to ischemic injury by independent pathogenic mechanisms (Figure 4.4A), then administration of COX-2 inhibitors to iNOS null mice should further reduce the damage. On the other hand, if the deleterious effects of NO are, in part, mediated through COX-2 reaction products (Figure 4.4B), then COX-2 inhibitors should not reduce the volume of damage in iNOS null mice. Accordingly, we administered NS-398 to iNOS null mice and wild-type controls [45]. We found that NS-398, while conferring neuroprotection in wild-type mice, did not reduce ischemic damage in iNOS null mice [45]. In contrast, the nNOS inhibitor 7-nitroindazole reduced the volume of injury in iNOS null mice, suggesting that the lack of effect of NS-398 was not due to the fact that iNOS null mice were maximally protected [45]. These findings suggest that iNOS-derived NO must be present in order for COX-2 to exert its deleterious effects after cerebral ischemia. Therefore, in this model, COX-2 reaction products are important mediators in the toxicity exerted by NO generated during postischemic inflammation.

While the interaction between iNOS and COX-2 provides additional evidence that COX-2 activity may be deleterious to the ischemic brain, the role of COX-2 in ischemic brain injury is far from clear. It has long been known that COX reaction products contribute to the regulation of cerebral circulation [46]. Recent data in COX-2 null mice indicate that COX-2 reaction products participate in the mechanisms coupling synaptic activity to blood flow in the somatosensory cortex [47]. Thus COX-2 inhibition might have effects on cerebrovascular regulation that could alter the outcome of cerebral ischemia. The cerebrovascular effects of COX-2's potential contribution to ischemic injury need to be assessed and characterized more extensively. Furthermore, COX-2 is expressed in excitatory neurons, wherein it is likely to play a role in synaptic transmission and plasticity [31]. Therefore, COX-2 inhibition may have effects on regenerative processes involved in functional recovery after stroke. Further studies addressing these issues are required to clarify, in full, the role of COX-2 in ischemic brain injury.

Conclusion

The data reviewed in this chapter suggest that iNOS and COX-2 play a critical role in the mechanisms of the delayed evolution of ischemic brain injury. However, iNOS and COX-2 do not produce damage by entirely separate mechanisms and, as such, they do not act as distinct pathogenic entities. Rather, NO generated by iNOS seems to be critical for the expression of the damage mediated by COX-2 reaction products. The evidence suggests that COX-2 reaction products are additional mechanisms by which NO exerts its cytotoxic actions. The findings reviewed here support the idea that there are important interactions among the multitude of pathogenic factors contributing to ischemic brain injury. These complex interactions should be taken into consideration in the development of treatment strategies combining multiple therapeutic approaches.

Acknowledgments

Supported by NIH/NINDS grants NS34179 and NS35806. C.I. is the recipient of a Javits Award from the NIH/NINDS. The excellent editorial assistance of Mrs. Deborah Kabes is gratefully acknowledged.

REFERENCES

1 Dirnagl U, Iadecola C & Moskowitz MA (1999) Pathobiology of ischaemic stroke: an integrated view. *Trends in Neurosciences*, 22, 373–416.

2 Lipton P (1999) Ischemic cell death in brain neurons. *Physiological Reviews*, 79, 1431–1568.

3 Iadecola C (1999) Overview: mechanisms of cerebral ischemic damage. In *Cerebral Ischemia: Molecular and Cellular Pathophysiology*, ed. W Walz, pp. 3–32. Totowa, NJ: Humana Press.

4 Clark RK, Lee EV, Fish CJ, White RF, Price WJ, Zonak ZL, Feuerstein GZ & Barone FC (1993) Development of tissue damage, inflammation and resolution following stroke: an immunohistochemical and quantitative planimetric study. *Brain Research Bulletin*, 31, 565–72.

5 Griffith OW & Stuehr DJ (1995) Nitric oxide synthases: properties and catalytic mechanism. *Annual Review of Physiology*, 57, 707–36.

6 Garthwaite J & Boulton CL (1995) Nitric oxide signaling in the central nervous system. *Annual Review of Physiology*, 57, 683–706.

7 Nathan C (1997) Inducible nitric oxide synthase: what difference does it make? *Journal of Clinical Investigation*, 100, 2417–23.

8 Vodovotz Y, Kwon NS, Pospischil M, Manning J, Paik J & Nathan C (1994) Inactivation of nitric oxide synthase after prolonged incubation of mouse macrophages with IFN-γ and bacterial lipopolysaccharide. *Journal of Immunology*, 152, 4110–18.

9 Gross SS & Wolin MS (1995) Nitric oxide: pathophysiological mechanisms. *Annual Review of Physiology*, 57, 737–69.

10 Iadecola C (1997) Bright and dark sides of nitric oxide in ischemic brain injury. *Trends in Neurosciences*, 20, 99–141.

11 Samdani AF, Dawson TM & Dawson VL (1997) Nitric oxide synthase in models of focal ischemia. *Stroke*, 28, 1283–8.

12 Huang Z, Huang PL, Ma J, Meng W, Ayata C, Fishman MC & Moskowitz MA (1996) Enlarged infarcts in endothelial nitric oxide synthase knockout mice are attenuated by nitro-L-arginine. *Journal of Cerebral Blood Flow & Metabolism*, 16, 981–7.

13 Feuerstein GZ, Wang X & Barone FC (1998) Inflammatory mediators and brain injury: the role of cytokines and chemokines in stroke and CNS diseases. In *Cerebrovascular Diseases*, eds. MD Ginsberg & J Bogousslavsky, pp. 507–31. Cambridge, MA: Blackwell Science.

14 Hallenbeck JM (1997) Cytokines, macrophages, and leukocytes in brain ischemia. *Neurology*, **49** (5 Suppl 4), S5–S9.

15 Iadecola C, Xu X, Zhang F, El-Fakahany EE & Ross ME (1995) Marked induction of calcium-independent nitric oxide synthase activity after focal cerebral ischemia. *Journal of Cerebral Blood Flow & Metabolism*, **15**, 52–9.

16 Iadecola C, Zhang F, Xu S, Casey R & Ross ME (1995) Inducible nitric oxide synthase gene expression in brain following cerebral ischemia. *Journal of Cerebral Blood Flow & Metabolism*, **15**, 378–84.

17 Grandati M, Verrecchia C, Revaud ML, Allix M, Boulu RG & Plotkine M (1997) Calcium-independent NO-synthase activity and nitrites/nitrates production in transient focal cerebral ischaemia in mice. *British Journal of Pharmacology*, **122**, 625–30.

18 Iadecola C, Zhang F, Casey R, Clark HB & Ross ME (1996) Inducible nitric oxide synthase gene expression in vascular cells after transient focal cerebral ischemia. *Stroke*, **27**, 1373–80.

19 Forster C, Clark HB, Ross ME & Iadecola C (1999) Inducible nitric oxide synthase expression in human cerebral infarcts. *Acta Neuropathologica*, **97**, 215–20.

20 Crow JP & Beckman JS (1995) Reactions between nitric oxide, superoxide and peroxynitrite: footprints of peroxynitrite in vivo. In *Nitric Oxide. Biochemistry, Molecular Biology and Therapeutic Implications*, eds. L Ignarro & F Murad, pp. 17–43. San Diego: Academic Press.

21 Iadecola C, Zhang F & Xu X (1995) Inhibition of inducible nitric oxide synthase ameliorates cerebral ischemic damage. *American Journal of Physiology*, **268**, R286–R292.

22 Parmentier S, Bohme GA, Lerouet D, Damour D, Stutzmann JM, Margaill I & Plotkine M (1999) Selective inhibition of inducible nitric oxide synthase prevents ischaemic brain injury. *British Journal of Pharmacology*, **127**, 546–52.

23 Nagayama M, Zhang F & Iadecola C (1998) Delayed treatment with aminoguanidine decreases focal cerebral ischemic damage and enhances neurologic recovery in rats. *Journal of Cerebral Blood Flow & Metabolism*, **18**, 1107–13.

24 MacMicking JD, Nathan C, Hom G, Chartrain N, Fletcher DS, Trumbauer M, Stevens K, Xie QW, Sokol K & Hutchinson N (1995) Altered responses to bacterial infection and endotoxic shock in mice lacking inducible nitric oxide synthase. *Cell*, **81**, 641–50.

25 Iadecola C, Zhang F, Casey R, Nagayama M & Ross ME (1997) Delayed reduction of ischemic brain injury and neurological deficits in mice lacking the inducible nitric oxide synthase gene. *Journal of Neuroscience*, **17**, 9157–64.

26 Zhao X, Haensel C, Ross ME & Iadecola C (1999) Gene-dosing effect of reduction of ischemic brain injury in mice lacking the inducible nitric oxide synthase gene. *Society for Neuroscience Abstract*, **25** (part 1), 793.

27 Nagayama M, Aber T, Nagayama T, Ross ME & Iadecola C (1999) Age-dependent increase in ischemic brain injury in wild-type mice and in mice lacking the inducible nitric oxide synthase gene. *Journal of Cerebral Blood Flow & Metabolism*, **19**, 661–6.

28 Wu KK (1995) Inducible cyclooxygenase and nitric oxide synthase. *Advances in Pharmacology*, **33**, 179–207.

29 Smith WL & DeWitt DL (1995) Biochemistry of prostaglandin endoperoxide H synthase-1 and synthase-2 and their differential susceptibility to nonsteroidal anti-inflammatory drugs. *Seminars in Nephrology*, **15**, 179–94.

30 Yamagata K, Andreasson KI, Kaufmann WE, Barnes CA & Worley PF (1993) Expression of a mitogen-inducible cyclooxygenase in brain neurons: regulation by synaptic activity and glucocorticoids. *Neuron*, **11**, 371–86.

31 Kaufmann WE, Worley PF, Pegg J, Bremer M & Isakson P (1996) COX-2, a synaptically induced enzyme, is expressed by excitatory neurons at postsynaptic sites in rat cerebral cortex. *Proceedings of the National Academy of Sciences, USA*, **93**, 2317–21.

32 Smith WL & Marnett LJ (1991) Prostaglandin endoperoxide synthase: structure and catalysis. *Biochimica et Biophysica Acta*, **1083**, 1–17.

33 Seibert K, Masferrer J, Zhang Y, Gregory S, Olson G, Hauser S, Leahy K, Perkins W & Isakson P (1995) Mediation of inflammation by cyclooxygenase-2. *Agents & Actions Supplement*, **46**, 41–50.

34 Planas AM, Soriano MA, Rodriguez-Farre E & Ferrer I (1995) Induction of cyclooxygenase-2 mRNA and protein following transient focal ischemia in the rat brain. *Neuroscience Letters*, **200**, 187–90.

35 Nogawa S, Zhang F, Ross ME & Iadecola C (1997) Cyclo-oxygenase-2 gene expression in neurons contributes to ischemic brain damage. *Journal of Neuroscience*, **17**, 2746–55.

36 Miettinen S, Fusco FR, Yrjänheikki J, Keinänen R, Hirvonen T, Roivainen R, Närhi M, Hökfelt T & Koistinaho J (1997) Spreading depression and focal brain ischemia induce cyclooxygenase-2 in cortical neurons through N-methyl-D-aspartic acid-receptors and phospholipase A2. *Proceedings of the National Academy of Sciences, USA*, **94**, 6500–5.

37 Iadecola C, Forster C, Nogawa S, Clark HB & Ross ME (1999) Cyclooxygenase-2 immunoreactivity in the human brain following cerebral ischemia. *Acta Neuropathologica*, **98**, 9–14.

38 Nakayama M, Uchimura K, Zhu RL, Stetler A, Isakson PC, Chen J & Graham SH (1998) Cyclooxygenase-2 inhibition prevents delayed death of CA1 hippocampal neurons following global ischemia. *Proceedings of the National Academy of Sciences, USA*, **95**, 10954–9.

39 Khayyam N, Thavendiranathan P, Carmichael FJ, Kus B, Jay V & Burnham WM (1999) Neuroprotective effects of acetylsalicylic acid in an animal model of focal brain ischemia. *Neuroreport*, **10**, 371–4.

40 Grilli M, Pizzi M, Memo M & Spano P (1996) Neuroprotection by aspirin and sodium salicylate through blockade of NF-κB activation. *Science*, **274**, 1383–5.

41 Nogawa S, Forster C, Zhang F, Nagayama M, Ross ME & Iadecola C (1998) Interaction between inducible nitric oxide synthase and cyclooxygenase-2 after cerebral ischemia. *Proceedings of the National Academy of Sciences, USA*, **95**, 10966–71.

42 Salvemini D & Masferrer JL (1996) Interactions of nitric oxide with cyclooxygenase: in vitro, ex vivo, and in vivo studies. *Methods in Enzymology*, **269**, 12–25.

43 Landino LM, Crews BC, Timmons MD, Morrow JD & Marnett LJ (1996) Peroxynitrite, the coupling product of nitric oxide and superoxide, activates prostaglandin biosynthesis. *Proceedings of the National Academy of Sciences, USA*, **93**, 15069–74.

44 Goodwin DC, Landino LM & Marnett LJ (1999) Effects of nitric oxide and nitric oxide-derived species on prostaglandin endoperoxide synthase and prostaglandin biosynthesis. *FASEB Journal*, **13**, 1121–36.

45 Nagayama M, Niwa K, Nagayama T, Ross ME & Iadecola C (1999) The cyclooxygenase-2 inhibitor NS-398 ameliorates ischemic brain injury in wild-type mice but not in mice with

deletion of the inducible nitric oxide synthase gene. *Journal of Cerebral Blood Flow & Metabolism,* **19,** 1213–19.

46 Pickard JD (1981) Role of prostaglandins and arachidonic acid derivatives in the coupling of cerebral blood flow to cerebral metabolism. *Journal of Cerebral Blood Flow & Metabolism,* **1,** 361–84.

47 Niwa K, Araki E, Morham SG, Ross ME & Iadecola C (2000) Cyclooxygenase-2 contributes to functional hyperemia in whisker-barrel cortex. *Journal of Neuroscience,* **20,** 763–70.

5

Mechanisms of ischemic tolerance

Valina L. Dawson[1] & Ted M. Dawson[2]

[1] Departments of Neurology, Neuroscience and Physiology, Johns Hopkins University School of Medicine, Baltimore, MD
[2] Departments of Neurology and Neuroscience, Johns Hopkins University School of Medicine, Baltimore, MD

Introduction

Preconditioning to ischemic tolerance is a phenomenon in which brief episodes of a subtoxic insult induce a robust protection against a lethal ischemic insult. The beneficial effects of preconditioning were first demonstrated in the heart. It is now clear that preconditioning can induce ischemic tolerance in a variety of organ systems, including the brain. Preconditioning stimuli are quite diverse, ranging from transient ischemic episodes, spreading depression [1], hypoxia [2], anoxia [3], chemical inhibition of oxidative phosphorylation [4] exposure to excitotoxins and cytokines [5–8].

There are two temporally and mechanistically distinct types of protection afforded by preconditioning stimuli; acute and delayed. Acute preconditioning is protein synthesis independent, mediated by post-translational protein modifications. Acute preconditioning is short lived, of the order of minutes to hours. Delayed preconditioning requires new protein synthesis and is sustained for days to weeks. Elucidation of the molecular mechanisms that are involved in preconditioning and ischemic tolerance might lead to the identification of drugs that mimic this protective response and improve the prognosis of patients at risk for ischemic injury.

Neuronal ischemic preconditioning was first reported by Kitagawa and co-workers [9] in gerbils subjected to sublethal transient global ischemia. CA1 hippocampal neurons exhibited reduced neuronal death after a severe ischemic insult 24 to 48 hours later. In the brain, ischemic preconditioning is mediated largely through the activation of the N-methyl-D-aspartate (NMDA) receptors through increases in intracellular calcium and requires new protein synthesis [10–14]. The acquisition of tolerance in the brain occurs over a relatively long period of time and persists for days. Requirements for the induction of tolerance depend, in part, on the experimental model, whether global or focal ischemia, and the animal species studied [9,15–19].

Changes in protein expression after preconditioning events

Many investigators have observed changes in protein expression or post-translational protein modifications after a preconditioning event. Preconditioning selectively induces a decrease in the levels of the NMDA receptor NR2A and NR2B subunits and a modest decrease in the levels of the NR1 subunit proteins in the synaptosomal fraction of the neocortex, but not the hippocampus [20]. Since ischemic tolerance is calcium dependent it is possible that restricted calcium influx through calcium channels may, in part, mediate the protective effects of preconditioning. RNA editing of the GluR2 subunit of α-amino-3-hydroxy-5-methyl-4-isoxazole propionic acid (AMPA) receptors determines receptor desensitization and calcium permeability. After ischemic tolerance, RNA editing of Q/R is unaltered but the R/G editing of the GluR2 subunit in the hippocampus is reduced by approximately 20% [21]. The effect of this reversible editing on the development of tolerance, if any, is not known.

In a rat model of focal ischemia, tolerance can be induced in the cortex [15,16] by the middle cerebral artery (MCA) suture method. Three 10 minute intervals of transient ischemia induce robust protection against subsequent 100 minute MCA occlusion, with a substantial reduction in infarct volumes measured 72 hours later. This approach does not induce significant changes in regional cerebral blood flow in the tolerant regions. In this model, the heat shock protein 70 (HSP70) is induced. Other stress proteins, such as grp75 and grp78 are not significantly altered [22]. Induction of HSP72 is also observed in hippocampal slices exposed to a preconditioning stimulus [23]. After transient global ischemia in rats and gerbils HSP27 and HSP70 are induced in the hippocampus, neocortex and thalamic nuclei [18,24,25]. It is not known whether induction of HSPs is necessary or sufficient to mediate the neuroprotection observed in tolerance. In the two-vessel occlusion model of global ischemia in the rat, protein kinase Cγ is translocated to cell membranes during preconditioning and is rapidly removed or degraded during the second otherwise lethal ischemic insult [26].

The induction of tolerance in CA1 neurons of the hippocampus may promote recovery of vulnerable cells from the initial responses to ischemia, which include blockade of protein synthesis, disaggregation of polysomes and dissolution of microtubules [27]. Preconditioning induced expression of Bcl-2 in the CA1 region of the hippocampus 30 hours after 2 minutes of ischemia in gerbils. The Bcl-2 protein was not detected at 12 hours and maximal expression was observed 4 days after the ischemic insult [28]. Although Bcl-2 can mediate neuroprotection, the role for Bcl-2 in tolerance is not yet clear. Cycloheximide induces a robust expression of Bcl-2 [29], but cycloheximide prevents the induction of tolerance in vitro [10]. Therefore, expression of the anti-apoptotic Bcl-2 protein may contribute to the induction of tolerance, but it may not be necessary for the expression of tolerance. Preconditioning markedly attenuates activation of p53 and its target genes p21 (WAF1/Cip1) and PAG608/Wig-1 [30], suggesting that repression of pro-apoptotic genes may also contribute to neuroprotection.

Mechanisms of ischemic tolerance

To gain a better understanding of signaling mechanisms, ischemia has been modeled in culture systems by combined oxygen glucose deprivation (OGD) [31]. Tolerance can be induced in vitro by brief OGD [10,11]. The salient features of ischemic tolerance observed in vivo [32] can be replicated in this culture model system: tolerance is dependent on NMDA receptor activation, but not on AMPA or kainate receptor activation, and requires calcium influx and new protein synthesis [10,11]. The demonstration of OGD-induced tolerance in vitro has provided a powerful means of determining which signaling pathways are activated during preconditioning exposure to OGD and assessing the functional significance of these signaling events.

Nitric oxide (NO)

In a newborn rat model of hypoxic preconditioning, exposure to sublethal hypoxia for 3 hours renders animals on postnatal day 6 resistant to cerebral hypoxic–ischemic insult imposed 24 hours later. In this model, preconditioning does not involve inducible nitric oxide synthase (NOS) or neuronal NOS (nNOS), but is dependent on NO produced by endothelial NOS to mediate protection [2]. In the rat hippocampal slice model, nNOS-derived NO is involved in neuroprotection mediated by anoxic preconditioning [3]. Preconditioning improves electrical recovery after anoxia in hippocampal slices, with no significant changes in reduced nicotinamide adenine dinucleotide hyperoxidation [3]. In culture models, a significant loss of neuroprotection occurs when NMDA receptor antagonists are present during the OGD preconditioning stimulus [10,11]. Application of the NOS inhibitor nitro-L-arginine during the preconditioning episode blocks the protective actions of preconditioning by ~70%, and coadministration of an excess of the NOS substrate L-arginine restores protection (Figure 5.1). NO donors induce tolerance in a dose-dependent manner, indicating that NO is a key mediator in processes leading to tolerance against lethal ischemia. The potent and selective inhibitor of guanylyl cyclase ODQ has no effect on ischemic preconditioning, nor does the cell-permeable cyclic GMP (cGMP) analog 8Br-cGMP elicit tolerance, thus ruling out a role for guanylyl cyclase in NO-mediated tolerance to OGD [10].

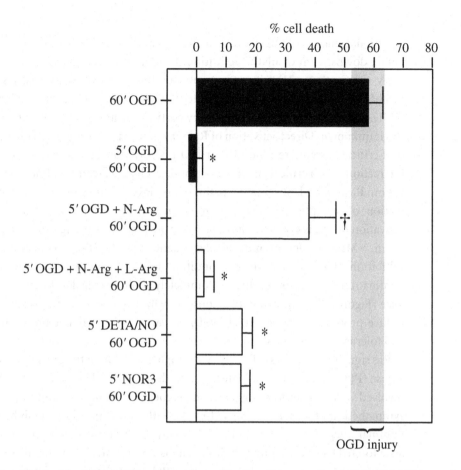

Figure 5.1   Nitric oxide (NO) mediates OGD preconditioning. Sixty minutes of OGD (60′ OGD) results
in approximately 60% neuronal cell death. Brief (5 minutes), sublethal OGD 24 hours
prior to exposure to 60 minutes of OGD (5′ OGD /60′OGD) results in survival of primary
cortical neurons. OGD tolerance is blocked by the NOS inhibitor nitro-L-arginine (N-Arg)
(100 μM) (5′ OGD + NArg/60′ OGD). Coadministration of excess NOS substrate L-Arg (1
mM) restores OGD tolerance (5′ OGD + N-Arg + L-Arg/60′ OGD). *$P < 0.001$ when
comparing 60′ OGD with 5′ OGD/60′ OGD, or 5′ + N-Arg + L-Arg/60′ OGD. Significance
was determined by a balanced two-way analysis of variance (ANOVA) with a Student's t
test at †$P < 0.001$ when comparing 5′ OGD/60′ OGD with 5′ OGD + N-Arg/60′ OGD. OGD
tolerance can be partially induced by 5 minutes of exposure to 10 μM of the NO donors
diethylenetriamine nitric oxide adduct (DETA/NO), or ethyl-2-hydroxyimino-5-nitro-3-
hexeneamide (NOR3). Significance was determined by a balanced two-way ANOVA with a
Student's t test at *$P < 0.001$ when comparing 60′ OGD to 5′ DETA/NO/60′ standard error
(SEM) OGD, or 5′ NOR3/60′ OGD. Each point is the mean ± standard error (SEM) ($n = 8$)
of at least two separate experiments. Each point reflects a minimum of 16 000 to 30 000
neurons counted. (The figure is modified from ref. 10 with permission. Copyright 2000
National Academy of Sciences, USA.)

p21 Ras

Functional analysis of OGD tolerance in cortical cultures has been extended to signaling downstream of nNOS activation. Lander and colleagues [33] have previously shown that p21 Ras is a target of NO and is activated by redox-sensitive mechanisms. Recently, we demonstrated NO-induced activation of p21 Ras after NMDA receptor stimulation in primary cortical cultures [34]. How NO activates Ras is unknown. Direct activation of Ras may occur via NO-mediated nitrosylation of a critical cysteine residue [33] or NO nitrosylation of Ras could promote an interaction with a critical guanine nucleotide exchange factor that leads to Ras activation. Ras-dependent signaling pathways are involved in gene transcription, regulation of synaptic plasticity, neuronal growth and survival [35,36]. Robust activation of Ras is observed during a 5 minute preconditioning exposure to OGD in an NMDA receptor- and NO-dependent, but cGMP-independent manner. Inhibition of Ras during the preconditioning event, pharmacologically or with dominant negative mutants to Ras, completely abolishes the development of tolerance (Figure 5.2). Expression of a constitutively active form of Ras is sufficient to induce protection against lethal OGD. Ras activation mediates preconditioning and tolerance to OGD [10].

Ras signaling mediates cell survival through activation of the phosphoinositol 3-kinase (PI3K)/Akt or Raf/Erk effector cascades [37–39]. The PI3K/Akt pathway is involved in anti-apoptotic signaling in cerebellar granule cells and in peripheral sympathetic and sensory neurons [40,41]. Neither pharmacological inhibition nor dominant negative mutants to PI3K have any effect on the development of tolerance to OGD, indicating that PI3K activity is not essential for ischemic preconditioning of cortical neurons [10]. However, PI3K/Akt-dependent signaling may be important for protection of peripheral neurons or spinal cord neurons.

Extracellular-signal-regulated kinases (Erks)

Ras also signals through the mitogen-activated protein kinase (MAPK)/Erk pathway. In this signaling cascade, Ras engages the serine/threonine kinase Raf, which activates Mek (MAPK/Erk kinase). Mek, in turn, phosphorylates and activates p42 and p44 Erks. The sequential interactions in the Ras/Erk signaling pathway permit regulation, integration and amplification of the initial signals to promote a graded temporal and spatial response. MAPK/Erk signaling cascades are linked to diverse neuronal processes, including long-term potentiation, synaptic plasticity, consolidation of memory, development, cell survival and cell death [35,42,43]. Ischemic preconditioning requires new protein synthesis and is sustained for long periods of time. It is a form of neuronal plasticity.

Recent reports indicate that Erk signaling may be important for the development of ischemic preconditioning. Hypoxia stimulates rapid Erk phosphorylation in the

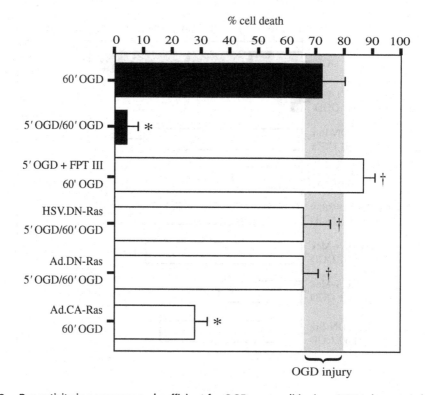

Figure 5.2   Ras activity is necessary and sufficient for OGD preconditioning. OGD tolerance is blocked
by the Ras inhibitor FPT Inh III (FPT III 250 μM) and by expression of a dominant negative
Ras mutant via adenovirus vector Ad.DN-Ras. Viruses containing the *lacZ* gene were used
to control for non-specific effects of the recombinant viral systems (data not shown). A
constitutively active form of Ras expressed by an adenoviral vector (Ad.CA-Ras) induces
neuroprotection against 60 minutes of OGD. Each point is the mean ± SEM ($n = 8$) of at
least two separate experiments. Each point reflects a minimum of 16 000 to 30 000
neurons counted. Significance was determined by a balanced two-way ANOVA with a
Student's *t* test at *$P < 0.001$ comparing 60′ OGD with 5′ OGD/60′ OGD, or Ad.CA-Ras-60′
OGD; †$P < 0.001$ when comparing 5′ OGD/60′ OGD with 5′ OGD + FPT III/60′ OGD, or
Ad.DNRas/5′ OGD/60′ OGD. (The figure is modified from ref. 10 with permission.
Copyright 2000 National Academy of Sciences, USA.)

cortex of rats in an NMDA receptor-dependent manner [44]. Increased phosphorylation of Mek and Erk has been observed in the CA1 region of the hippocampus
in a rat model of global cerebral ischemic preconditioning [45]. We have recently
demonstrated a functional requirement for the Ras/Erk signaling pathway in the
acquisition of tolerance in vitro. Dominant negative mutants to Raf, Mek and Erk2
all blocked the development of tolerance to OGD and the OGD-induced activation
of Erk in primary cortical cultures (Figure 5.3). Conversely, constitutively active Raf

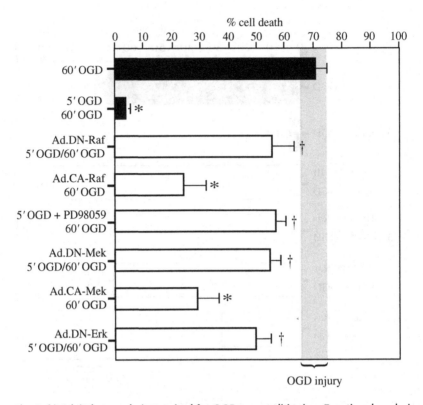

Figure 5.3   The Raf/Mek/Erk cascade is required for OGD preconditioning. Functional analysis of the
role of Raf/Mek/Erk signaling in OGD preconditioning. Expression of a dominant negative
mutant to Raf (Ad.DN-Raf) in primary cortical neurons blocks the development of OGD
tolerance, and a constitutively active Raf (Ad.CA-Raf) is capable of conferring
neuroprotection against lethal OGD. Significance was determined by a balanced two-way
ANOVA with a Student's t test at *$P<0.001$ when comparing 60′ OGD with 5′ OGD/60′
OGD or with Ad.CARaf/60′ OGD; †$P<0.001$ when comparing 5′ OGD/60′ OGD with
Ad.DNRaf-5′ OGD/60′ OGD. Pharmacological inhibition of Mek with PD98059 (50 μM) or
expression of a dominant negative mutant to Mek (Ad.DN-Mek) prevents OGD tolerance,
and constitutively active Mek (Ad.CA-Mek) induces protection against 60 minutes of OGD.
*$P<0.001$ when comparing 60′ OGD with 5′ OGD/60′ OGD or Ad.CAMek/60′ OGD;
†$P<0.001$ when comparing 5′ OGD/60′ OGD with Ad.DNMek-5′/60′ OGD. Expression of
a dominant negative mutant to Erk (Ad.DN-Erk2) blocks OGD tolerance in a manner
similar to its upstream signaling mediators. †$P<0.001$ when comparing 5′ OGD/60′ OGD
to Ad.DNErk-5′ OGD/60′ OGD. Each point is the mean ± SEM ($n=8$) of at least two
separate experiments. Each data point reflects a minimum of 16 000 to 30 000 neurons
counted. (The figure is modified from ref. 10 with permission. Copyright 2000 National
Academy of Sciences, USA.)

and Mek mutants induced neuroprotection against 60 minutes of OGD and were capable of activating similar levels of Erk phosphorylation. Our results indicate that all of these signaling mediators, Ras, Raf, Mek and Erk are required for the development of tolerance [10].

Since induction of neuronal ischemic tolerance is dependent on new protein synthesis, and the development of tolerance is blocked by cycloheximide [10], the profound protection derived from preconditioning may result from transcriptional activation of neuroprotective proteins by the NMDA/NO/p21^{Ras}/Erk pathway (Figure 5.4). Erk activation can stimulate nuclear transcription factors such as Elk-1 and the cyclic AMP response element binding protein (CREB) [46]. These transcription factors stimulate the transcription of immediate early response genes, which, in turn, induce the delayed response genes that influence neuronal activity including growth factors, enzymes that synthesize neurotransmitters, synaptic vesicle proteins, ion channels and structural proteins [47,48]. Elk-1 and CREB are attractive candidate molecules for mediating the effects of preconditioning.

Alternate activators of neuronal preconditioning

Glutamate receptor activation can elicit the production and release of brain-derived neurotrophic factor (BDNF) [49], which can signal through activation of the Ras/Erk pathway [50]. However, BDNF administration for 5 minutes does not induce OGD tolerance in primary cortical cultures and specific anti-BDNF antibodies or TrkB receptor bodies failed to block tolerance to OGD, thus ruling out a significant role for BDNF in OGD tolerance [10]. BDNF may, however, play a role in spreading depression-induced tolerance [1,51] and recent studies have ascribed a role for nNOS in mediating the neuroprotection induced by cortical spreading depression [52,53]. BDNF is markedly neuroprotective against neonatal hypoxic-ischemic brain injury in vivo [54]. In this model, intracerebroventricular administration of BDNF to rats on postnatal day 7 results in phosphorylation of extracellular signal regulated kinase (ERK)1/2, and pharmacological inhibition of ERK reversed the neuroprotective effects of BDNF on hypoxic–ischemic brain injury [54].

As in cardiac preconditioning, adenosine may play a role in neuronal preconditioning and acute ischemic tolerance [55,56]. Activation of adenosine receptors confers a wide time window of ischemic tolerance, lasting up to 72 hours, the early (immediate) part of which depends on the opening of K_{ATP} channels [55,57,58]. It is not yet known whether there is a signaling pathway similar to that observed in the heart, and whether there is interaction of this pathway with the NO, Ras/Erk signaling pathway.

Tumor necrosis factor-alpha (TNF-α) is a preconditioning stimulus that can induce ischemic tolerance. A transient 10 minute occlusion of the MCA induces

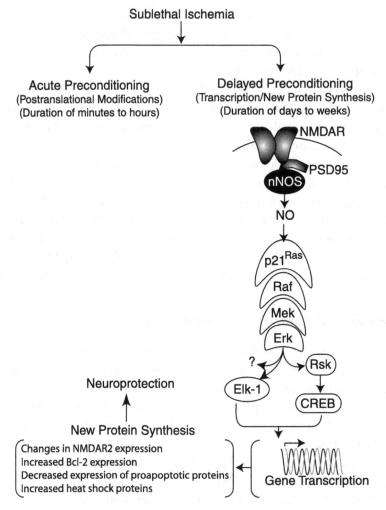

Figure 5.4   Ischemic preconditioning. Preconditioning can occur in two phases, acute and delayed. Acute preconditioning is due to post-translational modification of proteins and has a brief duration of minutes to hours. Delayed preconditioning requires new protein synthesis and is sustained for days to weeks. Delayed neuronal ischemic preconditioning is mediated largely through the activation of the NMDA receptors (NMDAR), involves increased intracellular calcium and requires new protein synthesis. The NMDA receptor is coupled to neuronal nitric oxide synthase (nNOS) via the scaffolding protein PSD-95 effectively coupling calcium influx with nNOS activation and NO production. In primary cortical cultures NMDA receptor stimulation leads to NO-induced activation of $p21^{Ras}$. Subsequently, Raf, Mek and Erk are activated. Inhibition of any of these steps during the preconditioning event is sufficient to prevent preconditioning from developing. It is yet unknown which transcriptional elements are activated or which protein(s) mediates tolerance; however, Elk-1 and CREB are attractive potential transcriptional candidates.

expression of TNF-α mRNA [59]. Exposure to TNF-α in vivo induced preconditioning in a time- and dose-dependent manner in mice that were subsequently subjected to MCA occlusion 48 hours after the preconditioning stimulus [7]. In vitro, TNF-α preconditions primary cortical cultures against subsequent hypoxia or OGD [6]. TNF-α exposure activates release of the second messenger, ceramide. Inhibition of ceramide synthase by fumonisin blocks preconditioning [5,6]. Thus an alternative preconditioning stimulus is stimulation of the ceramide second messenger system. Ceramide has been implicated in intracellular signal transduction systems regulating such diverse activities as cellular differentiation, activation, survival and apoptosis. As such, this is another attractive signaling pathway for eliciting long-term neuronal plasticity.

Conclusion

Preconditioning sets in motion a series of signaling cascades that ultimately result in profound neuroprotection due to expression of newly synthesized proteins. Preconditioning leading to tolerance is a novel form of neuronal plasticity that may share common signaling pathways with other forms of neuronal plasticity including long-term potentiation, long-term depression and hyperalgesia. However, the challenge in harnessing the preconditioning pathways is that glutamate, NO or cytokines, including TNF-α, play an important role in acute stroke in promoting ischemic damage [15]. In order to develop new therapeutic strategies it is important to separate the neuroprotective pathways from the neurotoxic pathways induced by these stimuli.

Acknowledgments

V.L.D. is supported by USPHS NS39148, and T.M.D. is supported by the American Heart Association and USPHS NS37090.

REFERENCES

1 Kawahara N, Croll SD, Wiegand SJ & Klatzo I (1997) Cortical spreading depression induces long-term alterations of BDNF levels in cortex and hippocampus distinct from lesion effects: implications for ischemic tolerance. *Neuroscience Research*, **29**, 37–47.

2 Gidday JM, Shah AR, Maceren RG, Wang Q, Pelligrino DA, Holtzman DM & Park TS (1999) Nitric oxide mediates cerebral ischemic tolerance in a neonatal rat model of hypoxic preconditioning. *Journal of Cerebral Blood Flow & Metabolism*, **19**, 331–40.

3 Centeno JM, Orti M, Salom JB, Sick TJ & Perez-Pinzon MA (1999) Nitric oxide is involved in anoxic preconditioning neuroprotection in rat hippocampal slices. *Brain Research*, **836**, 62–9.

4 Riepe MW, Esclaire F, Kasischke K, Schreiber S, Nakase H, Kempski O, Ludolph AC, Dirnagl U & Hugon J (1997) Increased hypoxic tolerance by chemical inhibition of oxidative phosphorylation: "chemical preconditioning". *Journal of Cerebral Blood Flow & Metabolism*, **17**, 257–64.

5 Ginis I, Schweizer U, Brenner M, Liu J, Azzam N, Spatz M & Hallenbeck JM (1999) TNF-α pretreatment prevents subsequent activation of cultured brain cells with TNF-α and hypoxia via ceramide. *American Journal of Physiology*, **276**, C1171–C1183.

6 Liu J, Ginis I, Spatz M & Hallenbeck JM (2000) Hypoxic preconditioning protects cultured neurons against hypoxic stress via TNF-α and ceramide. *American Journal of Physiology*, **278**, C144–C153.

7 Nawashiro H, Tasaki K, Ruetzler CA & Hallenbeck JM (1997) TNF-α pretreatment induces protective effects against focal cerebral ischemia in mice. *Journal of Cerebral Blood Flow & Metabolism*, **17**, 483–90.

8 Ohtsuki T, Ruetzler CA, Tasaki K & Hallenbeck, JM (1996) Interleukin-1 mediates induction of tolerance to global ischemia in gerbil hippocampal CA1 neurons. *Journal of Cerebral Blood Flow & Metabolism*, **16**, 1137–42.

9 Kitagawa K, Matsumoto M, Tagaya M, Hata R, Ueda H, Niinobe M, *et al.* (1990) "Ischemic tolerance" phenomenon found in the brain. *Brain Research*, **528**, 21–4.

10 Gonzalez-Zulueta M, Feldman AB, Klesse LJ, Kalb RG, Dillman JF, Parada LF, Dawson TM & Dawson VL (2000) Requirement for nitric oxide activation of p21(ras)/extracellular regulated kinase in neuronal ischemic preconditioning. *Proceedings of the National Academy of Sciences, USA*, **97**, 436–41.

11 Grabb MC & Choi DW (1999) Ischemic tolerance in murine cortical cell culture: critical role for NMDA receptors. *Journal of Neuroscience*, **19**, 1657–62.

12 Kasischke K, Ludolph AC & Riepe MW (1996) NMDA-antagonists reverse increased hypoxic tolerance by preceding chemical hypoxia. *Neuroscience Letters*, **214**, 175–8.

13 Kato H, Liu Y, Araki T & Kogure K (1992) MK-801, but not anisomycin, inhibits the induction of tolerance to ischemia in the gerbil hippocampus. *Neuroscience Letters*, **139**, 118–21.

14 Roth S, Li B, Rosenbaum PS, Gupta H, Goldstein IM, Maxwell KM & Gidday JM (1998) Preconditioning provides complete protection against retinal ischemic injury in rats. *Investigative Ophthalmology & Visual Science*, **39**, 777–85.

15 Barone FC, White RF, Spera PA, Ellison J, Currie RW, Wang X & Feuerstein GZ (1998) Ischemic preconditioning and brain tolerance: temporal histological and functional outcomes, protein synthesis requirement, and interleukin-1 receptor antagonist and early gene expression. *Stroke*, **29**, 1937–50.

16 Chen J & Simon R (1997) Ischemic tolerance in the brain. *Neurology*, **48**, 306–11.

17 Heurteaux C, Lauritzen I, Widmann C & Lazdunski M (1995) Essential role of adenosine, adenosine A1 receptors, and ATP-sensitive K^+ channels in cerebral ischemic preconditioning. *Proceedings of the National Academy of Sciences, USA*, **92**, 4666–70.

18 Kato H, Kogure K, Liu Y, Araki T & Itoyama Y (1994) Induction of NADPH-diaphorase activity in the hippocampus in a rat model of cerebral ischemia and ischemic tolerance. *Brain Research*, **652**, 71–5.

19 Kogure K & Kato H (1993) Altered gene expression in cerebral ischemia. *Stroke*, **24**, 2121–7.

20 Shamloo M & Wieloch T (1999) Changes in protein tyrosine phosphorylation in the rat brain after cerebral ischemia in a model of ischemic tolerance. *Journal of Cerebral Blood Flow & Metabolism*, **19**, 173–83.

21 Yamaguchi K, Yamaguchi F, Miyamoto O, Hatase O & Tokuda M (1999) The reversible change of GluR2 RNA editing in gerbil hippocampus in course of ischemic tolerance. *Journal of Cerebral Blood Flow & Metabolism*, **19**, 370–5.

22 Chen J, Graham SH, Zhu RL & Simon RP (1996) Stress proteins and tolerance to focal cerebral ischemia. *Journal of Cerebral Blood Flow & Metabolism*, **16**, 566–77.

23 Pringle AK, Thomas SJ, Signorelli F & Iannotti F (1999) Ischaemic pre-conditioning in organotypic hippocampal slice cultures is inversely correlated to the induction of the 72 kDa heat shock protein (HSP72). *Brain Research*, **845**, 152–64.

24 Aoki M, Abe K, Kawagoe J, Sato S, Nakamura S & Kogure K (1993) Temporal profile of the induction of heat shock protein 70 and heat shock cognate protein 70 mRNAs after transient ischemia in gerbil brain. *Brain Research*, **601**, 185–92.

25 Liu Y, Kato H, Nakata N & Kogure K (1993) Temporal profile of heat shock protein 70 synthesis in ischemic tolerance induced by preconditioning ischemia in rat hippocampus. *Neuroscience*, **56**, 921–7.

26 Shamloo M & Wieloch T (1999) Rapid decline in protein kinase Cγ levels in the synaptosomal fraction of rat hippocampus after ischemic preconditioning. *Neuroreport*, **10**, 931–5.

27 Furuta S, Ohta S, Hatakeyama T, Nakamura K & Sakaki S (1993) Recovery of protein synthesis in tolerance-induced hippocampal CA1 neurons after transient forebrain ischemia. *Acta Neuropathologica*, **86**, 329–36.

28 Shimazaki K, Ishida A & Kawai N (1994) Increase in bcl-2 oncoprotein and the tolerance to ischemia-induced neuronal death in the gerbil hippocampus. *Neuroscience Research*, **20**, 95–9.

29 Furukawa K, Estus S, Fu W, Mark RJ & Mattson MP (1997) Neuroprotective action of cycloheximide involves induction of bcl-2 and antioxidant pathways. *Journal of Cell Biology*, **136**, 1137–49.

30 Tomasevic G, Shamloo M, Israeli D & Wieloch T (1999) Activation of p53 and its target genes p21(WAF1/Cip1) and PAG608/Wig-1 in ischemic preconditioning. *Molecular Brain Research*, **70**, 304–13.

31 Monyer H, Giffard RG, Hartley DM, Dugan LL, Goldberg MP & Choi DW (1992) Oxygen or glucose deprivation-induced neuronal injury in cortical cell cultures is reduced by tetanus toxin. *Neuron*, **8**, 967–73.

32 Bond A, Lodge D, Hicks CA, Ward MA & O'Neill MJ (1999) NMDA receptor antagonism, but not AMPA receptor antagonism attenuates induced ischaemic tolerance in the gerbil hippocampus. *European Journal of Pharmacology*, **380**, 91–9.

33 Lander HM, Ogiste JS, Pearce SF, Levi R & Novogrodsky A (1995) Nitric oxide-stimulated guanine nucleotide exchange on p21ras. *Journal of Biological Chemistry*, **270**, 7017–20.

34 Yun HY, Gonzalez-Zulueta M, Dawson VL & Dawson TM (1998) Nitric oxide mediates N-methyl-D-aspartate receptor-induced activation of p21ras. *Proceedings of the National Academy of Sciences, USA,* **95,** 5773–8.

35 Curtis J & Finkbeiner S (1999) Sending signals from the synapse to the nucleus: possible roles for CaMK, Ras/ERK, and SAPK pathways in the regulation of synaptic plasticity and neuronal growth. *Journal of Neuroscience Research,* **58,** 88–95.

36 Manabe T, Aiba A, Yamada A, Ichise, T, Sakagami H, Kondo H & Katsuki M (2000) Regulation of long-term potentiation by H-Ras through NMDA receptor phosphorylation. *Journal of Neuroscience,* **20,** 2504–11.

37 Bading H & Greenberg ME (1991) Stimulation of protein tyrosine phosphorylation by NMDA receptor activation. *Science,* **253,** 912–4.

38 Downward J (1998) Mechanisms and consequences of activation of protein kinase B/Akt. *Current Opinion in Cell Biology,* **10,** 262–7.

39 Rosen LB, Ginty DD, Weber MJ & Greenberg ME (1994) Membrane depolarization and calcium influx stimulate MEK and MAP kinase via activation of Ras. *Neuron,* **12,** 1207–21.

40 Bonni A, Brunet A, West AE, Datta SR, Takasu MA & Greenberg ME (1999) Cell survival promoted by the Ras-MAPK signaling pathway by transcription-dependent and independent mechanisms. *Science,* **286,** 1358–62.

41 Dudek H, Datta SR, Franke TF, Birnbaum MJ, Yao R, Cooper GM, Segal RA, Kaplan DR & Greenberg ME (1997) Regulation of neuronal survival by the serine-threonine protein kinase Akt. *Science,* **275,** 661–5.

42 Impey S, Obrietan K & Storm DR (1999) Making new connections: role of ERK/MAP kinase signaling in neuronal plasticity. *Neuron,* **23,** 11–14.

43 Orban PC, Chapman PF & Brambilla R (1999) Is the Ras-MAPK signalling pathway necessary for long-term memory formation? *Trends in Neurosciences,* **22,** 38–44.

44 Gozal E, Simakajornboon N, Dausman JD, Xue YD, Corti M, El-Dahr SS & Gozal D (1999) Hypoxia induces selective SAPK/JNK-2–AP-1 pathway activation in the nucleus tractus solitarii of the conscious rat. *Journal of Neurochemistry,* **73,** 665–74.

45 Shamloo M, Rytter A & Wieloch T (1999) Activation of the extracellular signal-regulated protein kinase cascade in the hippocampal CA1 region in a rat model of global cerebral ischemic preconditioning. *Neuroscience,* **93,** 81–8.

46 Vanhoutte P, Barnier JV, Guibert B, Pages C, Besson MJ, Hipskind RA & Caboche J (1999) Glutamate induces phosphorylation of Elk-1 and CREB, along with c-fos activation, via an extracellular signal-regulated kinase-dependent pathway in brain slices. *Molecular and Cellular Biology,* **19,** 136–46.

47 De Cesare D, Fimia GM & Sassone-Corsi P (1999) Signaling routes to CREM and CREB: plasticity in transcriptional activation. *Trends in Biochemical Sciences,* **24,** 281–5.

48 Siegelbaum SA (1999) CREB can get you depressed. *Neuron,* **23,** 414–15.

49 Marini AM, Rabin SJ, Lipsky RH & Mocchetti I (1998) Activity-dependent release of brain-derived neurotrophic factor underlies the neuroprotective effect of N-methyl-D-aspartate. *Journal of Biological Chemistry,* **273,** 29394–9.

50 Riccio A, Ahn S, Davenport CM, Blendy JA & Ginty DD (1999) Mediation by a CREB family transcription factor of NGF-dependent survival of sympathetic neurons. *Science,* **286,** 2358–61.

51 Matsushima K, Schmidt-Kastner R, Hogan MJ & Hakim AM (1998) Cortical spreading depression activates trophic factor expression in neurons and astrocytes and protects against subsequent focal brain ischemia. *Brain Research*, **807**, 47–60.

52 Caggiano AO & Kraig RP (1998) Neuronal nitric oxide synthase expression is induced in neocortical astrocytes after spreading depression. *Journal of Cerebral Blood Flow & Metabolism*, **18**, 75–87.

53 Shen PJ & Gundlach AL (1999) Prolonged induction of neuronal NOS expression and activity following cortical spreading depression (SD): implications for SD- and NO-mediated neuroprotection. *Experimental Neurology*, **160**, 317–32.

54 Han BH & Holtzman DM (2000) BDNF protects the neonatal brain from hypoxic-ischemic injury in vivo via the ERK pathway. *Journal of Neuroscience*, **20**, 5775–81.

55 Plamondon H, Blondeau N, Heurteaux C & Lazdunski M (1999) Mutually protective actions of kainic acid epileptic preconditioning and sublethal global ischemia on hippocampal neuronal death: involvement of adenosine A1 receptors and K(ATP) channels. *Journal of Cerebral Blood Flow & Metabolism*, **19**, 1296–308.

56 Reshef A, Sperling O & Zoref-Shani E (1998) Adenosine-induced preconditioning of rat neuronal cultures against ischemia-reperfusion injury. *Advances in Experimental Medicine & Biology*, **431**, 365–8.

57 Reshef A, Sperling O & Zoref-Shani E (1996) Preconditioning of primary rat neuronal cultures against ischemic injury: characterization of the "time window of protection". *Brain Research*, **741**, 252–7.

58 Reshef A, Sperling O & Zoref-Shani E (1998) Opening of ATP-sensitive potassium channels by cromakalim confers tolerance against chemical ischemia in rat neuronal cultures. *Neuroscience Letters*, **250**, 111–14.

59 Wang X, Li X, Erhardt JA, Barone FC & Feuerstein GZ (2000) Detection of tumor necrosis factor-α mRNA induction in ischemic brain tolerance by means of real-time polymerase chain reaction. *Journal of Cerebral Blood Flow & Metabolism*, **20**, 15–20.

6

Clinically tolerated NMDA receptor antagonists and newly cloned NMDA receptor subunits that mimic them

Stuart A. Lipton

Center for Neuroscience and Aging, The Burnham Institute, La Jolla, CA

Excitotoxic and free radical injury to cerebrocortical neurons

In recent years, excitotoxic (glutamate-related) and free radical-mediated injury/cell death of neurons has been recognized as an important final common pathway in a variety of neurological diseases, ranging from acute ischemic stroke and trauma, to chronic neurodegenerative conditions such as Huntington's disease, amyotrophic lateral sclerosis, Alzheimer's disease and human immunodeficiency virus-associated dementia [1–5]. Many laboratories, including our own, have shown that neuronal cell death in these maladies is all due at least in part to the excitotoxic and free radical nature of the insult. We have further demonstrated that fulminant insults with glutamate and free radicals lead to severe energy depletion with resultant loss of ionic homeostasis. This produces swelling and cell lysis or necrosis. Conversely, more mild insults produce only transient energy loss and result in neuronal apoptosis [6,7]. Moreover, the existence of a final common pathway for neuronal damage means that a similar therapeutic approach may possibly be effective for each of these varied insults.

Therapeutic approaches to preventing cerebrocortical neuron injury: glutamate receptor antagonists

A major type of glutamate receptor-mediated cerebrocortical neuron injury is due to overstimulation of the N-methyl-D-aspartate (NMDA) subtype of receptor [8,9]. Although other glutamate receptors can contribute to excitotoxicity, the NMDA receptor is particularly important because of its extreme permeability to Ca^{2+}, which in excess can overload mitochondria and lead to excessive enzyme activity and free radical formation. Previously, multiple attempts to develop clinically tolerated NMDA receptor antagonists have failed because of problems with side effects [5,10]. After all, the NMDA receptor is important in normal functioning of the nervous system, for example, in many central nervous system pathways mediating long-term potentiation, thought to represent a cellular correlate of learning and memory.

NMDA receptor antagonists: open-channel block and S-nitrosylation

We have developed a series of drugs that interfere only with excessive activation of NMDA receptor-operated ion channels and leave relatively spared normal, physiological activity [11–13]. In this manner, side effects are avoided. Interestingly, one such agent that we have developed, the open-channel blocker memantine, is of relatively low affinity and thus spares normal function. However, it is of high selectivity so it does not block the functioning of other receptor types. Our laboratory has used this therapeutic approach to prevent apoptosis and necrosis in various neuronal cell types bearing NMDA receptors, including cerebrocortical neurons. In fact, memantine recently passed a series of five phase III clinical trials for vascular (multi-infarct) dementia and Alzheimer's disease in both Europe and the USA. The drug is now marketed in Europe as a neuroprotectant and is being considered for approval by the Food and Drug Administration in the USA.

We have also described redox modulatory sites, consisting of several critical cysteine residues on the NMDA receptor that appear to act biophysically as they gain control of the receptor. In simple terms, these sites, similar to memantine blocking the NMDA receptor-operated ion channel only when it is open for excessively long (pathological) periods of time, act like a volume control on your television set. By turning down the volume, we can avoid excessive stimulation of the cell by NMDA receptors, thus avoiding excitotoxic cell death. Reduction–oxidation (redox)-related forms of nitric oxide (NO) can react with some of these cysteine residues by a novel chemical reaction that we and our colleagues have characterized, known as S-nitrosylation (representing transfer of the NO group to a cysteine sulfhydryl). This reaction affords neuroprotection to cerebrocortical neurons as well as to other types of neuron [4,14,15]. We have also combined these redox-active drugs with channel blockers such as memantine to produce new therapeutic agents, called nitro-memantines, that act as if they modulate two volume control knobs on your television set (see Figure 6.1 for sites of action). In this manner, we can not only target the NO group to the NMDA receptor using memantine, thus avoiding systemic side effects such as hypotension, but also fine tune receptor activity even more precisely to prevent neuronal cell damage. By combining structure/function information about the NMDA receptor in this manner and by obtaining crystal structure information at the sites of drug interaction, we hope to design even better and safer therapeutic reagents.

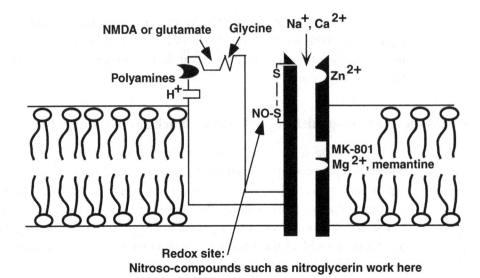

Figure 6.1   Schematic drawing of the NMDA receptor–channel complex, which is stimulated (left) by NMDA or glutamate. Glycine acts as a coagonist. There are several modulatory sites that regulate the degree of cation (Na^+ and Ca^{2+}) influx. These modulatory sites include: (i) the channel, where Mg^{2+} or various drugs such as MK-801, phencyclidine and memantine bind; (ii) a pH-sensitive region where H^+ exerts an effect; (iii) a polyamine binding site; (iv) a Zn^{2+} binding site; (v) a redox site consisting of at least five critical thiol (-SH) groups, one of which reacts predominantly with an oxidized congener of NO (supplied, for example, by nitroglycerin) and, in some cases, may facilitate disulfide bond formation.

A new family of NMDA receptor subunits that act as modulatory agents

Recently, while studying drug–receptor interactions, we cloned and characterized a new family of NMDA receptor subunits, termed NR3. In the case of NR3A, the first family member that we cloned, the subunit acts in a novel manner somewhat akin to that of memantine and NO-related species to downmodulate NMDA receptor activity by acting as a "volume control". In this case, when expressed in conjunction with the previously known NR1 and NR2 subunits of the NMDA receptor, NR3A decreases the unitary current and the degree of Ca^{2+} permeability of the channels [16,17]. This is the first ligand-gated channel subunit to be found to manifest this type of regulatory behavior. This new family of subunits may therefore be of therapeutic importance, and indeed preliminary evidence obtained from NR3A knockout mice that we have generated suggests that NR3A may protect the young nervous system from excitotoxic damage during development.

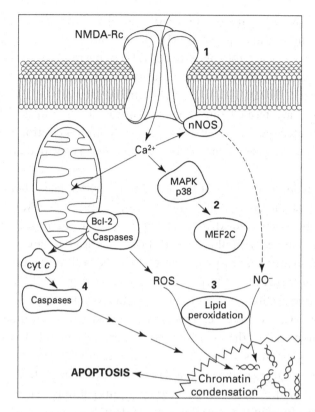

Figure 6.2   Schematic illustration of the signaling pathways discovered or characterized in the Lipton laboratory that can be targeted to prevent neuronal apoptosis in a variety of neurological diseases, including stroke. Drug or molecular therapies are being developed: (1) to antagonize NMDA receptors (NMDA-Rc), (2), to modulate activation of the p38 MAPK-MEF2 transcription factor pathway, (3) to prevent toxic reactions of free radicals such as •NO and reactive oxygen species including superoxide anion, and (4) to inhibit apoptosis-inducing enzymes including caspases. nNOS, neuronal NO synthetase; MAPK, mitogen-activated protein kinase; ROS, reactive oxygen species; cyt c, cytochrome c.

Events downstream to the NMDA receptor

Additional studies in our laboratory have characterized a series of downstream signaling pathways that lead to apoptosis and are triggered by excessive stimulation of NMDA receptors in cerebrocortical neurons (Figure 6.2). These pathways include (i) mitochondrial Ca^{2+} overload with subsequent cytochrome c release [18], (ii) free radical production (reactive nitrogen intermediates, such as NO, and reactive oxygen species, such as superoxide anion) [4,6], (iii) p38 mitogen-activated protein kinase (MAPK) -induced phosphorylation/activation of myocyte enhancer factor 2 (MEF2) transcription factor [19,20] and (iv) caspase activation with DNA fragmentation and apoptosis [21,22]. Interestingly, we have shown that NO-related species can react not only with critical cysteine residues on the NMDA receptor but also with a cysteine residue in the active site of caspases to downregulate excessive enzymatic activity and prevent neuronal apoptosis [15,23]. As mentioned above, we have termed this reaction S-nitrosylation, and it consists of transfer of NO-related species (specifically NO^+, with one less electron than ˙NO) to the thiol group of critical cysteine residues on proteins to control their function [24].

MEF2C, the predominant form of the MEF2 transcription factor family in the cerebral cortex, was initially cloned in our laboratory [19]. Recently, it has been found that the stress-activated MAPK p38 can activate MEF2 in an apparently Ca^{2+}-dependent manner, and that this pathway can lead to apoptosis [25]. Preliminary data suggest that caspase activation can be both upstream (initiator caspases) and downstream (effector caspases) in the p38/MEF2 pathway. Interestingly, in transfecting dominant interfering and constitutively active forms of p38 and MEF2C, we have recently demonstrated that activation of the p38/MEF2 pathway exerts the opposite effect during neuronal development, namely preventing apoptosis. In fact, transfection with MEF2C can drive precursor cells into a neuronal phenotype, acting as a master switch in controlling neuronal differentiation [20]. A better understanding of this pathway may well lead to new antiapoptotic drugs in the central nervous system. For example, p38 antagonists are already in advanced clinical trials for a variety of degenerative conditions such as arthritis, and our preliminary work suggests that they may be useful in protecting neurons from excitotoxic and traumatic insults [25].

Conclusions and future perspectives

After a series of highly publicized failed clinical trials, NMDA receptor antagonists were all but given up for dead with regard to neuroprotection in stroke and other neurological disorders. Recently, we discovered that drugs thought not to work so well because of their low affinity could be harnessed as neuroprotectants if they were of high selectivity. In fact, our group has shown that one such drug, memantine, acts only to block excessive (pathological) glutamate effects and leaves relatively spared normal neurotransmission. This drug has now passed five phase III clinical trials for vascular (multi-infarct) dementia and Alzheimer's disease and holds promise for acute stroke therapy as well. Newer drugs using these principles of clinically tolerated neuroprotection appear to be even more promising in preclinical work. Additionally, we have cloned a new family of NMDA receptor subunits that mimic the effects of these drugs by downregulating excessive NMDA receptor activity. These new developments have rekindled interest in the NMDA receptor and have shown that clinical treatment with these drugs, if done in a manner that avoids the side effects of high affinity agents, can be realized.

REFERENCES

1 Choi DW (1988) Glutamate neurotoxicity and diseases of the nervous system. *Neuron*, **1**, 623–34.

2 Meldrum B & Garthwaite J (1990) Excitatory amino acid neurotoxicity and neurodegenerative disease. *Trends in Pharmacological Sciences*, **11**, 379–87.

3 Dawson VL, Dawson TM, London ED, Bredt DS & Snyder SH (1991) Nitric oxide mediates glutamate neurotoxicity in primary cortical cultures. *Proceedings of the National Academy of Sciences, USA*, **88**, 6368–71.

4 Lipton SA, Choi Y-B, Pan Z-H, Lei SZ, Chen HS, Sucher NJ, Loscalzo J, Singel DJ & Stamler JS (1993) A redox-based mechanism for the neuroprotective and neurodestructive effects of nitric oxide and related nitroso-compounds. *Nature*, **364**, 626–32.

5 Lipton SA & Rosenberg PA (1994) Mechanisms of disease: excitatory amino acids as a final common pathway for neurologic disorders. *New England Journal of Medicine*, **330**, 613–22.

6 Bonfoco E, Krainc D, Ankarcrona M, Nicotera P & Lipton SA (1995) Apoptosis and necrosis: two distinct events induced, respectively, by mild and intense insults with N-methyl-D-aspartate or nitric oxide/superoxide in cortical cell cultures. *Proceedings of the National Academy of Sciences, USA*, **92**, 7162–6.

7 Ankarcrona M, Dypbukt JM, Bonfoco E, Zhivotovsky B, Orrenius S, Lipton SA & Nicotera P (1995) Glutamate-induced neuronal death: a succession of necrosis or apoptosis depending on mitochondrial function. *Neuron*, **15**, 961–73.

8 Hahn JS, Aizenman E & Lipton SA (1988) Central mammalian neurons normally resistant to glutamate toxicity are made sensitive by elevated extracellular Ca^{2+}: toxicity is blocked by the N-methyl-D-aspartate antagonist MK-801. *Proceedings of the National Academy of Sciences, USA*, **85**, 6556–60.

9 Sucher NJ, Aizenman E & Lipton SA (1991) N-methyl-D-aspartate antagonists prevent kainate neurotoxicity in rat retinal ganglion cells in vitro. *Journal of Neuroscience*, **11**, 966–71.

10 Lipton SA (1993) Prospects for clinically tolerated NMDA antagonists: open-channel blockers and alternative redox states of nitric oxide. *Trends in Neurosciences*, **16**, 527–32.

11 Chen H-SV, Pellegrini JW, Aggarwal SK, Lei SZ, Warach S, Jensen FE & Lipton SA (1992) Open-channel block of N-methyl-D-aspartate (NMDA) responses by memantine: therapeutic advantage against NMDA receptor-mediated neurotoxicity. *Journal of Neuroscience*, **12**, 4427–36.

12 Chen H-SV & Lipton SA (1997) Mechanism of memantine block of NMDA-activated channels in rat retinal ganglion cells: uncompetitive antagonism. *Journal of Physiology*, **499**, 27–46.

13 Chen H-SV, Wang YF, Rayudu PV, Edgecomb P, Neill JC, Segal MM, Lipton SA & Jensen FE (1998) Neuroprotective concentrations of the *N*-methyl-D-aspartate open-channel blocker memantine are effective without cytoplasmic vacuolation following post-ischemic administration and do not block maze learning or long-term potentiation. *Neuroscience*, **86**, 1121–32.

14 Kim W-K, Choi Y-B, Rayudu PV, Das P, Asaad W, Arnelle DR, Stamler JS & Lipton SA (1999) Attenuation of NMDA receptor activity and neurotoxicity by nitroxyl anion, NO$^-$. *Neuron*, **24**, 461–9.

15 Choi Y-B, Tenneti L, Le DA, Ortiz J, Bai G, Chen HS & Lipton SA (2000) Molecular basis of NMDA receptor-coupled ion channel modulation by *S*-nitrosylation. *Nature Neuroscience*, **3**, 15–21.

16 Sucher NJ, Akbarian S, Chi CL, Leclerc CL, Awobuluyi M, Deitcher DL, Wu MK, Yuan JP & Jones EG (1995) Developmental and regional expression pattern of a novel NMDA receptor-like subunit (NMDAR-L) in the rodent brain. *Journal of Neuroscience*, **15**, 6509–20.

17 Das S, Sasaki YF, Rothe T, Premkumar LS, Takasu M, Crandall JE, Dikkes P, Conner DA, Rayudu PV, Cheung W, Chen HS, Lipton SA & Nakanishi N (1998) Increased NMDA current and spine density in mice lacking the NMDA receptor subunit NR3A. *Nature*, **393**, 377–81.

18 Budd SL, Tenneti L, Lishnak T & Lipton SA (2000) Mitochondrial and extramitochondrial apoptotic signaling pathways in cerebrocortical neurons. *Proceedings of the National Academy of Sciences, USA*, **97**, 6161–6.

19 Leifer D, Krainc D, Yu Y-T, McDermott J, Breitbart RE, Heng J, Neve RL, Kosofsky B & Nadal-Ginard B (1993) MEF2C, a MADS/MEF2-family transcription factor expressed in a laminar distribution in cerebral cortex. *Proceedings of the National Academy of Sciences, USA*, **90**, 1546–50.

20 Okamoto S, Krainc D, Sherman K & Lipton SA (2000) Antiapoptotic role of the p38 mitogen-activated protein kinase-myocyte enhancer factor 2 transcription factor pathway during neuronal differentiation. *Proceedings of the National Academy of Sciences, USA*, **97**, 7561–6.

21 Tenneti L, D'Emilia DM, Troy CM & Lipton SA (1998) Role of caspases in *N*-methyl-D-aspartate-induced apoptosis in cerebrocortical neurons. *Journal of Neurochemistry*, **71**, 946–59.

22 Tenneti L & Lipton SA (2000) Involvement of activated caspase-3-like proteases in *N*-methyl-D-aspartate-induced apoptosis in cerebrocortical neurons. *Journal of Neurochemistry*, **74**, 134–42.

23 Tenneti L, D'Emilia DM & Lipton SA (1997) Suppression of neuronal apoptosis by *S*-nitrosylation of caspases. *Neuroscience Letters*, **236**, 139–42.

24 Stamler JS, Toone EJ, Lipton SA & Sucher NJ (1997) (S)NO signals: translocation, regulation, and a consensus motif. *Neuron*, **18**, 691–6.

25 Kikuchi M, Tenneti L & Lipton SA (2000) Role of p38 mitogen-activated protein kinase in axotomy-induced apoptosis of rat retinal ganglion cells. *Journal of Neuroscience*, **20**, 5037–44.

Part III

Apoptosis

Co-Chairs: Robert M. Sapolsky & Chung Y. Hsu

7

Cell death programs in neural development and disease

Sabina Sperandio[1], Ian deBelle[2], Susana Castro-Obregon[3],
Gabriel del Rio[4] & Dale E. Bredesen[5]

[1, 3, 4, 5] Buck Institute for Age Research, Novato, CA, [2] Burnham Institute, La Jolla, CA
[5] Department of Neurology, University of California, San Francisco, San Francisco, CA

Extensive research over the past several years has led to the elucidation of genetic and biochemical pathways involved in apoptosis (from the Greek *apo* = away from, and *ptosis* = falling), which is often referred to as the program for cell death. Concurrently, studies in stroke and degenerative diseases have sought to address the underlying mechanisms of neural cell death in these disease states. Interestingly, initial attempts to map the results from apoptosis mechanistic studies onto the patterns observed in neurological diseases have resulted in something of a paradox. On the one hand, the expression of genes associated with neurodegenerative diseases, such as mutants of *sod1* associated with amyotrophic lateral sclerosis or mutants of β-amyloid precursor protein associated with Alzheimer's disease, has been shown to induce apoptosis in cultured cells [1,2]; on the other hand, studies in vivo have not disclosed classic apoptosis as the major route of neuronal cell death in any of the major neurodegenerative diseases [3–5]. Initially, it was thought that this may simply be because the rate of cell death in neurodegenerative diseases is slow enough that it is difficult to capture enough neurons in the act of apoptosis (which is typically a relatively rapid program, occurring over minutes to a few hours in cultured cells) to demonstrate a clear increase in disease states. However, accurate transgenic models of these diseases have allowed a careful enough evaluation to identify many dying neurons, with the resultant demonstration that these do not display the morphological features of apoptosis [3–5].

What are the potential resolutions to this apparent paradox? Several possibilities exist, none of which is mutually exclusive. For example, several recent reports have demonstrated that at least some features of the apoptotic program can be activated at the synapse [6–8]. This phenomenon has been referred to as "synaptosis", although it is not yet clear whether neurite retraction actually results from this

Table 7.1. Comparison of different types of developmental neuronal cell death

	Type 1	Type 2	Type 3
Morphologically similar designations	Nuclear; apoptosis	Autophagic	Cytoplasmic; paraptosis
Morphological features	Chromatin condensation, nuclear fragmentation, apoptotic bodies	Autophagosomes	Cytoplasmic vacuoles derived predominantly from ER and mitochondria
Examples of inhibitors	Caspase inhibitors; some Bcl-2 family members	3-Methyladenine	?
References	11,23	10,16	11,12,17

Notes:
ER, endoplasmic reticulum.

process [9]. Nonetheless, the identification of apoptotic biochemistry in the synaptic regions raises the possibility that classic apoptosis may be largely lacking in some neurological conditions because the apoptotic program may be activated at the synapse but not the soma. However, this would then lead to the question of why the apoptotic program is not activated in the soma under these conditions.

Another possibility is that the analysis of apoptosis may fail to take into account alternative, non-apoptotic programs of cell death. Is there any basis on which to believe that such alternative programs may exist? If one assumes that developmental neuronal cell death is programmatic, and that different morphologies reflect different biochemical mechanisms, then there is: developmental neuronal cell death has been described as being of type 1, 2 or 3 [10] (Table 7.1). Type 1 cell death, also referred to as the nuclear form [11], demonstrates all of the morphological features of apoptosis. Type 2 cell death, also referred to as autophagic cell death, features autophagosomes apparently derived from lysosomes. Type 3 cell death has been divided into two subtypes, type 3A and type 3B [12]. Type 3B, which appears to be much more common than type 3A, has also been referred to as the cytoplasmic form [11]. This form of cell death has been described in developing chick spinal cord motor neurons, duck trochlear nucleus and neonatal rat superior colliculus, among other locations. It features cytoplasmic vacuolation, derived predominantly from the endoplasmic reticulum and, later during the process, from the mitochondria.

The molecular mechanisms underlying apoptosis have been increasingly well defined over the past several years. At the heart of the process are the caspases, a family of cysteine proteases that cleaves at specific aspartate residues [13]. These proteases have been divided into three groups, based on their substrate preference: although all groups cleave with Asp in the P1 position, the effector caspases such as caspase-3 and caspase-7 tend to prefer Asp in the P4 position (i.e., three residues amino-terminal to the P1 position, after which cleavage occurs) [14]. In contrast, the initiator caspases such as caspase-8 and caspase-9 tend to prefer aliphatic amino acids such as Val in the P4 position. The inflammation-associated caspases such as caspase-1, caspase-4 and caspase-5 tend to prefer large residues such as Trp or Tyr in the P4 position.

In contrast to apoptosis, the molecular mechanisms underlying types 2 and 3 cell death are virtually unknown. Recent work has suggested that type 2 (autophagic) cell death may be mediated in at least some cases by Ras [15,16].

We have recently been studying a programmed form of cell death that is non-apoptotic by its lack of terminal deoxynucleotidyl transferase-mediated uridine 5'-triphosphate-biotin nick end labeling staining, lack of apoptotic morphology at the light and electron microscopic levels, lack of caspase activity (measured as cleavage of a synthetic substrate, DEVD-AFC (Asp-Glu-Val-Asp-aminofluorocoumarin)), lack of internucleosomal DNA cleavage, lack of phosphatidylserine flipping (measured as Annexin-V staining) and lack of inhibition by apoptosis inhibitors including p35 (a general caspase inhibitor), zVAD.fmk (a general caspase inhibitor), Boc-aspartyl-fluoromethylketone (a general caspase inhibitor), and Bcl-x$_L$ [17] (S. Castro-Obregon et al., unpublished data). Morphologically, it is indistinguishable from the type 3B, or cytoplasmic, form of cell death, featuring cytoplasmic vacuolation that appears to derive primarily from endoplasmic reticulum and mitochondria. Because of this cytoplasmic vacuolation, it resembles cell deaths labeled as necrotic, but it is programmed, on the basis of its block by inhibitors of transcription and translation. These findings raise the question of whether some cell deaths previously labeled necrotic (e.g., some ischemic neuronal cell deaths), on the basis of morphology, may in fact be due to an alternative, non-apoptotic program of cell death. If so, it will be of interest to characterize this alternative program and develop effective inhibitors.

Our studies began with the evaluation of dependence receptors [18–20], which are receptors that induce cell death when expressed in their unliganded state, but inhibit cell death when bound by their ligands. Although most of these appear to induce apoptosis, we found that one of the candidate dependence receptors, insulin-like growth factor I receptor (IGFIR), may induce non-apoptotic cell death [17]. Surprisingly, despite its lack of morphological similarity to apoptosis and its lack of inhibition by broad caspase inhibitors, we found that IGFIR-induced non-apoptotic programmed cell death could be blocked by a catalytic mutant of caspase-9 that functions as a dominant negative (but not by other catalytic mutant caspases). Furthermore, the expression of caspase-9 was found to induce both apoptotic and non-apoptotic cell death, and these two forms could be dissected by the use of caspase inhibitors such as zVAD.fmk and BAF, which blocked caspase-9-induced apoptosis but not caspase-9-induced non-apoptotic cell death.

Furthermore, we identified mutations within caspase-9 that blocked apoptosis but enhanced non-apoptotic cell death [17]. Additional support for a separation of apoptosis from non-apoptotic programmed cell death was provided by DNA microarray analysis, which showed almost no overlap between the genes differentially expressed in these two forms of cell death (S. Castro-Obregon et al., unpublished data).

These results suggest that a form of programmed cell death that is non-apoptotic by criteria of morphology and biochemistry may nonetheless be mediated by a caspase. Because of the relationship of this form of cell death to apoptosis, we dubbed this *paraptosis*, from *para* (related to) and *apoptosis*. Despite the overlap of paraptosis and apoptosis based on caspase-9 involvement, however, paraptosis does not appear to be induced by classic, apoptotic caspase-9 activity: as noted above, the two effects could be separated both by caspase inhibitors and by mutations in caspase-9. These results suggest that caspase-9 may actually display two separable activities, although it is as yet unclear whether the pro-paraptotic activity is proteolytic, and, if so, whether it is due to cleavage with Asp in the P1 position of substrates that mediate paraptosis or whether it is due to cleavage at residues other than Asp.

It is of interest to ask under what conditions cell deaths with morphological similarity to paraptosis may occur. Of course, morphological similarity does not necessarily imply biochemical similarities; however, in the case of apoptosis, morphologically similar cell deaths have typically turned out to have similar underlying proteolytic activation. In the case of paraptosis, morphologically similar cell deaths have been described during neuronal development [11], in a transgenic model of amyotrophic lateral sclerosis [3,5], and in some cases of cell death in simple organisms [21,22]. These latter findings raise the question of whether paraptosis may have preceded apoptosis evolutionarily. In addition, as noted above, some cell deaths assumed to be necrotic, based on morphological criteria, may turn out to be programmed.

REFERENCES

1 Lu DC, Rabizadeh S, Chandra S, Shayya RF, Ellerby LM, Ye X, Salvesen GS, Koo EH & Bredesen DE (2000) A second cytotoxic proteolytic peptide derived from amyloid beta-protein precursor. *Nature Medicine*, **6**, 397–404.

2 Rabizadeh S, Gralla EB, Borchelt DR, Gwinn R, Valentine JS, Sisodia S, Wong P, Lee M, Hahn H & Bredesen DE (1995) Mutations associated with amyotrophic lateral sclerosis convert superoxide dismutase from an antiapoptotic gene to a proapoptotic gene: studies in yeast and neural cells. *Proceedings of the National Academy of Sciences, USA*, **92**, 3024–8.

3 Dal Canto MC & Gurney ME (1994) Development of central nervous system pathology in a murine transgenic model of human amyotrophic lateral sclerosis. *American Journal of Pathology*, **145**, 1271–9.

4 Turmaine M, Raza A, Mahal A, Mangiarini L, Bates GP & Davies SW (2000) Nonapoptotic neurodegeneration in a transgenic mouse model of Huntington's disease. *Proceedings of the National Academy of Sciences, USA*, **97**, 8093–7.

5 Migheli A, Atzori C, Piva R, Tortarolo M, Girelli M, Schiffer D & Bendotti C (1999) Lack of apoptosis in mice with ALS. *Nature Medicine*, **5**, 966–7 (Letter).

6 Ivins KJ, Bui ET & Cotman CW (1998) Beta-amyloid induces local neurite degeneration in cultured hippocampal neurons: evidence for neuritic apoptosis. *Neurobiology of Disease*, **5**, 365–78.

7 Mattson MP, Keller JN & Begley JG (1998) Evidence for synaptic apoptosis. *Experimental Neurology*, **153**, 35–48.

8 Mattson MP, Partin J & Begley JG (1998) Amyloid beta-peptide induces apoptosis-related events in synapses and dendrites. *Brain Research*, **807**, 167–76.

9 Raff MC (1992) Social controls on cell survival and cell death. *Nature*, **356**, 397–400.

10 Schweichel JU & Merker HJ (1973) The morphology of various types of cell death in prenatal tissues. *Teratology*, **7**, 253–66.

11 Pilar G & Landmesser L (1976) Ultrastructural differences during embryonic cell death in normal and peripherally deprived ciliary ganglia. *Journal of Cell Biology*, **68**, 339–56.

12 Clarke PG (1990) Developmental cell death: morphological diversity and multiple mechanisms. *Anatomy & Embryology*, **181**, 195–213.

13 Salvesen GS & Dixit VM (1997) Caspases: intracellular signaling by proteolysis. *Cell*, **91**, 443–6.

14 Thornberry NA, Rano TA, Peterson EP, Rasper DM, Timkey T, Garcia-Calvo M, Houtzager VM, Nordstrom PA, Roy S, Vaillancourt JP, Chapman KT & Nicholson DW (1997) A combinatorial approach defines specificities of members of the caspase family and granzyme B. Functional relationships established for key mediators of apoptosis. *Journal of Biological Chemistry*, **272**, 17907–11.

15 Chi S, Kitanaka C, Noguchi K, Mochizuki T, Nagashima Y, Shirouzu M, Fujita H, Yoshida M, Chen W, Asai A, Himeno M, Yokoyama S & Kuchino Y (1999) Oncogenic Ras triggers cell suicide through the activation of a caspase-independent cell death program in human cancer cells. *Oncogene*, **18**, 2281–90.

16 Kitanaka C & Kuchino Y (1999) Caspase-independent programmed cell death with necrotic morphology. *Cell Death & Differentiation*, **6**, 508–15.

17 Sperandio S, deBelle I & Bredesen DE (2000) An alternative, non-apoptotic form of programmed cell death. *Proceedings of the National Academy of Sciences, USA*, **97**, 14376–81.

18 Bredesen DE, Ye X, Tasinato A, Sperandio S, Wang JJ, Assa-Munt N & Rabizadeh S (1998) p75NTR and the concept of cellular dependence: seeing how the other half die. *Cell Death & Differentiation*, **5**, 365–71.

19 Mehlen P, Rabizadeh S, Snipas SJ, Assa-Munt N, Salvesen GS & Bredesen DE (1998) The DCC gene product induces apoptosis by a mechanism requiring receptor proteolysis. *Nature*, **395**, 801–4.

20 Rabizadeh S, Oh J, Zhong LT, Yang J, Bitler CM, Butcher LL & Bredesen DE (1993) Induction of apoptosis by the low-affinity NGF receptor. *Science*, **261**, 345–8.

21 Cornillon S, Foa C, Davoust J, Buonavista N, Gross JD & Golstein P (1994) Programmed cell death in *Dictyostelium. Journal of Cell Science*, **107**, 2691–704.

22 Jurgensmeier JM, Krajewski S, Armstrong RC, Wilson GM, Oltersdorf T, Fritz LC, Reed JC & Ottilie S (1997) Bax- and Bak-induced cell death in the fission yeast Schizosaccharomyces pombe. *Molecular Biology of the Cell*, **8**, 325–39.

23 Kerr JF, Wyllie AH & Currie AR (1972) Apoptosis: a basic biological phenomenon with wide-ranging implications in tissue kinetics. *British Journal of Cancer*, **26**, 239–57.

8

Apoptotic gene expression in brain ischemia and ischemic tolerance

Roger P. Simon

R. S. Dow Center for Neurobiology, Legacy Research, Portland, OR

Introduction

It is now clear that the process of apoptotic cell death plays a major role in the outcome of acute ischemic injury in the brain, and there is evidence that these gene families may play a role in the phenomenon of ischemic tolerance as well. These genes and their translated proteins are widely distributed throughout the body and diffusely represented in the brain. Thus, while their overall death modulatory role is known, precisely what the activity of a particular apoptotic or anti-apoptotic gene product might be in a particular cell type in a specific paradigm of ischemia is not clear, clouding the pathway to therapeutic translation. A few of these central issues are reviewed below.

Anti-apoptotic gene expression in ischemia and tolerance are not cell-type specific

These features are clearly demonstrated in focal ischemia. Using the intraluminal suture method, one can produce ischemic infarction in the caudate putamen while producing a penumbral effect in the cortex. In such a situation there is widespread induction of the prosurvival gene product, Bcl-2. However, expression in the penumbral cortex is almost entirely neuronal, while in the ventral-cortical regions close to the ischemic core, the predominant cell type expressing Bcl-2 is astroglial. Bcl-2 is expressed in the infarct core as well where neither neurons nor glia survive. The cells expressing Bcl-2 there are the endothelial cells of the surviving blood vessels (Figure 8.1) [1]. Virtually the identical picture is seen in experiments investigating a newly described Bcl-2 family member with a 46% homology to Bcl-2: Bcl-w. Thus, cell survival genes are seen in cells in the ischemic brain which will survive regardless of their cell type. Cells that are committed to die, such as those in the CA1 sector in global ischemia, express the death modulatory gene *bax* [2].

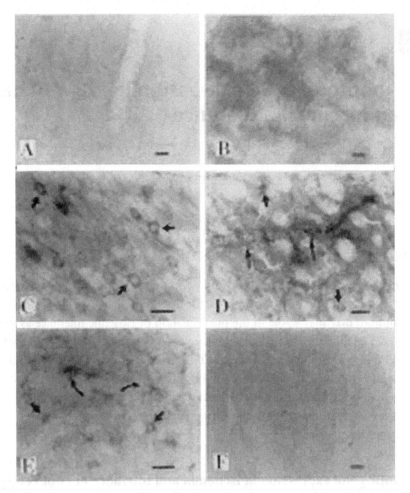

Figure 8.1   Bcl-2 immunostaining in coronal brain sections from rats 24 hours after 60 minutes of middle cerebral artery occlusion. (A) Contralateral cortex; (B) contralateral caudate; (C) Bcl-2 induction in neurons (arrows) in frontoparietal cortex; (D) Bcl-2 induction in a few neurons (short arrows) and vessels (long arrows) in the caudate; (E) Bcl-2 induction in a few neurons (straight arrows) and mainly in microglia (curved arrows) in the infarct border zone; (F) the cortical section incubated in the absence of primary antibody for Bcl-2. Bars = 20 μm. (Data from ref. 1.)

Thus, while dying cells express a gene product that induces death and surviving cells produce a gene product that is pro-survival, a pure cause and effect relationship has a component of retrospective deduction. The question of cause and effect is illustrated in ischemic tolerance. In the model of transient focal ischemia inducing tolerance to subsequent prolonged focal ischemia, the tolerance phenomenon is not seen during the first 24 hours but is present subsequently and is maximal at

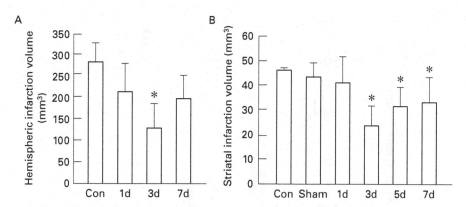

Figure 8.2   (A) Ischemic tolerance. Preconditioning (Con) ischemia (30 minutes) significantly reduced ($P<0.05$) the volume of hemispheric damage when performed 3 days (d) before 100 minutes of ischemia. (Data from ref 3.) (B) Striatal tolerance. Preconditioning ischemia (20 minutes) conferred protection against 60 minutes of middle cerebral artery occlusion (MCAO) when performed 3, 5 or 7 days previously (S. Shimuzu, S.H. Graham & R.L. Zhu, unpublished data).

3 days (Figure 8.2A) [3]. If one looks for the presence of a putative neuroprotective protein in this model, its expression should follow the time course of the induction of tolerance. In this regard the neuroprotective chaperone protein HSP70 fails such a test as it is robustly induced in cortical neurons by 24 hours. However, if the effector cell producing the phenomenon of tolerance were to be shown to be astroglial, then HSP70 is a candidate as its expression in glia is not seen until 48 hours [3].

Apoptotic gene expression in ischemia and tolerance are not regionally specific

In focal ischemia with reperfusion, the caudate infarcts and the cortex become penumbral. The cell survival proteins (Bcl-2 and Bcl-w) are induced in cortical neurons, presumably providing protection. That neuroprotection is being provided by Bcl-2 is supported by an increase in the infarction size in the setting of Bcl-2 antisense administration in vivo (Figure 8.3), which results in an attenuation of the expression of this anti-apoptotic gene product [4] . If one reduces the duration of transient focal ischemia in this model, then tolerance is induced in the striatum (Figure 8.2B). In this circumstance, Bcl-2 (the presumed neuroprotective element) is shown to be expressed in neurons within the striatum. The tolerance phenomenon, to subsequent severe transient focal ischemia, can be blocked in the striatum with Bcl-2 antisense (S. Shimuzu, S.H. Graham & R.L. Zhu, unpublished data).

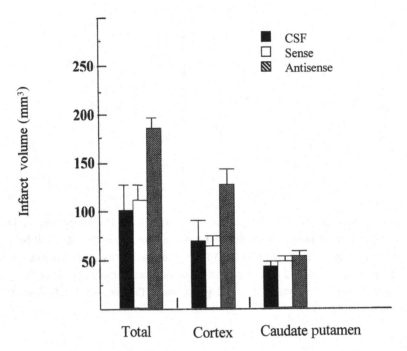

Figure 8.3   The effect of Bcl-2 antisense oligo on infarct volume in rat brains after 1 hour of ischemia and 72 hours of reperfusion. Antisense, but not sense, oligo increases infarct volume in both the cortex and caudate putamen, compared with cerebrospinal fluid (CSF)-treated brains. (Data from ref. 4).

Apoptotic gene expression in ischemia and tolerance are not injury-type specific

The phenomenon of apoptotic gene expression is one that is found in multiple organ systems. The phenomenon of tolerance is also broadly represented and perhaps most prominently investigated in the heart [5]. Both apoptotic gene expression and tolerance occur in paradigms other than focal ischemia. In ischemia per se the paradigms to induce tolerance are multiple and include focal ischemia protecting against global ischemia, global ischemia protecting against focal ischemia, focal ischemia protecting against focal ischemia, and global ischemia protecting against global ischemia [5]. Ischemic tolerance has also been demonstrated in the spinal cord [6].

Epilepsy is another acute circumstance in which anti- and pro-apoptotic gene expression is upregulated. In epilepsy, the CA3 sector of the hippocampus is the most vulnerable and the CA1 less so. In this circumstance the pro-apoptotic gene

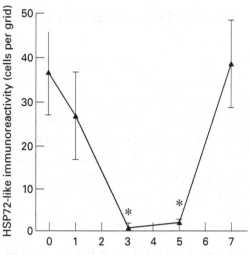

Figure 8.4   Epileptic tolerance. Effects of prior, bicuculline-induced seizures on the expression of HSP72-like immunoreactivity in the CA3c sector of the hippocampus. (Data from ref. 8.)

Bax is expressed in the CA3 sector while the anti-apoptotic gene *bcl-2* has its expression in the CA1 sector [7]. This is the opposite circumstance to the pyramidal cell regions expressing the genes in ischemia, demonstrating that a given hippocampal sector is not vulnerable because of the apoptotic gene (pro- or anti-apoptotic) it is solely capable of inducing, but rather that multiple gene products can be induced from the same cell population. In epilepsy acute cell injury and death occurs. If one quantifies this effect in the highly vulnerable CA3 sector using a marker of injury (HSP70 expression) and cell death (acid fuchsin staining), a dose–response curve between the seizure duration and these markers can be found. If one then pretreats the animal with an epileptic stimulus and subsequently repeats the epileptic event one can show the development of a marked degree of tolerance against epileptic brain injury [8]. As in ischemia, this tolerance is not present in the first 24 hours but is maximally induced at 3 days and persists through 5 days (Figure 8.4).

Additionally, hyperthermic or hypoxic treatment of neonatal rats protects the brain from subsequent ischemia. Interestingly, neither of the preparatory stimuli inducing tolerance produced HSP70 expression [9]. An additional example is the cross-protection of kainic acid-induced seizures and global ischemia upon neuronal injury from either stressor [10]. Remarkably, ischemic preconditioning protects against traumatic brain injury as well [11].

Apoptotic gene expression in ischemia (and perhaps tolerance) is not protein specific

A host of proteins are upregulated in ischemia and are candidates for programmed cell death effectors and cell survival proteins in the setting of ischemia and the induction of tolerance phenomena. Proteins are likely to be responsible in substantial measure as their modulation can alter the outcome of ischemic injury [4] and protein-sensitive inhibitors block the induction of the phenomenon of tolerance. In focal ischemia, *bcl-2* is upregulated in neurons, glia and endothelial cells that survive [1]. When one looks at surviving cells in focal ischemia with attention to the *bcl-2* family gene product, Bcl-w, one sees exactly the same pattern; neurons in penumbral cortex, astrocytes in the transition zone and endothelial cells in the ischemic core express the survival factor. Further, the survival protein is expressed in noninjured neurons, i.e., those which do not show DNA fragmentation. Within a given neuron the Bcl-2 protein is found in the cytosol, but with ischemia it colocalizes with a marker for the mitochondrial membrane. Bcl-2 and Bcl-w (and perhaps Bcl-x$_L$, which has a 42% homology to Bcl-2) function similarly in ischemia because they share the BH1–3 binding domains that are essential for heterodimerization with pro-apoptotic Bcl-2 family members. In addition, they contain the transmembrane C-terminal domain, which allows translocation to the mitochondrial membrane. Why this redundancy of function among Bcl family members exists is unknown. However, the similarity of these proteins does not completely explain their effect in the ischemic neuron. For example, it has been shown that Bcl-w protects against apoptosis induced by overexpression of Bax or Bad, but not that induced by the pro-apoptotic Bcl-2 family member Bak or Bik, even though Bcl-w is able to heterodimerize with all four proteins [12]. On the other hand, A1 protein, a Bcl-w homologue, although unable to bind to either Bax or Bad remains capable of blocking Bax- and Bad-induced cytotoxicity [12]. In addition, certain BH mutants of Bcl-x$_L$ that do not bind Bax, retain anti-apoptotic activity [13,14]. Therefore, alternative mechanisms for apoptosis regulation by Bcl-2 family members exist that are independent of simple binding domains. One such mechanism is the stabilization of the mitochondrial membrane (Figure 8.5), perhaps by inhibiting the opening of the mitochondrial transition pore, which attenuates cytochrome *c* release (Figure 8.6) and resultant caspase induction [15,16].

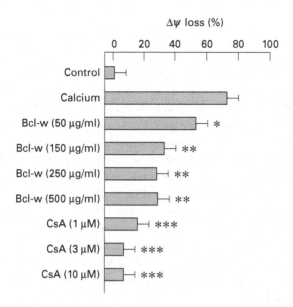

Figure 8.5   Effects of Bcl-w and cyclosporin A (CsA) on calcium-induced (100 μmol/l) loss of
mitochondrial transmembrane potential ($\Delta\Psi$) in isolated brain mitochondria. $\Delta\Psi$ was
determined by measuring the uptake of rhodamine-123 fluorescence. The protonophore
CCCP (10 μmol/l), served as the positive control (100%) for $\Delta\Psi$ loss. Data are mean ± SD of
three different experiments. *$P < 0.05$, **$P < 0.01$, ***$P < 0.0001$ vs. calcium-treated group
without inhibitors (analysis of variance and post hoc Fisher's t tests). (Data from ref. 16)

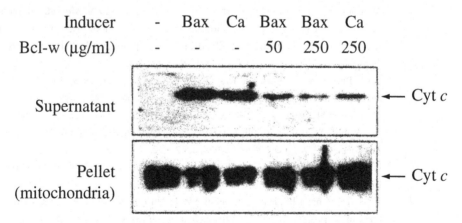

Figure 8.6   Effects of Bcl-w on cytochrome c (Cyt c) release from isolated brain mitochondria induced
by Bax or calcium (Ca). Mitochondria were incubated with the recombinant Bax protein
(50 μg/ml) or calcium (100 μmol/l) for 1 hour in the presence or absence of Bcl-w at the
indicated concentrations and then centrifuged. The supernatant and pellet were subjected
to Western blot analysis for cytochrome c. Note that Bcl-w inhibits Bax- or calcium-
induced cytochrome c release. Results are representative of two independent
experiments. (Data from ref. 16.)

REFERENCES

1 Chen J, Graham SH, Chan PH, Lan J, Zhou RL & Simon RP (1995) bcl-2 is expressed in neurons that survive focal ischemia in the rat. *Neuroreport*, **6**, 394–8.

2 Chen J, Zhu RL, Nakayama M, Kawaguchi K, Jin K, Stetler RA, Simon RP & Graham SH (1996) Expression of the apoptosis-effector gene, Bax, is up-regulated in vulnerable hippocampal CA1 neurons following global ischemia. *Journal of Neurochemistry*, **67**, 64–71.

3 Chen J, Graham SH, Zhu RL & Simon RP (1996) Stress proteins and tolerance to focal cerebral ischemia. *Journal of Cerebral Blood Flow & Metabolism*, **16**, 566–77.

4 Chen J, Simon RP, Nagayama T, Zhu R, Loeffert JE, Watkins SC & Graham SH (2000) Suppression of endogenous bcl-2 expression by antisense treatment exacerbates ischemic neuronal death. *Journal of Cerebral Blood Flow & Metabolism*, **20**, 1033–9.

5 Chen J & Simon R (1997) Ischemic tolerance in the brain. *Neurology*, **48**, 306–11.

6 Zvara DA, Colonna DM, Deal DD, Vernon JC, Gowda M & Lundell JC (1999) Ischemic preconditioning reduces neurologic injury in a rat model of spinal cord ischemia. *Annals of Thoracic Surgery*, **68**, 874–80.

7 Graham SH, Chen J, Stetler RA, Zhu RL, Jin KL & Simon RP (1996) Expression of the proto-oncogene bcl-2 is increased in the rat brain following kainate-induced seizures. *Restorative Neurology and Neuroscience*, **9**, 243–50.

8 Sasahira M, Lowry T, Simon RP & Greenberg DA (1995) Epileptic tolerance: prior seizures protect against seizure-induced neuronal injury. *Neuroscience Letters*, **185**, 95–8.

9 Wada T, Kondoh T & Tamaki N (1999) Ischemic "cross" tolerance in hypoxic ischemia of immature rat brain. *Brain Research*, **847**, 299–307.

10 Plamondon H, Blondeau N, Heurteaux C & Lazdunski M (1999) Mutually protective actions of kainic acid epileptic preconditioning and sublethal global ischemia on hippocampal neuronal death: involvement of adenosine A1 receptors and K(ATP) channels. *Journal of Cerebral Blood Flow & Metabolism*, **19**, 1296–308.

11 Perez-Pinzon MA, Alonso O, Kraydieh S & Dietrich WD (1999) Induction of tolerance against traumatic brain injury by ischemic preconditioning. *Neuroreport*, **10**, 2951–4.

12 Holmgreen SP, Huang DC, Adams JM & Cory S (1999) Survival activity of Bcl-2 homologs Bcl-w and A1 only partially correlates with their ability to bind pro-apoptotic family members. *Cell Death & Differentiation*, **6**, 525–32.

13 Cheng EH, Levine B, Boise LH, Thompson CB & Hardwick JM (1996) Bax-independent inhibition of apoptosis by Bcl-X_L. *Nature*, **379**, 554–6.

14 Kelekar A, Chang BS, Harlan JE, Fesik SW & Thompson CB (1997) Bad is a BH3 domain-containing protein that forms an inactivating dimer with Bcl-X_L. *Molecular and Cellular Biology*, **17**, 7040–6.

15 Green DR (2000) Apoptotic pathways: paper wraps stone blunts scissors. *Cell*, **102**, 1–4.

16 Yan C, Chen J, Chen D, Minami M, Pei W, Yin XM & Simon RP (2000) Overexpression of the cell death suppressor Bcl-w in ischemic brain: implications for a neuroprotective role via the mitochondrial pathway. *Journal of Cerebral Blood Flow & Metabolism*, **20**, 620–30.

9

Cellular mechanisms of white matter ischemia: what can we learn from culture models?

Suzanne Underhill[1], Selva Baltan Tekkök[2], M. Josh Hasbani[3] &
Mark P. Goldberg[4]

[1–4] Department of Neurology, Washington University School of Medicine, St. Louis, MO

Introduction

Ischemic brain disease is a serious cause of neurological disability, with profound social and economic consequences. Ischemic strokes in large-vessel territories damage both gray and white matter. In addition, white matter may be preferentially injured by infarcts in the distribution of small penetrating arteries [1]. The pathophysiology of hypoxic–ischemic injury of white matter can be expected to have unique features in comparison to gray matter because white matter contains no synapses or neuronal soma, but instead has myelinated axons and oligodendrocytes. One of the important lessons learned is that energy deprivation engages different mechanisms of injury in glial cells as compared with neuronal cell bodies or axonal processes [2–4]. A detailed understanding of the mechanisms of central nervous system white matter injury would be of central importance in designing more effective neuroprotective and therapeutic strategies for this injury. To fully protect brain function against anoxia/ischemia, it is necessary to preserve the functional integrity of white matter as well as gray matter. Surviving neuronal populations whose axonal connections have been destroyed or disabled would be functionally useless.

Although white matter is most often severely affected in human stroke, studies of rodent stroke models rarely note white matter injury. In part this is because a considerably smaller proportion of the mouse or rat brain comprise white matter. The mature human brain is approximately 50% white matter [5] whereas far less of the rodent brain is white matter. In the lissencephalic brain, cerebral infarction may indeed be confined to the cortical gray matter. Furthermore, special histological techniques are required to detect injury to white matter components. Therefore, therapies targeting gray matter may appear especially effective in rodents. Ischemic brain injury in humans might be minimized by therapeutic strategies designed to reduce white as well as gray matter damage. To develop such approaches, we need more information about the cellular mechanisms of white matter ischemic injury.

Cell culture approaches to white matter injury

In vitro models are often used to generate hypotheses about brain injury mechanisms and to develop new therapeutic approaches. The major cellular elements of white matter in the central nervous system are axons, oligodendrocytes, astrocytes, microglia and endothelial cells. Since each of these cell types is readily isolated, their vulnerability to hypoxic and toxic insults can be modeled in vitro. This chapter will focus on current information obtained from culture models that examine hypoxic injury of white matter cellular elements.

Advantages and disadvantages of cell culture approaches

Cell culture models offer obvious advantages for cell biological studies. Cells may be examined before, during and after carefully controlled toxicity paradigms. Direct tissue effects of hypoxia–ischemia can be isolated from effects on the brain vasculature. Some, but not all aspects of tissue ischemia can be modeled in culture by energy depletion caused by oxygen–glucose deprivation (OGD) in a sealed chamber, or by chemically induced energy depletion caused by agents such as cyanide or 2-deoxyglucose. In vitro models allow more precise control of the duration and severity of this exposure. Since cells in a tissue culture dish are accessible, observations can be made of several attributes during an experiment. These parameters may be as diverse as electrophysiology, morphology, membrane integrity and ion, molecule and even organelle changes and movement. Cell culture allows the control of the extracellular medium and ionic environment as well as direct cellular drug delivery at specified concentrations, without regard to permeability of the blood–brain barrier.

Cell culture approaches also allow study of highly purified cellular elements in isolation. For investigation of white matter injury, relevant cultures include astrocytes, oligodendrocytes, microglia, endothelial cells and neuronal axons. Cultures can be prepared from specified brain regions and from purified cells with specific phenotypes and maturational stages. Such specificity assists collection of biochemical or molecular data that would be difficult to interpret in more intact tissue. In common with cell lines, primary cell cultures can be valuable because they allow a large number of experiments while minimizing the use of experimental animals.

It is important to keep in mind the substantial limitations of cell culture approaches. Tissue dissociation removes all of the three-dimensional cell–cell interactions that may prove critical in mechanisms of hypoxic death. In white matter, this applies most immediately to the relationship between white matter axons, oligodendrocytes and their myelin. Primary cultures are most often derived from fetal or neonatal tissue, and therefore the maturational properties of cultured cells may not be representative of those found in the mature brain. There are other serious potential concerns with the phenotypes and functional properties of cultured cells. For example, astrocytes in culture can be classified as type I and type II, but type II astrocytes have not yet been identified in vivo. It was recently demonstrated that oligodendrocyte precursor cells, sometimes used as a source of oligodendrocyte cultures, can become multipotential precursor cells with the addition of certain growth factors [6]. This could hypothetically lead to the presence of unexpected cell types, even neurons, in cultures originating from a defined glial cell type. The complexity of the intact biological system cannot be directly modeled in vitro. Despite these limitations, in vitro models often provide useful mechanistic data that can form the basis for in vivo approaches.

Assessing cellular injury in culture models

Most investigations of ischemic injury in cell culture are concerned with death or damage of a single cell type. Therefore, it is essential to identify the cells of interest. The cell types derived from white matter can generally be distinguished using phase-contrast morphological criteria. However, these definitions are not absolute, and it is always appropriate to confirm cellular identity with more definitive immunocytochemical markers (Table 9.1). Most of these require tissue fixation and permeabilization, although some (e.g., O1 [7]) recognize extracellular epitopes that can be labeled in living cells. The use of immunocytochemical markers for cellular identification can be difficult if the specific protein is no longer expressed after cellular injury.

The next technical challenge is defining the end-points. Cell death is an obvious end-point, which can be measured in a number of ways. Compromise in membrane integrity is often an early and irreversible manifestation of cell death. This may be identified using exclusion dyes, such as trypan blue and propidium iodide. Release of endogenous intracellular proteins such as lactate dehydrogenase (LDH) is a measure of overall culture vulnerability. Conversely, cell survival can be assessed by uptake of fluorescent cytosolic dyes bound to charged groups (such as acetate or methyl esters) that are cleaved by endogenous esterase and concentrated only in living cells. Cell death by apoptosis may not involve early disruption of cell membranes. Apoptotic morphology can be demonstrated by transmission electron microscopy, fluorescence microscopy with nuclear dyes and terminal deoxynucleotidyl transferase-mediated uridine 5'-triphosphate-biotin nick end labeling

Table 9.1. Morphological and immunocytochemical recognition of white matter cellular elements in primary cultures

Cell type	Phase criteria	Morphology	Markers
Type 1 astrocyte	Light	Flat, polygonal	Anti-GFAP
Type 2 astrocyte	Light	Flat with long processes	Anti-GFAP and A2B5
Oligodendrocyte	Dark	Round with extensively branched processes	Anti-Gal-C, O4, O1, anti-MBP
Non-reactive microglia	Dark	Angular with short filopodia (increased movement)	Isolectin B4 (less than reactive counterparts), OX42
Reactive microglia	Light	Round, sometimes with rough edges (increased movement)	Isolectin B4, OX6
Endothelial cell	Light	Flat, oval	Factor VIII
Neuronal axon	Dark	Round phase bright halo around cell body, with long, smooth, thin process; axon may originate from cell body or proximal dendrite	SMI31, anti-neurofilament

Notes:
GFAP, glial fibrillary acidic protein; Gal-C, galactocerebroside; MBP, myelin basic protein.

(although this is not entirely specific to apoptosis). Apoptotic cell death is also documented by DNA laddering and cellular activation of caspases.

Most microscopic techniques require that the cells of interest remain adherent to the substrate at the end of the experiment. Glial cells commonly detach from culture substrates and therefore may potentially be incorrectly scored as dead. Another problem commonly encountered in assessment of glial, but not neuronal, cultures is that cell division may continue during culture. Net cell death must be balanced against the possibility of increased proliferation after insults. Cell division can be assessed with uptake and immunocytochemistry for bromodeoxyuridine.

Vulnerability of individual white matter components

Biochemically, white matter has a three-fold higher lipid content than protein content, reflecting the fact that the bulk of this tissue is myelin provided by oligodendrocytes [8]. The major cellular components of white matter are similar to those of gray matter, with the exception that neuronal cell bodies are not present. Generally speaking, the glial components provide the necessary environment for axons to function optimally. Compromise of any of these individual components

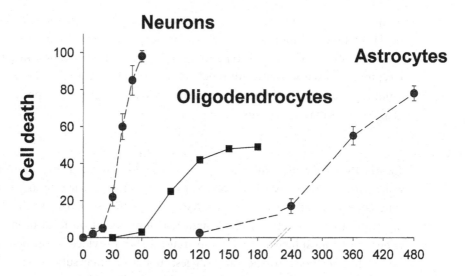

Figure 9.1   Comparison of cellular vulnerability to oxygen–glucose deprivation (OGD). Cortical cultures were exposed to OGD for the duration indicated, and cell death was assessed 1 day later by measurement of LDH release (neurons, astrocytes) or cell counts (oligodendrocytes). Neuronal and oligodendrocyte cultures included an astrocyte monolayer. The oligodendrocyte experiments were not continued beyond 3 hours to avoid possible confusion with astrocyte death. (Neuron and astrocyte data are from ref. 40; oligodendrocyte data are from S.P. Althomsons and M.P. Goldberg (unpublished).)

will affect the overall function of white matter. The intimate relationship of astrocytes with the blood supply makes the role of these cells during ischemic injury particularly important. Endothelial cells comprising this blood supply may also play an integral role in white matter integrity during ischemic injury. Microglia serve as the brain's immune system and their role during any injury is key to maintaining a stable environment. The role of each of these components in normal brain function is so important that injury of any of these cell types in white matter may have a profound effect upon the function of the brain.

In vitro approaches have been used to examine the vulnerability of each of these components to ischemic injury. Current evidence from this and other laboratories suggests different vulnerabilities of each of these components, indicating the most likely cell targets for treatment. Figure 9.1 shows the relative vulnerability of cultured cortical neurons, oligodendrocytes and astrocytes to OGD. Although these experiments were performed under very similar conditions, it is apparent that these cell types differ substantially in vulnerability. Lethal durations of OGD ranged from about 60 minutes for neurons, to 6 to 8 hours for astrocytes. Mechanisms of these injuries are also beginning to be elucidated and suggest future directions for particular therapeutic approaches. These approaches also allow direct assessment of the vulnerability of each cell type to injury by excessive activation of glutamate receptors or excitotoxicity. Although excitotoxicity is traditionally a problem unique to neuronal cell bodies, increasing evidence suggests the possibility that glial elements may also be susceptible.

Axons

Clearly, the important functional property of white matter is to transmit action potentials. Axons often extend for great distances from their cell bodies through different extracellular environments. Axons are highly specialized so that they can accomplish their functions. For instance, axons depend on local production of adenosine triphosphate, as energy substrates are not provided by the neuronal cell body. This metabolic isolation also suggests that axons may suffer energy deprivation in a manner independent of neuronal cell bodies [3]. Damage to the axon is especially important because the axon is the only component of central white matter that does not regenerate.

Few cell culture investigations have examined injury of neuronal axons in isolation from their cell bodies. Some methods are available for this task. Variations of the Campenot chamber [9] have been used extensively to study axon trophism and metabolism. These models most often use sympathetic or dorsal root ganglion cells because of their extensive axon elaboration, particularly in the presence of nerve growth factor. For example, Sattler and colleagues [10] used a Campenot chamber to observe the pharmacology of intracellular calcium elevation after axon transection. Ivins [11] used a modified Campenot chamber to observe β-amyloid toxicity in hippocampal neurites. Smith et al. [12] developed a trauma model of axonal stretch. In this model, axons are physically separated from cell bodies, though exposed to the same environment. Cells exposed to axonal stretch were found to be morphologically highly resilient, though cytoskeletal rearrangements persisted and may have long-term effects. These models support the significance of axonal insult upon the integrity of neuronal function, but have not been applied to questions of ischemic injury.

Recent experiments in our laboratory have examined the vulnerability of cortical neuronal axons to excitotoxic and hypoxic insults. These experiments have been performed in cultures that include axons together with neuronal cell bodies and dendrites. Axons were strikingly resistant to exposure to the excitotoxins N-methyl-D-aspartate (NMDA) and kainate. Drug applications that caused immediate cellular swelling and spine loss in neuronal dendrites resulted in no detectable morphological change in axons (Figure 9.2) [13], assessed by fluorescent labeling with DiI or neuronal transfection with derivatives of green fluorescent protein.

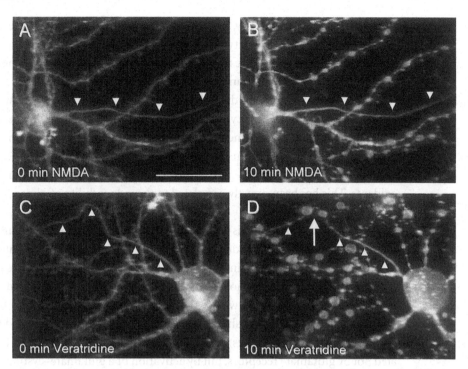

Figure 9.2   Axons are injured by activation of voltage-gated sodium channels, but not NMDA receptors. Confocal images show single, cultured cortical neurons labeled with the fluorescent tracer, DiI. Application of NMDA (30 μm for 10 minutes) caused widespread beading and spine loss of neuronal dendrites, but did not affect the axon (arrowheads). In contrast, application of the sodium channel activator, veratridine, caused beading in both axons and dendrites (arrow). (From ref. 13, with permission.)

Axons were not uniformly resistant to this form of injury, as they were readily damaged by application of veratridine, a toxin that activates voltage-gated sodium channels. Despite their resistance to glutamate receptor agonists, axons in cortical neuronal culture can be damaged by prolonged OGD, and this injury can be reduced by application of the voltage-gated sodium channel blocker, tetrodotoxin (M. J. Hasbani et al., unpublished data). These data suggest that non-myelinated axons are not directly vulnerable to excitotoxic damage, but are vulnerable to hypoxic–ischemic injury. In agreement with the studies of Stys and colleagues [14], these results suggest an important role for the activation of voltage-gated sodium channels in axonal hypoxic injury.

Oligodendrocytes

While the susceptibility of neurons to ischemic injury has been a central focus of much research, glial cell vulnerability is also critical. Oligodendrocytes are also vulnerable to ischemic injury, and investigations in cell culture have established susceptibility through a variety of pathways. The mechanisms of this toxicity are largely related to oxidative stress and elevated extracellular glutamate; however, the details of each of these mechanisms are still under investigation.

Free radicals are generated during ischemic injury in the brain (reviewed by ref. 15). In culture, oligodendrocytes are substantially compromised by exposure to free radicals [16,17]. Heightened vulnerability is thought to be due to the low glutathione content and high iron content of oligodendrocytes [18]. Glutathione is an endogenous free radical scavenger and iron can mediate the formation of strong oxidants. This has been directly correlated to the vulnerability of oligodendrocytes to OGD [19,20].

Cerebral ischemia in vivo is accompanied by an increase in extracellular glutamate [21,22]. In such high concentrations, this amino acid can mediate mechanisms of cell death. Once again, investigations of glutamate toxicity have generally focused on neuronal injury; however, some investigators have found that glial cells are also vulnerable in similar ways.

Volpe and colleagues [20] showed that oligodendrocytes can be killed by exposure to glutamate. These investigators reported that glutamate toxicity was mediated not by glutamate receptors, but by activation of a glutamate–cystine exchange mechanism. This exchanger is chloride dependent, energy independent and utilizes the natural gradient of higher intercellular glutamate to bring cystine into the cell. Under normal conditions, cystine is then converted into glutathione, a potent free radical scavenger. Under conditions of elevated extracellular glutamate the transporter effluxes cystine from the cell, creating a depletion of glutathione. This reduces the cell's natural mechanisms for coping with the generation of free radicals. In fact, even basal levels of free radical formation can kill cells deprived of cystine. In combination with increased free radical formation caused by other forms of oxidative stress, oligodendrocytes are increasingly compromised by ischemic injury.

Increasing evidence indicates that receptor-mediated glutamate toxicity can also occur. Oligodendrocytes express functional non-NMDA glutamate receptors, as demonstrated by protein, mRNA and electrophysiological assays [23–29]. The physiological significance of glutamate receptors on glial cells is not fully established. Recently, actual glutamatergic synapses were reported on oligodendrocyte precursor cells in the CA1 region of the hippocampus [30], although the role of synaptic glial communication is not yet established.

The presence of these receptors on oligodendrocytes makes them vulnerable to glutamate toxicity. It appears that only non-NMDA ionotropic receptors are relevant to oligodendrocyte glutamate excitotoxicity. Although metabotropic glutamate receptors may be present on a subset of oligodendrocytes, they do not play a large role in glutamate toxicity, as distinguished by pharmacology [31,32]. Also, while NMDA receptor-mediated toxicity is a large field of study, oligodendrocytes do not exhibit any properties of having these receptors and thus these are not a likely mechanism of oligodendrocyte vulnerability [31–35].

Current data suggest that glutamate toxicity of immature and mature oligodendrocytes is mediated largely by the α-amino-3-hydroxy-5-methyl-4-isoxazole propionic acid (AMPA) subclass of receptors [25,32–34,36]. This laboratory and others have demonstrated that AMPA is toxic and that injury can be blocked by selective AMPA antagonists such as NBQX and GYKI52466, and enhanced by the AMPA activator cyclothiazide. Further, this pharmacological profile may be seen under conditions of OGD, indicating its relevance under ischemic conditions [33].

It is not yet known how AMPA/kainate receptor activation kills oligodendrocytes. Calcium entry may be a key component [32,37]. Putative intercellular cascades may include calpain activation, cyclic AMP activation [38] or apoptosis. Evidence from this laboratory suggests that an end-point of glutamate receptor stimulation may actually be free radical formation, thus potentiating the free radical overload on these cells [39].

Oligodendrocytes are vulnerable to ischemic injury in many of the same ways that neurons are. Tissue culture investigations have demonstrated that oxidative stress increases the formation of free radicals, that elevated glutamate initiates excitotoxicity, further potentiating the formation of free radicals, and that the ability of the cell to scavenge these free radicals is greatly compromised. All of these factors lead to loss or impairment of a major component of white matter.

Astrocytes

Cultured astrocytes are strikingly less vulnerable than neurons to hypoxic injury (Figure 9.1) [40]. Astrocytes are killed in the ischemic core (an area of pan-necrosis), but may respond by proliferation and enhanced activity surrounding an infarct. Although astrocytes express non-NMDA receptors, they are not vulnerable to glutamate toxicity [41]. This resistance may be due to the very rapid desensitization of AMPA receptors on cultured astrocytes [42]. In the presence of cyclothiazide, which blocks AMPA receptor desensitization, AMPA or kainate triggers intracellular calcium elevation and astrocyte death within hours. Free radical-mediated damage may also be less in astrocytes as compared with other cell types. Astrocytes have substantially more ability to scavenge free radicals through glutathione pathways than do oligodendrocytes [18].

The method of assessing astrocyte injury in tissue culture may be relevant, as well as the propensity of astrocytes to proliferate. Counts of live and dead cells are a common method of assessing cell viability. This method often does not account for proliferation, particularly over a long time course. Since astrocyte proliferation is particularly prominent after injury, a more accurate assessment would make use of bromodeoxyuridine labeling, indicating the production of new cells. LDH release is a common indicator of cell viability. This method is particularly useful since the supernatant is analyzed and the health of the same culture may be monitored over a number of hours. Lyons and Kettenmann [43] found an increase in LDH release in astrocytes 1 to 7 days after a 2-deoxyglucose OGD paradigm. This did not agree, however, with the maintenance of cell number.

Microglia

Microglia, like astrocytes, have also been seen to increase around areas of ischemic injury in the intact brain [44]. The role of microglia in pathological paradigms is generally assessed as an increase in reactive microglia after injury. The reactive form of microglia releases a number of factors, particularly inflammatory cytokines, that affect the injury environment.

Lyons and Kettenmann [43] reported an intermediate vulnerability of microglia to OGD between astrocytes and oligodendrocytes. The mechanisms of this toxicity, however, are unclear. However, microglia express functional glutamate receptors [45]. This indicates a potential for glutamate excitotoxicity, though this has not been reported.

Endothelial cells

Endothelial cells are also vulnerable to ischemic injury. The initial cause of a stroke may produce irreversible damage to these cells by physical means, but in cell culture, intermediate vulnerability to OGD has also been determined [46]. The death of endothelial cells during OGD is accompanied by fragmentation of DNA, suggesting apoptotic mechanisms. This event is also accompanied by a significant increase in inducible nitric oxide synthase. Blocking nitric oxide synthase is partially protective, suggesting that endothelial cells die by a nitric oxide-dependent mechanism.

Putting white matter back together: studying cellular interactions in culture

Comparing different types of cell in culture provides clues as to what may occur in vivo (Table 9.2). We have reviewed experiments performed with individual cell types in isolation. While such studies provide useful information, they do not directly examine cellular interactions that might contribute to ischemic white matter injury.

Understanding these interactions requires either intact tissue or cell culture models that combine more than one cell type. For example, several studies have examined interactions between astrocytes and oligodendrocytes. These cells are

Table 9.2. Vulnerability to hypoxic or excitotoxic insults in vitro. Relative comparison of response of white matter components to oxygen–glucose deprivation (OGD) and glutamate toxicity. Cell body responses are a reflection of viability while dendrite and axon data, to date, reflect morphological changes

Cell type	OGD	NMDA	AMPA/KA
Neuronal cell bodies	+++	+++	+
Dendrites	+++	++	++
Axons	+	−	−
Astrocytes	+	−	−
Oligodendrocytes	++	−	+

Notes:

+++, the greatest response seen; −, no or very little response; NMDA, *N*-methyl-D-aspartate; AMPA, α-amino-3-hydroxy-5-methyl-4-isoxazole propionic acid; KA, kainic acid.

readily maintained in coculture and the presence of astrocytes greatly extends the survival of purified oligodendrocytes under baseline conditions (e.g., see ref. 47). Because astrocytes play a major role in regulating the extracellular milieu, they may be expected to modify the vulnerability of other cells during conditions of energy depletion. Astrocytes have more than twice the glutathione content of oligodendrocytes [18]. In coculture, this increased glutathione content in astrocytes may help to protect oligodendrocytes from events that generate free radicals, such as cystine deprivation or epinephrine and norepinephrine toxicity [17,48]. This may also apply to the free radicals generated during OGD. Astrocytes also play an important role in maintaining the extracellular glutamate concentration. Cultured oligodendrocyte precursors can release toxic glutamate concentrations during OGD [36] and axon cylinders may also efflux glutamate [49]. Astrocytes function to remove extracellular glutamate under baseline conditions through sodium-dependent glutamate transporters. These transporters may protect the brain during glutamate elevation during stroke or contribute by effluxing glutamate to pathological levels. In the white matter, it is not yet known whether astrocytes reduce extracellular glutamate or increase it.

Microglia contribute to myelin damage in models of multiple sclerosis, and it would be valuable to know whether this occurs in ischemic injury as well. Oligodendrocytes and microglia colocalize in the postischemic brain in vivo [44]. Cell culture investigation has demonstrated that microglia can lyse oligodendrocytes via nitric oxide production [50]. Nitric oxide production in endothelial cells might further potentiate this mechanism of injury. Coculture of these two types of cell has not been reported. Microglia can contribute to cellular injury in additional ways, such as by the release of tissue plasminogen activator [51].

Perhaps one of the most interesting and as yet uninvestigated scenarios is the effect of glial cell compromise upon axons. Astrocyte regulation of extracellular free radicals and glutamate during energy depletion could be important in axonal survival. Recent evidence from an optic nerve model suggests that increasing astrocyte glycogen can protect axonal conduction during glucose deprivation, perhaps by transport of lactate from astrocytes to axons [52]. Another important intercellular interaction is the effect of oligodendrocyte damage on neighboring axons. In a cortical brain slice OGD model, protection of oligodendrocytes by glutamate receptor blockade also reduced axonal injury [53]. It remains to be determined whether this occurs because dying oligodendrocytes release toxic substances or fail to provide normally protective functions. Because oligodendrocytes can myelinate axons in culture [54,55], it may be possible to examine these interactions in vitro.

Beyond cell culture

Ultimately, detailed cellular interactions of ischemic white matter must be assessed in more intact model systems. The isolated optic nerve [56] and acute brain [53] or spinal cord slice [49] preparations offer valuable tools for such investigation. A key feature is the ability to monitor signal conduction in myelinated axons. Most of these models involve axon transection and can be maintained for only a few hours after preparation. These models offer access to cells for monitoring activity in much the same way as cell culture. They also provide control of the extracellular medium and delivery of pharmacological agents, although to a more limited extent than in culture because of diffusion barriers in thick tissue.

Preclinical testing of potential therapeutic effects on white matter requires suitable in vivo models. As yet, there are no widely used models of selective injury to the brain white matter. Many rodent stroke models include damage to both gray and white matter. The proportion of white matter is small and special histological techniques are required to note damage to white matter elements. For example, increased immunocytochemical staining for tau and amyloid precursor proteins is a sensitive indicator of damage to oligodendrocytes and axons, respectively [57].

The goal of studying white matter ischemia in tissue culture is to divulge what is injured, how it is injured and, ultimately, how we may intervene and prevent this damage. Many answers about white matter ischemia have been found using tissue culture of astrocytes, oligodendrocytes, microglia and axons. This approach allows for detailed investigation of each component of white matter. The answers that we may have, however, are not applicable without testing in vivo. Ultimately, the intact system is the only way to actually test how all of the components interact and affect one another. Hopefully, answers from tissue culture may be applied to in vivo systems and lead to therapeutic interventions for stroke and other excitotoxic diseases.

Acknowledgments

S.B.T. is supported by a fellowship from the American Heart Association. This work was supported by National Institutes of Health grants NS36265, NS37230, and NS32636.

REFERENCES

1 Fisher CM (1979) Capsular infarcts: the underlying vascular lesions. *Archives of Neurology*, **36**, 65–73.

2 Choi DW (1988) Glutamate neurotoxicity and diseases of the nervous system. *Neuron*, **1**, 623–34.

3 Ransom BR, Waxman SG & Stys PK (1993) Anoxic injury of central myelinated axons: ionic mechanisms and pharmacology. *Research Publications – Association for Research in Nervous & Mental Disease*, **71**, 121–51.

4 Stys PK (1998) Anoxic and ischemic injury of myelinated axons in CNS white matter: from mechanistic concepts to therapeutics. *Journal of Cerebral Blood Flow & Metabolism*, **18**, 2–25.

5 Miller AK, Alston RL & Corsellis JA (1980) Variation with age in the volumes of grey and white matter in the cerebral hemispheres of man: measurements with an image analyser. *Neuropathology and Applied Neurobiology*, **6**, 119–32.

6 Kondo T & Raff M (2000) Oligodendrocyte precursor cells reprogrammed to become multi-potential CNS stem cells. *Science*, **289**, 1754–7.

7 Sommer I & Schachner M (1981) Monoclonal antibodies (O1 to O4) to oligodendrocyte cell surfaces: an immunocytological study in the central nervous system. *Developmental Biology*, **83**, 311–27.

8 Raval-Fernandes S, Sawant LA, Aebersold RH, Ducret A & Rome LH (1997) Axonal proteins involved in myelination: characterization of a collagen-like protein. *Developmental Neuroscience*, **19**, 421–9.

9 Campenot RB (1982) Development of sympathetic neurons in compartmentalized cultures. II. Local control of neurite survival by nerve growth factor. *Developmental Biology*, **93**, 13–21.

10 Sattler R, Tymianski M, Feyaz I, Hafner M & Tator CH (1996) Voltage-sensitive calcium channels mediate calcium entry into cultured mammalian sympathetic neurons following neurite transection. *Brain Research*, **719**, 239–46.

11 Ivins KJ, Bui ET & Cotman CW (1998) Beta-amyloid induces local neurite degeneration in cultured hippocampal neurons: evidence for neuritic apoptosis. *Neurobiology of Disease*, **5**, 365–78.

12 Smith DH, Wolf JA, Lusardi TA, Lee VM & Meaney DF (1999) High tolerance and delayed elastic response of cultured axons to dynamic stretch injury. *Journal of Neuroscience*, **19**, 4263–9.

13 Hasbani MJ, Hyrc KL, Faddis BT, Romano C & Goldberg MP (1998) Distinct roles for sodium, chloride, and calcium in excitotoxic dendritic injury and recovery. *Experimental Neurology*, **154**, 241–58.

14 Stys PK & Lopachin RM (1998) Mechanisms of calcium and sodium fluxes in anoxic myelinated central nervous system axons. *Neuroscience*, **82**, 21–32.

15 Phillis JW (1994) A "radical" view of cerebral ischemic injury. *Progress in Neurobiology*, **42**, 441–8.

16 Kim YS & Kim SU (1991) Oligodendroglial cell death induced by oxygen radicals and its protection by catalase. *Journal of Neuroscience Research*, **29**, 100–6.

17 Noble PG, Antel JP & Yong VW (1994) Astrocytes and catalase prevent the toxicity of catecholamines to oligodendrocytes. *Brain Research*, **633**, 83–90.

18 Juurlink BH, Thorburne SK & Hertz L (1998) Peroxide-scavenging deficit underlies oligodendrocyte susceptibility to oxidative stress. *Glia*, **22**, 371–8.

19 Yoshioka A, Yamaya Y, Saiki S, Kanemoto M, Hirose G, Beesley J & Pleasure D (2000) Non-*N*-methyl-D-aspartate glutamate receptors mediate oxygen–glucose deprivation-induced oligodendroglial injury. *Brain Research*, **854**, 207–15.

20 Oka A, Belliveau MJ, Rosenberg PA & Volpe JJ (1993) Vulnerability of oligodendroglia to glutamate: pharmacology, mechanisms, and prevention. *Journal of Neuroscience*, **13**, 1441–53.

21 Benveniste H, Drejer J, Schousboe A & Diemer NH (1984) Elevation of the extracellular concentrations of glutamate and aspartate in rat hippocampus during transient cerebral ischemia monitored by intracerebral microdialysis. *Journal of Neurochemistry*, **43**, 1369–74.

22 Hagberg H, Lehmann A, Sandberg M, Nystrom B, Jacobson I & Hamberger A (1985) Ischemia-induced shift of inhibitory and excitatory amino acids from intra- to extracellular compartments. *Journal of Cerebral Blood Flow & Metabolism*, **5**, 413–19.

23 Patneau DK, Wright PW, Winters C, Mayer ML & Gallo V (1994) Glial cells of the oligodendrocyte lineage express both kainate- and AMPA-preferring subtypes of glutamate receptor. *Neuron*, **12**, 357–71.

24 Puchalski RB, Louis JC, Brose N, Traynelis SF, Egebjerg J, Kukekov V, Wenthold RJ, Rogers SW, Lin F & Moran T (1994) Selective RNA editing and subunit assembly of native glutamate receptors. *Neuron*, **13**, 131–47.

25 Yoshioka A, Hardy M, Younkin DP, Grinspan JB, Stern JL & Pleasure D (1995) Alpha-amino-3-hydroxy-5-methyl-4-isoxazolepropionate (AMPA) receptors mediate excitotoxicity in the oligodendroglial lineage. *Journal of Neurochemistry*, **64**, 2442–8.

26 Ong WY, Leong SK, Garey LJ & Reynolds R (1996) A light- and electron-microscopic study of GluR4-positive cells in cerebral cortex, subcortical white matter and corpus callosum of neonatal, immature and adult rats. *Experimental Brain Research*, **110**, 367–78.

27 Matute C, Sanchez-Gomez MV, Martinez-Millan L & Miledi R (1997) Glutamate receptor-mediated toxicity in optic nerve oligodendrocytes. *Proceedings of the National Academy of Sciences, USA*, **94**, 8830–5.

28 Chew LJ, Fleck MW, Wright P, Scherer SE, Mayer ML & Gallo V (1997) Growth factor-induced transcription of GluR1 increases functional AMPA receptor density in glial progenitor cells. *Journal of Neuroscience*, **17**, 227–40.

29 Furuta A & Martin LJ (1999) Laminar segregation of the cortical plate during corticogenesis is accompanied by changes in glutamate receptor expression. *Journal of Neurobiology*, **39**, 67–80.

30 Bergles DE, Roberts JD, Somogyi P & Jahr CE (2000) Glutamatergic synapses on oligodendrocyte precursor cells in the hippocampus. *Nature*, **405**, 187–91.

31 Holtzclaw LA, Gallo V & Russell JT (1995) AMPA receptors shape Ca^{2+} responses in cortical oligodendrocyte progenitors and CG-4 cells. *Journal of Neuroscience Research*, **42**, 124–30.

32 Sanchez-Gomez MV & Matute C (1999) AMPA and kainate receptors each mediate excitotoxicity in oligodendroglial cultures. *Neurobiology of Disease*, **6**, 475–85.

33 McDonald JW, Althomsons SP, Hyrc KL, Choi DW & Goldberg MP (1998) Oligodendrocytes from forebrain are highly vulnerable to AMPA/kainate receptor-mediated excitotoxicity. *Nature Medicine*, **4**, 291–7.

34 McDonald JW, Levine JM & Qu Y (1998) Multiple classes of the oligodendrocyte lineage are highly vulnerable to excitotoxicity. *Neuroreport*, **9**, 2757–62.

35 Liu HN, Molina-Holgado E & Almazan G (1997) Glutamate-stimulated production of inositol phosphates is mediated by Ca^{2+} influx in oligodendrocyte progenitors. *European Journal of Pharmacology*, **338**, 277–87.

36 Fern RJ, Yesko CM, Thornhill BA, Kim HS, Smithies O & Chevalier RL (1999) Reduced angiotensinogen expression attenuates renal interstitial fibrosis in obstructive nephropathy in mice. *Journal of Clinical Investigation*, **103**, 39–46.

37 Yoshioka A, Ikegaki N, Williams M & Pleasure D (1996) Expression of *N*-methyl-D-aspartate (NMDA) and non-NMDA glutamate receptor genes in neuroblastoma, medulloblastoma, and other cell lines. *Journal of Neuroscience Research*, **46**, 164–78.

38 Yoshioka A, Shimizu Y, Hirose G, Kitasato H & Pleasure D (1996) Cyclic AMP-elevating agents prevent oligodendroglial excitotoxicity. *Journal of Neurochemistry*, **70**, 2416–23.

39 Althomsons S P, McDonald JW, Hyrc KH, Dugan LL, Choi DW & Goldberg MP (1997) AMPA receptor activation mediates hypoxic oligodendrocyte death in vitro. *Society for Neuroscience Abstract*.

40 Goldberg MP & Choi DW (1993) Combined oxygen and glucose deprivation in cortical cell culture: calcium-dependent and calcium-independent mechanisms of neuronal injury. *Journal of Neuroscience*, **13**, 3510–24.

41 Choi DW, Maulucci-Gedde M & Kriegstein AR (1987) Glutamate neurotoxicity in cortical cell culture. *Journal of Neuroscience*, **7**, 357–68.

42 David JC, Yamada KA, Bagwe MR & Goldberg MP (1996) AMPA receptor activation is rapidly toxic to cortical astrocytes when desensitization is blocked. *Journal of Neuroscience*, **16**, 200–9.

43 Lyons SA & Kettenmann H (1998) Oligodendrocytes and microglia are selectively vulnerable to combined hypoxia and hypoglycemia injury in vitro. *Journal of Cerebral Blood Flow & Metabolism*, **18**, 521–30.

44 Mabuchi T, Kitagawa K, Ohtsuki T, Kuwabara K, Yagita Y, Yanagihara T, Hori M & Matsumoto M (2000) Contribution of microglia/macrophages to expansion of infarction and response of oligodendrocytes after focal cerebral ischemia in rats. *Stroke*, 31, 1735–43.

45 Noda M, Nakanishi H, Nabekura J & Akaike N (2000) AMPA-kainate subtypes of glutamate receptor in rat cerebral microglia. *Journal of Neuroscience*, 20, 251–8.

46 Xu J, He L, Ahmed SH, Chen SW, Goldberg MP, Beckman JS & Hsu CY (2000) Oxygen-glucose deprivation induces inducible nitric oxide synthase and nitrotyrosine expression in cerebral endothelial cells. *Stroke*, 31, 1744–51.

47 Gard AL, Burrell MR, Pfeiffer SE, Rudge JS & Williams WC II (1995) Astroglial control of oligodendrocyte survival mediated by PDGF and leukemia inhibitory factor-like protein. *Development*, 121, 2187–97.

48 Yonezawa M, Back SA, Gan X, Rosenberg PA & Volpe JJ (1996) Cystine deprivation induces oligodendroglial death: rescue by free radical scavengers and by a diffusible glial factor. *Journal of Neurochemistry*, 67, 566–73.

49 Li S, Mealing GA, Morley P & Stys PK (1999) Novel injury mechanism in anoxia and trauma of spinal cord white matter: glutamate release via reverse Na^+-dependent glutamate transport. *Journal of Neuroscience*, 19, RC16.

50 Merrill JE, Ignarro LJ, Sherman MP, Melinek J & Lane TE (1993) Microglial cell cytotoxicity of oligodendrocytes is mediated through nitric oxide. *Journal of Immunology*, 151, 2132–41.

51 Rogove AD & Tsirka SE (1998) Neurotoxic responses by microglia elicited by excitotoxic injury in the mouse hippocampus. *Current Biology*, 8, 19–25.

52 Wender R, Brown AM, Fern R, Swanson RA, Farrell K & Ransom BR (2000) Astrocytic glycogen influences axon function and survival during glucose deprivation in central white matter. *Journal of Neuroscience*, 20, 6804–10.

53 Tekkök SB & Goldberg MB (2001) Ampa/kainate receptor activation mediates hypoxic oligodendrocyte death and axonal injury in cerebral white matter. *Journal of Neuroscience*, 21, 4237–48.

54 Peterson ER & Murrary MR (1955) Myelin sheath formation of avian spinal ganglia. *American Journal of Anatomy*, 96, 319.

55 Lubetzki C, Demerens C, Anglade P, Villarroya H, Frankfurter A, Lee VM & Zalc B (1993) Even in culture, oligodendrocytes myelinate solely axons. *Proceedings of the National Academy of Sciences, USA*, 90, 6820–4.

56 Stys PK, Ransom BR & Waxman SG (1990) Effects of polyvalent cations and dihydropyridine calcium channel blockers on recovery of CNS white matter from anoxia. *Neuroscience Letters*, 115, 293–9.

57 Dewar D, Yam P & McCulloch J (1999) Drug development for stroke: importance of protecting cerebral white matter. *European Journal of Pharmacology*, 375, 41–50.

Part IV

Hot topics

Co-Chairs: Rona G. Giffard & Myron D. Ginsberg

10

Astrocytes in ischemic stroke

Jane H.-C. Lin[1] & Maiken Nedergaard[2]

[1] Department of Pathology, New York Medical College, Valhalla, New York
[2] Department of Cell Biology and Anatomy, New York Medical College, Valhalla, New York

Astrocytes are active participants in brain function

Astrocytes are electrically unexcitable cells that traditionally are regarded as the brain's support cells. A chief function of astrocytes is to maintain an optimal environment for synaptic transmission by tightly regulating interstitial ion and neurotransmitter concentrations. Other functions include production of neurotrophins and cytokines, and astrocytic endfeet are an essential part of the blood–brain barrier. In development, radial glial cells direct and support the migration of immature neurons [1]. Several lines of work within the last few years have shown that astrocytes also participate more directly in neurotransmission [2]. Astrocytes communicate with one another by calcium signaling and these calcium signals are transmitted to neurons [3,4]. As such, astrocytes contribute to synaptic transmission [5]. Recent reports have gone on to demonstrate that astrocytes are potent modulators of inhibitory transmission in the hippocampus and function as a necessary intermediary in long-term potentiation of GABAergic synapses (GABA is γ-aminobutyric acid) [6].

Astrocytes have traditionally received little attention in the stroke field

Stroke research has paid little attention to astrocytes. During the last decade, the excitotoxin hypothesis has dominated the field [7,8]. Since astrocytes are not sensitive to glutamate and survive exposure to 10 mM glutamate [9], it is not surprising that astrocytes have been regarded as minor players in the process of ischemic infarction. Also, astrocytes are highly resistant to ischemic conditions, whereas the viability of neurons is compromised within minutes [9]. In addition, loss of astrocytes during ischemia is in principle not irreversible, since astrocytes may regenerate in adults [10]. In fact, the postischemic brain is packed with reactive hypertrophic astrocytes, though it remains unknown whether these reactive astrocytes have the same functional characteristics as non-reactive astrocytes [11].

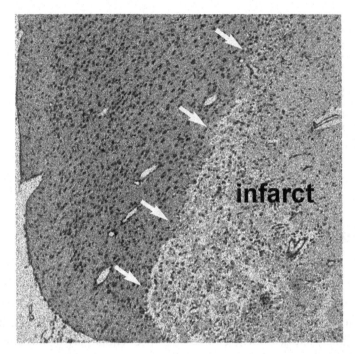

Figure 10.1   A sharp transition separates an ischemic infarct from its surroundings. Hematoxylin and eosin-stained section of a cortical infarct 4 days after occlusion of the middle cerebral artery in a rat [14]. The infarct appears pale and all cell types, including neurons and astrocytes, have lost viability. The peri-infarct tissue is structurally preserved with only dispersed neuronal damage.

The excitotoxin hypothesis revised

According to the excitotoxin hypothesis, ischemic neuronal death is a consequence of the excessive amounts of glutamate released during brain ischemia [12]. Astrocytes are not directly incorporated into the hypothesis owing to their resistance to glutamate, but it is generally thought that the observed loss of astrocytes within ischemic lesions is a result of low blood flow [13]. One would therefore predict that ischemic infarcts might be surrounded by broad border zones of selective neuronal injury. However, this pattern of injury is not observed. Rather, ischemic infarcts are characterized by sharp transitions between necrotic tissue (infarct) and structurally intact tissue with little cellular damage [14] (Figure 10.1). Several neuropathological studies have in the past searched for the existence of selective neuronal injury in the infarct surroundings, the ischemic penumbra. The results have been disappointing in that, although dead neurons can be found in the penumbra, they are too infrequent and dispersed to support a glutamatergic mechanism of ischemic damage [15].

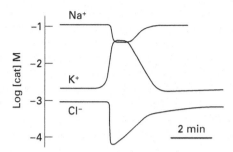

Figure 10.2 Interstitial ion changes in spreading depression [23].

The relatively all-or-none pattern of cellular damage in focal stroke constitutes an informative paradox to the excitotoxin hypothesis, which cannot be explained within its framework. In fact, since astrocytes are more resistant to ischemia than neurons, the scarcity of dead neurons outside the infarct indicates that neurons die to a significant extent only in areas where astrocytes are killed. In this chapter, we will discuss the importance of spreading depression and astrocytic signaling in the pathogenesis of ischemic stroke. Spreading depression waves are mediated by calcium signaling in astrocytes [16,17] and contribute to ischemic injury [18,19].

Definition of spreading depression

Spreading depression, classically described as the spreading depression of Leão, is a generalized response of vertebrate gray matter to a variety of noxious influences [20]. It constitutes a slowly moving wave of tissue depolarization in the intact brain [21]. Spreading depression is experimentally evoked by applying potassium chloride (KCl) or the excitatory neurotransmitter glutamate to exposed cortical tissue, or by traumatic injury [22]. Spreading depression is characterized by a reversible cessation of neuronal activity that propagates slowly (20 to 80 μm/s), and is accompanied by a loss of membrane potential and transmembrane ionic gradients [23] (Figure 10.2). In the neocortex, the propagation of spreading depression can be tracked by inserting ion- or potential-sensitive electrodes at various distances from the focus of initiation [23]. Another preparation, the isolated chick retina, has the distinct advantage of permitting direct visual observation of individual waves of spreading depression, each of which can be followed under low-power microscopy as an enlarging dark circle with its center at the site of stimulation [24,25] (Figure 10.3). The reflectance changes that accompany retinal spreading depression are believed to result from the transient decrease in interstitial volume that accompanies it [26]. This preparation has been used to show that gap junction coupling is required for propagation of spreading depression [25].

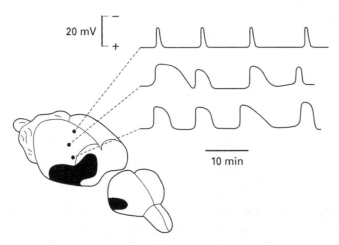

Figure 10.3 Spontaneous waves of spreading depression after occlusion of the middle cerebral artery. Three K$^+$ electrodes were inserted in the cortical peri-infarct zone [28].

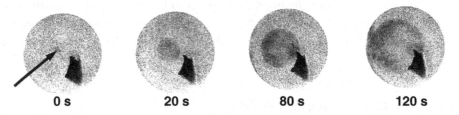

Figure 10.4 Spreading depression in the retina ex vivo [25].

Spreading depression is spontaneously evoked in focal stroke and head injury

When focal ischemia is induced by occlusion of the middle cerebral artery in rats, spontaneous waves of spreading depression are generated within the ischemic tissue [18,27] (Figure 10.4). What triggers these repeated waves of spreading depression in focal stroke is not established, but increased levels of extracellular K$^+$ and glutamate, known to evoke spreading depression in the normal non-ischemic brain, are characteristically found in the permanently depolarized ischemic core region. Spreading depression might thus be initiated by K$^+$ and/or glutamate diffusion from the ischemic core into the immediate surroundings. Alternatively, waves of depolarization can be generated from transient ischemic foci within the border zone itself [28]. We have previously shown that tissue swelling and hypoglycemia lower the threshold for eliciting spreading depression [15]. Since brain ischemia is associated with edema and a decrease in brain glucose content, it is likely that the threshold for generation of spreading depression is lower in ischemic than in normal brain.

Before   During SD   After

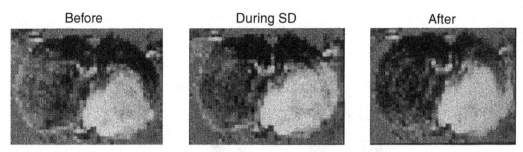

Figure 10.5   Spreading depression (SD) evoked expansion of ischemic injury visualized by T_2 nuclear magnetic resonance imaging. The middle cerebral artery was occluded 30 minutes earlier. The first panel illustrates the ischemic lesion 30 minutes after artery occlusion. The middle panel maps the same lesion during a KCl-evoked wave of spreading depression, whereas the last panel illustrates the lesion after recovery from spreading depression. Spreading depression caused a stepwise increase in lesion size that only partially recovered. As a result, the lesion was permanently enlarged. The ischemic lesion appears white, whereas the normal tissue is dark [31].

Spreading depression increases lesion size

Several lines of evidence have supported the view that spreading depression increases tissue damage in stroke. First, inhibition of spreading depression decreases the volume of infarction [18,29]. Second, stroke volume enlarges if additional waves of spreading depression are experimentally increased in the ischemic brain [30]. Third, nuclear magnetic resonance (T_2-weighted) imaging of experimental stroke has revealed that the infarct expands stepwise during each wave of spreading depression [19,31] (Figure 10.5). The contribution of spreading depression to injury is significant. It is estimated that final infarct size increases by 23% for each wave of spreading depression generated in the ischemic brain [29].

Spreading depression evokes a widespread inflammatory response

A growing body of work has shown that spreading depression is also associated with a widespread increase in expression of glial fibrillary acidic protein, microglial activation and immediate early gene expression [32–34]. The inflammatory response includes most of the same, but not the opposite hemisphere. In accordance with this, spreading depression cannot cross from one hemisphere to the other (Figure 10.6). The inflammatory response has been linked to secondary injury in both stroke and trauma [19].

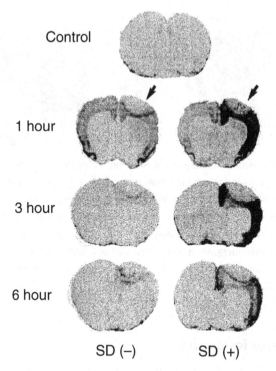

Figure 10.6   *c-fos* gene expression is increased in the ipsilateral cortex after traumatic brain injury (arrow) in animals with spontaneous spreading depression waves (SD+), but only in a small rim around the lesion in animals without (SD−) [32].

Astrocytic calcium signaling as a tool to study spreading depression

The propagation of calcium increments that spread from cell to cell constitute a newly described manner of intercellular signaling. These calcium waves can spread over long distances within a population of astrocytes and are transmitted to neurons [3,4] and endothelial cells [35]. A variety of electrical, mechanical or physiological stimuli, including exposure to glutamate, can act as triggers for the induction of astrocytic calcium waves. These stimuli activate phospholipase C, which in turn promotes an increase in inositol 3-phosphate (IP_3) levels and the subsequent release of calcium from intracellular stores [36]. It is generally believed that the presence of gap junctions is required for the propagation of the wave, and in fact, it has been assumed that the passage of Ca^{2+} and/or IP_3 through the gap junction channel may contribute to the spread of the calcium signal. However, studies from our group and others have shown that, in addition to a gap junction-mediated pathway, the calcium wave travels from cell to cell by the release of a purinergic compound, probably adenosine triphosphate, which activates purinergic receptors and the IP_3/Ca^{2+} cascade in neighboring cells [37,38] (Figure 10.7).

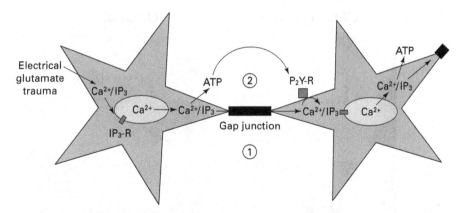

Figure 10.7 Coexistence of two intercellular signaling pathways in astrocytes. Astrocytic calcium waves are mediated by either (1) diffusion of Ca^{2+}/IP_3 via gap junction channels or (2) release of adenosine triphosphate (ATP) and activation of purinergic receptors [37,38]. Both signaling mechanisms coexist in astrocytes, but purinergic signaling can be selectively upregulated after, for example, inflammatory responses. IP_3-R, inositol 3-phosphate (IP_3) receptor; P_2Y-R, purinergic receptor.

The calcium waves travel with the same velocity of propagation as spreading depression and are triggered by identical stimulation paradigms. It has been suggested that calcium signaling represents the in vitro expression of spreading depression. Experimental evidence now supports the contention that astrocytic calcium waves constitute the leading edge of a propagating spreading depression wave. In particular, astrocytic calcium increments precede the depolarizing wave of spreading depression by several seconds in acutely prepared hippocampal slices [17,39]. Also, spreading depression is highly sensitive to gap junction inhibitors both in the isolated chicken retina and in the neocortex of live rats. The sensitivity to N-methyl-D-aspartate (NMDA) receptor antagonists of spreading depression suggests that glutamate-induced depolarization is a secondary amplification step required for long-distance propagation of spreading depression as compared with the small radius of calcium waves. Calcium waves migrate a maximum of 300 μm as compared with spreading depression, which can expand over the entire span of neocortex [16].

Astrocytic gap junctions propagate or amplify ischemic injury

For decades it was assumed that dying astrocytes uncouple during the process of cell death. We challenged this view by demonstrating functional coupling among ischemic dying astrocytes both in vivo and in vitro [40] (Figure 10.8). Using the fluorescence recovery after a photobleach technique, we found that astrocytes

82 min anoxia   **Octanol**

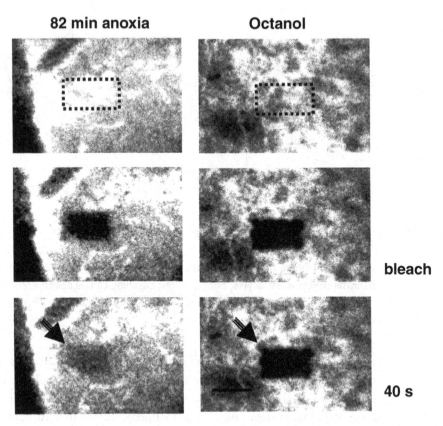

bleach

40 s

Figure 10.8   Gap junctions remain functional in the exposed rat parietal cortex for more than 1 hour after cardiac arrest. The parietal cortex was loaded with a gap junction-permeable fluorescence indicator, CDCF. The fluorescence recovery after the photobleach technique was used to study gap junction coupling in the ischemic brain. Shortly after obtaining a baseline image of CDCF fluorescence, an argon–krypton laser was used to bleach fluorescence in a rectangle. The rate of refill of fluorescence is a measure of gap junction coupling. Left panel, parietal cortex of a rat killed 83 minutes earlier; right panel, cortex of the same rat exposed to 1 mM octanol (octanol, bleached 76 minutes after cardiac arrest). Rectangles (dotted lines) in upper panels delineate area selected for photobleach. Middle panels illustrate the same field immediately after photobleach. Recovery of fluorescence 40 seconds after photobleach is shown in lower panels (arrows). Rapid refill is evident in the left panel, indicating that gap junctions remained functional 83 minutes after cardiac arrest. In contrast, the gap junction inhibitor, octanol, efficiently reduced coupling in the same animal [41]. Bar = 20 μm.

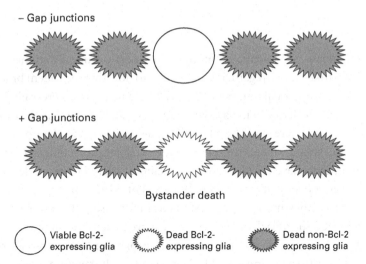

Figure 10.9. Gap junction can propagate injury to include otherwise viable glia cells. A coculture system of Bcl-2-expressing (which increases the cellular resistance to injury) and Bcl-2-negative C6 glioma cells was used to define the role of gap junctions in bystander death. Resistant Bcl-2-expressing glial cells survive injury in the absence of gap junction coupling, whereas less resistant Bcl-2-negative cells die after the same insult. If the Bcl-2-expressing and Bcl-2-negative cells are coupled by gap junctions, injury expands to include the otherwise viable Bcl-2-expressing cells. The bystander killing of gap junction-coupled, Bcl-2-expressing cells is delayed and can be reduced by gap junction inhibitors [41].

remained coupled for several hours after cardiac arrest. The implication of this observation is that astrocytes in the ischemic penumbra are linked by gap junctions to astrocytes within the ischemic core. Intracellular intermediates, including IP_3 and Ca^{2+} can thereby freely diffuse from dying to viable astrocytes and vice versa.

These studies served as a basis for demonstrating that gap junctions can propagate and amplify injury to include otherwise viable bystander glial cells [41]. Using a coculture model, we showed that dying glial cells can kill neighboring glial cells by a gap junction-mediated pathway (Figure 10.9). We proposed that gap junction-mediated propagation or amplification of injury might contribute to secondary injury in ischemia and tested the effects of gap junction blockade in a rat focal ischemic model. We found that a reduction in gap junction coupling was associated with both a significant decrease in infarct size and the frequency of spreading depression [42]. Propagation of spreading depression involves gap junction-mediated calcium signaling [16]. Thus, spreading depression may mediate bystander death by mechanisms involving astrocytic signaling.

Conclusion

The mechanisms of ischemic brain injury are most commonly studied in rodent models of stroke. In this regard, it is important to note that the rodent brain is composed of a roughly equal number of glial cells and neurons, whereas glial cells outnumber neurons 10 to 1 in the human brain [43]. Thus more than 90% of the cells in the human brain are glia. The relatively higher ratio of glia to neurons in humans may help to explain why agents that provide excellent protection against ischemic injury in rodents have failed so notably in clinical trials. For example, an impressive literature documents the beneficial effects of NMDA receptor antagonists in experimental stroke models; yet most clinical trials using these same agents have failed, whether due to lack of efficacy or excessive toxicity. From the perspective of parenchymal astrocytes, this should not be surprising: NMDA receptors are not expressed by astrocytes and an NMDA antagonist will therefore target a relatively smaller population of cells in humans as compared with rats or mice. Indeed, stroke therapy may benefit from a stronger focus upon glial cells and in particular upon glial gap junctions.

Acknowledgment

This work was supported by NIH/NINDS grants NS30007 and NS35011.

REFERENCES

1 Kettenmann H & Ransom BR (1995) *Neuroglia*. New York: Oxford University Press.

2 Smith SJ (1994) Neuromodulatory astrocytes. *Current Biology,* **4**, 807–10.

3 Nedergaard M (1994) Direct signaling from astrocytes to neurons in cultures of mammalian brain cells. *Science,* **263**, 1768–71.

4 Parpura V, Basarsky TA, Liu F, Jeftinija K, Jeftinija S & Haydon PG (1994) Glutamate-mediated astrocyte-neuron signalling. *Nature,* **369**, 744–7.

5 Araque A, Parpura V, Sanzgirl RP & Haydon PG (1999) Tripartite synapses: glia, the unacknowledged partner. *Trends in Neuroscience,* **22**, 208–15.

6 Kang J, Jiang L, Goldman SA & Nedergaard M (1998) Astrocyte-mediated potentiation of inhibitory synaptic transmission. *Nature Neuroscience,* **1**, 683–92.

7 Sattler R & Tymianski M (2000) Molecular mechanisms of calcium-dependent excitotoxicity. *Journal of Molecular Medicine,* **78**, 3–13.

8 Meldrum BS (2000) Glutamate as a neurotransmitter in the brain: review of physiology and pathology. *Journal of Nutrition,* **130** (4S Suppl), 1007S-1015S.

9 Goldberg WJ, Kadingo RM & Barrett JN (1986) Effects of ischemia-like conditions on cultured neurons: protection by low Na^+, low Ca^{2+} solutions. *Journal of Neuroscience,* **6,** 3144–51.

10 Levison SW & Goldman JE (1997) Multipotential and lineage restricted precursors coexist in the mammalian perinatal subventricular zone. *Journal of Neuroscience Research,* **48,** 83–94.

11 Clark RK, Lee EV, Fish CJ, White RF, Price WJ, Jonak ZL, Feuerstein GZ & Barone FC (1993) Development of tissue damage, inflammation and resolution following stroke: an immuno-histochemical and quantitative planimetric study. *Brain Research Bulletin,* **31,** 565–72.

12 Choi D (1998) Antagonizing excitotoxicity: a therapeutic strategy for stroke? *Mt Sinai Journal of Medicine,* **65,** 133–8.

13 Hossmann KA (1996) Excitotoxic mechanisms and focal ischemia. In *Cellular and Molecular Mechanisms of Ischemic Brain Damage,* vol. 71, eds. B. Siesjö & T. Wieloch, pp. 69–74. Philadelphia: Lippincott-Raven.

14 Nedergaard M (1987) Neuronal injury in the infarct border: a neuropathological study in the rats. *Acta Neuropathologica,* **73,** 131–7.

15 Nedergaard M & Diemer NH (1987) Focal ischemia of the rat brain with special reference to the influence of plasma glucose concentration. *Acta Neuropathologica,* **73,** 131–7.

16 Nedergaard M & Goldman S (1996) Spreading depression – a gap junction mediated event? In *Gap Junctions in the Nervous System,* eds. D. Spray & R. Dermietzel, pp. 75–84. Austin, TX: RG Landes.

17 Kunkler PE & Kraig RP (1998) Calcium waves precede electrophysiological changes of spreading depression in hippocampal organ cultures. *Journal of Neuroscience,* **18,** 3416–25.

18 Nedergaard M & Astrup J (1986) Infarct rim: effects of hyperglycemia on direct current potential and ^{14}C 2-deoxyglucose phosphorylation. *Journal of Cerebral Blood Flow & Metabolism,* **6,** 607–15.

19 Hossmann KA (1999) The hypoxic brain. Insights from ischemia research. *Advances in Experimental Medicine and Biology,* **474,** 155–69.

20 Leao A (1944) Spreading depression of activity in the cerebral cortex. *Journal of Neurophysiology,* **7,** 359–90.

21 Nedergaard M (1988) Mechanism of brain injury in focal cerebral ischemia. *Acta Neurologica Scandinavica,* **77,** 63–85.

22 Nicholson C & Kraig RP (1981) The behavior of extracellular ions during spreading depression. In *The Application of Selective Microelectrodes,* ed. T. Zeuthen, pp. 217–38. Amsterdam: Elsevier.

23 Hansen AJ (1988) Brain ion homeostasis in cerebral ischemia. *Neurochemical Pathology,* **9,** 195–209.

24 Martin-Ferreira H & Oliveira-Castro Gd (1966) Light scattering changes accompanying spreading depression in isolated retina. *Journal of Neurophysiology,* **29,** 715–26.

25 Nedergaard M, Cooper A & Goldman S (1995) Gap junctions are required for the propagation of spreading depression. *Journal of Neurobiology,* **28,** 433–44.

26 Martins-Ferreira H, Nedergaard M & Nicholson C (2000) Perspectives on spreading depression. *Brain Research Reviews,* **32,** 215–34.

27 Iijima T, Mies G & Hossmann K-A (1992) Repeated negative DC deflections in rat cortex following middle cerebral artery occlusion are abolished by MK-801: effect on volume of ischemic injury. *Journal of Cerebral Blood Flow & Metabolism*, **12**, 727–33.

28 Nedergaard M & Hansen AJ (1993) Characterization of cortical depolarization evoked in focal cerebral ischemia. *Journal of Cerebral Blood Flow & Metabolism*, **13**, 568–74.

29 Mies G, Iijima T & Hossmann K-A (1993) Correlation between peri-infarct DC shifts and ischaemic neuronal damage in rats. *Neuroreport*, **4**, 709–11.

30 Takano K, Latour LL, Formato JE, Carano RAD, Helmer KG, Hasegawa Y, Sotak CH & Fisher M (1996) The role of spreading depression in focal ischemia evaluated by diffusion mapping. *Annals of Neurology*, **39**, 308–18.

31 Busch E, Gyngell ML, Eis M, Hoehn-Berlage M & Hossmann K-A (1996) Potassium-induced cortical spreading depressions during focal cerebral ischemia in rats: contribution to lesion growth assessed by diffusion-weighted NMR and biochemical imaging. *Journal of Cerebral Blood Flow & Metabolism*, **16**, 1090–9.

32 Hermann DM, Mies G & Hossmann K-A (1999) Expression of c-*fos*, *jun*B, c-*jun*, *MKP*-1 and *hsp*72 following traumatic neocortical lesions in rats – relation to spreading depression. *Neuroscience*, **88**, 599–608.

33 Kraig RP, Dong LM, Thisted R & Jaeger CB (1991)Spreading depression increases immuno-histochemical staining of glial fibrillary acidic protein. *Journal of Neuroscience*, **11**, 2187–98.

34 Gehrmann J, Mies G, Bonnekoh P, Banati R, Iijima T, Kreutzberg GW & Hossmann KA (1993) Microglial reaction in the rat cerebral cortex induced by cortical spreading depression. *Brain Pathology*, **3**, 11–17.

35 Leybaert L, Paemeleire K, Strahonja A & Sanderson MJ (1998) Inositol-trisphosphate-dependent intercellular calcium signaling in and between astrocytes and endothelial cells. *Glia*, **24**, 398–407.

36 Berridge MJ (1993) Inositol trisphosphate and calcium signalling. *Nature*, **361**, 315–25.

37 Cotrina ML, Lin JH-C, Alves-Rodrigues A, Liu S, Li J, Azmi-Ghadimi H, Kang J, Naus CCG & Nedergaard M (1998) Connexins regulate calcium signaling by controlling ATP release. *Proceedings of the National Academy of Sciences, USA*, **95**, 15735–40.

38 Guthrie PB, Knappenberger J, Segal M, Bennett MVL, Charles AC & Kater SB (1999) ATP released from astrocytes mediates glial calcium waves. *Journal of Neuroscience*, **19**, 520–8.

39 Basarsky TA, Duffy SN, Andrew RD & MacVicar BA (1998) Imaging spreading depression and associated intracellular calcium waves in brain slices. *Journal of Neuroscience*, **18**, 7189–99.

40 Cotrina ML, Kang J, Lin JH-C, Bueno E, Hansen TW, He L, Liu Y & Nedergaard M (1998) Astrocytic gap junctions remain open during ischemic conditions. *Journal of Neuroscience*, **18**, 2520–37.

41 Lin JH-C, Weigel H, Cotrina ML, Liu S, Bueno E, Hansen AJ, Hansen TW, Goldman S & Nedergaard M (1998) Gap-junction-mediated propagation and amplification of cell injury. *Nature Neuroscience*, **1**, 494–500.

42 Rawanduzy A, Hansen A, Hansen TW & Nedergaard M (1997) Effective reduction of infarct volume by gap junction blockade in a rodent model of stroke. *Journal of Neurosurgery*, **87**, 916–20.

43 Kandel E (1991) In *Nerve Cell and Behavior*, eds. E Kandel, J Schwart & T Jessel, pp. 18–32. New York: Elsevier Science.

11

Aquaporin-4 water channels and brain edema

Geoffrey T. Manley[1], Miki Fujimura[2], Tonghui Ma[3], Nobuo Noshita[4], Ferda Filiz[5], Andrew W. Bollen[6], Pak H. Chan[7] & Alan S. Verkman[8]

[1] Department of Neurological Surgery, University of California, San Francisco, CA
[2,7] Department of Neurosurgery, Stanford University School of Medicine, Stanford, CA
[3,5,8] Departments of Medicine and Physiology, Cardiovascular Research Institute, University of California, San Francisco, CA
[6] Department of Pathology, University of California, San Francisco, CA

Introduction

Abnormalities in brain water balance, such as edema and increased intracranial pressure, play an important role in the pathophysiology of acute head trauma, stroke and a variety of neurological disorders [1,2]. However, little is known about the molecular mechanisms responsible for these alterations in cerebral water balance. Consequently, at present the therapeutic options are limited to neurosurgical decompression, intravenous administration of hyperosmolar agents and steroids, therapies that were introduced more than 40 years ago [3]. There is recent evidence that molecular water channels called aquaporins, which have recently been identified in mammals [4,5], may play an important role in brain edema, thus offering therapeutic alternatives.

Aquaporins are small integral membrane proteins that function primarily as bidirectional water-selective transporters in many cell types in the kidney, lung and other fluid-transporting tissues where water flow is driven by osmotic gradients and hydrostatic pressure differences. The brain expresses at least two members of the aquaporin family in areas that are known to participate in the production and absorption of brain fluid. Aquaporin-1 is selectively expressed on the ventricular surface of choroid plexus epithelium where it may play a role in cerebrospinal fluid (CSF) production [6,7]. Aquaporin-4 (AQP4) is abundantly expressed throughout the brain, particularly at the blood–brain and brain–CSF interfaces. AQP4 is expressed to a much lesser extent in tissue outside of the nervous system [8]. AQP4 expression is seen in astrocytes adjacent to the ependymal and pial surfaces that are in contact with CSF in the ventricular system and subarachnoid space [9]. Highly polarized AQP4 expression is also found in astrocytic foot processes near, or in direct contact with, blood vessels [10].

The specific localization of AQP4 to these anatomical and cellular regions of the central nervous system suggests a role for AQP4 in cerebral water balance. The purpose of this study was to test the hypothesis that AQP4 is involved in cerebral edema. Well-characterized experimental models of water intoxication [11] and ischemic stroke [12,13] were used to produce cerebral edema in wild-type ($AQP4^{+/+}$) and AQP4 null ($AQP4^{-/-}$) mice. The results indicate that AQP4 deletion in mice is associated with greatly reduced cerebral edema in response to water intoxication and stroke, with improved clinically relevant indices including survival and neurological status. These results implicate a key role for AQP4 in modulating brain water transport, and suggest that AQP4 inhibition may provide a new therapeutic option for reducing brain edema and other pathological alterations in brain water transport in a wide variety of neurological disorders [14].

Methods

Transgenic mice

AQP4 null mice were generated as previously described [8]. All experiments were performed on weight-matched littermates produced by intercrossing of CD1 heterozygotes. The investigators were blinded to the genotype for all experiments. All protocols were approved by the University of California at San Francisco (UCSF) or Stanford Committees on Animal Research.

Water intoxication

$AQP4^{+/+}$ and $AQP4^{-/-}$ mice received intraperitoneal injections of distilled water equal to 20% of body weight with desmopressin (0.4 µg/kg). For analysis of morbidity, the mice were evaluated using a 100-point neurological deficit scale, with a score of zero being normal and 100 representing brain death [14,15]. The time of death was recorded for Kaplan–Meier survival analysis.

Electron microscopy

Brain ultrastructure was evaluated 30 minutes after water intoxication. Animals were sacrificed and perfused with 2.0% (v/v) paraformaldehyde and 2.0% (v/v) glutaraldehyde in a 0.1 M sodium cacodylate buffer. The brains were then removed, sectioned, postfixed in osmium tetroxide and then embedded in epoxy resin. Ultrathin sections (60 to 90 nm) were stained with 2% (w/v) uranyl acetate and lead citrate and examined with a 100s JEOL electron microscope. An astrocytic foot process cross-sectional area was determined using randomly selected transmission electron micrographs containing astrocytic foot processes adjacent to brain capillaries from wild-type and AQP4-deficient mice ($n=6$ each). Images were digitized and the area of the pericapillary foot processes was measured using the NIH Image software.

Tissue-specific gravity

Brain tissue water was measured using a gravimetric column as described by Marmarou et al. [16]. The mice were sacrificed at 0, 15 and 30 minutes after water intoxication. Multiple 5 mm^3 brain samples were obtained from coronal sections from the frontal ($n=6$) and parietal ($n=8$) regions. Portions of the liver were also obtained for comparison of tissue edema. Specific gravities were calculated using the regression line from the standards. Specific gravity values for all samples were averaged for each mouse. Specific gravity was converted to percentage of brain water using reported specific gravity data on mouse brain solids [17].

Permanent focal cerebral ischemia

Adult male AQP4$^{-/-}$ mice ($n=10$) and the wild-type littermates ($n=10$) (35 to 45 g) were subjected to permanent focal middle cerebral artery occlusion (MCAO) as previously described [18]. Neurological deficits of the experimental animals were graded on a scale of 0 to 4 as described [19], with minor modification. The criteria were as follows; grade $0=$ no observable neurological deficits, grade $1=$ failed to extend right forepaw, grade $2=$ circled to the right, grade $3=$ fell to the right, grade $4=$ could not walk spontaneously, grade $5=$ dead. Neurological deficits were evaluated 24 hours after MCAO.

For histological assessment, the brains were removed, rapidly frozen, sectioned at 500 μm intervals and then stained with cresyl violet. The slides were scanned with a GS-700 imaging densitometer (Bio-Rad, Hercules, CA) and then the unstained area, ipsilateral hemisphere or contralateral hemisphere was analyzed using Multi-Analyst software (Bio-Rad). The volumes of the ipsilateral hemisphere and contralateral hemisphere were calculated by multiplying each area by the distance [20]. Hemisphere enlargement (percentage of hemisphere enlargement), which represents the amount of edema formation, was expressed as [(ipsilateral hemisphere volume – contralateral hemisphere volume) / contralateral hemisphere volume] × 100.

Statistical analysis

Data are presented as the mean ± standard error of the mean (SEM). Statistical analyses of the neurological deficit scores, tissue-specific gravity, percentage of hemisphere enlargement and infarct volume were compared between the AQP4$^{-/-}$ and AQP4$^{+/+}$ mice using t tests. The Wilcoxon signed rank test was used for the

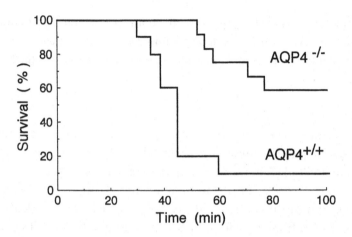

Figure 11.1   Effect of water intoxication on survival in AQP4[+/+] and AQP4[-/-] mice (*n* = 12 each group). The percentage of surviving AQP4[+/+] and AQP4[-/-] mice is shown for each time point.

non-parametric comparison of neurological deficit scores. $P < 0.05$ was considered statistically significant.

Results

To evaluate the effect of AQP4 deletion on the development of cerebral edema, we first used the well-established model of water intoxication [3,21]. Water intoxication was produced in the mice by intraperitoneal infusion of distilled water and desmopressin. In this model, rapid water infusion causes serum hyponatremia, which creates an osmotic gradient to drive water entry into the brain to produce cellular (cytotoxic) edema. The degree of hyponatremia (110 ± 5 vs. 109 ± 6 mEq/l) did not differ between the AQP4[-/-] and AQP4[+/+] mice. After the water infusion, the experimental animals exhibited signs of neurological dysfunction secondary to brain swelling, with a substantial mortality rate (Figure 11.1). The AQP4[+/+] mice became uncoordinated with rapid progression to paralysis. In contrast, the AQP4[-/-] mice remained mildly lethargic, with significantly better neurological deficit scores. By 45 minutes, many of the AQP4[+/+] mice became comatose and died. At 60 minutes, only 8% of the AQP4[+/+] mice were alive compared with 76% of the AQP4[-/-] mice.

To determine whether the improvement in outcome was due to differences in brain tissue water content, the specific gravity of brain fragments was measured. After water intoxication, specific gravity decreased in both groups indicating increased tissue water content (Figure 11.2B). At 15 minutes there was a significantly greater reduction in specific gravity of brain fragments from the

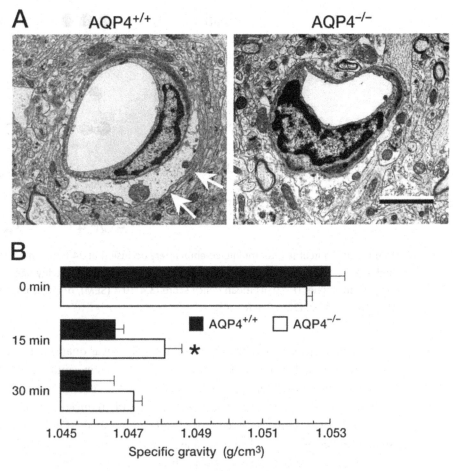

Figure 11.2 Localization and quantification of cerebral edema after water intoxication.
(A) Transmission electron micrographs showing edematous cerebral cortex at 30 minutes. Note the swollen astrocytic foot process in the brain from AQP4$^{+/+}$ and AQP4$^{-/-}$ mice (arrows). (B) Specific gravity determination of brain tissue from untreated AQP4$^{+/+}$ and AQP4$^{-/-}$ mice. After 15 and 30 minutes of water intoxication, there was a significantly greater reduction (*$P < 0.02$) in tissue-specific gravity in the AQP4$^{+/+}$ mice, indicating a substantial increase in brain water content compared with the AQP4$^{-/-}$ mice.

AQP4$^{+/+}$ mice. At 30 minutes there was a 2.4% increase in water content in AQP4$^{+/+}$ mice vs. a 1.6% increase in the AQP4$^{-/-}$ mice. Given the highly polarized expression of AQP4 in the astrocytic foot processes surrounding the brain capillary [9] and their proposed role in cerebral water transport, these structures were examined using transmission electron microscopy (Figure 11.2A). Consistent with previous reports [22], all AQP4$^{+/+}$ mice had evidence of widespread pericapillary

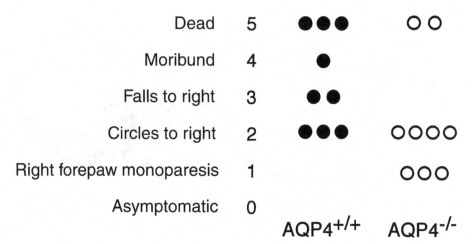

		AQP4+/+	AQP4-/-
Dead	5	●●●	○ ○
Moribund	4	●	
Falls to right	3	● ●	
Circles to right	2	●●●	○○○○
Right forepaw monoparesis	1		○○○
Asymptomatic	0		

Figure 11.3 Neurological outcome after middle cerebral artery occlusion at 24 hours in AQP4+/+ and AQP4−/− mice. The AQP4+/+ mice (●) had a slightly higher mortality rate and a significantly higher ($P<0.01$) mean deficit score (3.4 ± 0.4 (SEM), $n=10$) compared with the AQP4−/− mice (2.2 ± 0.5, $n=10$).

astrocytic foot process swelling by 30 minutes. This was quantified by calculating the cross-sectional area of foot processes adjacent to brain capillaries. Water intoxication increased the average foot process area in the AQP4+/+ mice from $0.73\pm 0.10\,mm^2$ to $5.78\pm1.01\,mm^2$. There was significantly reduced ($P<0.005$) swelling of the astrocytic foot processes in the water-intoxicated AQP4−/− mice. Only a small number of minimally enlarged astrocytic foot processes could be identified in the AQP4−/− mice at 30 minutes, as shown in Figure 11.2A.

We next used a model of focal cerebral ischemia that results in both cellular and vasogenic edema. The permanent MCAO model was chosen because of its relevance to ischemic hemispheric stroke in humans [12]. The neurological evaluation of AQP4+/+ and AQP4−/− mice after 24 hours of permanent MCAO is summarized in Figure 11.3. AQP4+/+ mice had a slightly higher mortality rate and a significantly ($P<0.01$) higher mean deficit score (3.4 ± 0.4) at 24 hours as compared with the AQP4−/− mice (2.2 ± 0.5).

Figure 11.4A shows the typical histological findings in AQP4+/+ and AQP4−/− mice 24 hours after permanent MCAO. Significantly less hemispheric enlargement resulting from brain edema was seen in the AQP4−/− mice. This was quantified by digitizing serial brain sections and calculating the cumulative area of hemispheric enlargement. Figure 11.4B shows a significant reduction ($P<0.0001$) in hemispheric enlargement in the AQP4−/− mice. The hemispheric enlargement was $67.5\pm3.6\%$ in the AQP4+/+ mice vs. $44.3\pm1.6\%$ in the AQP4−/− mice (Figure 11.4C).

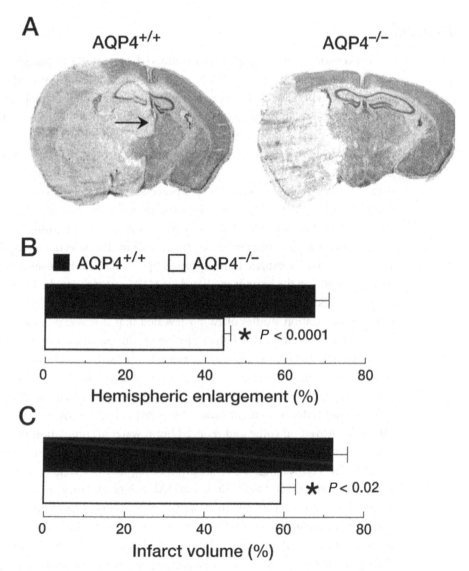

Figure 11.4   Histological analysis of AQP4$^{+/+}$ and AQP4$^{-/-}$ mice after ischemia. (A) Representative low magnification images of cresyl violet-stained brain 24 hours after permanent middle cerebral artery occlusion. Note the increased swelling and hemispheric enlargement in the AQP4$^{+/+}$ mouse brain section. (B) Hemispheric enlargement, determined by quantitative image analysis, was significantly lower in the AQP4$^{-/-}$ mice ($P<0.0001$, $n=7$). (C) Infarct volume, determined by quantitative image analysis, was significantly lower in the AQP4$^{-/-}$ mice ($P<0.02$, $n=7$).

Discussion

The expression of AQP4 in glial cells at blood–brain interfaces probably accounts for the glial-specific swelling after acute water intoxication. Most of the previous studies on cerebral edema focused on ionic mechanisms that regulate the osmotic equilibrium between brain tissue and plasma where an acute decrease in plasma osmolality creates a concentration gradient causing cerebral edema. As seen here and in other experimental studies, the swelling is predominantly localized to the glial processes around the capillaries with sparing of the neurons [22,23]. This characteristic swelling of astrocytic foot processes is also found in brain tissue from head-injured patients [24]. This raises the question as to why there is selective astrocytic swelling after a systemic perturbation in brain osmolality. Several complex theories have been proposed to account for this selectivity [23]. However, a simple alternative explanation suggested by our data is that osmotically driven water transport in the brain is mediated by AQP4 water channels. The existence of a glial-specific water transporter has been hypothesized for many years [25]. Immunolocalization studies of AQP4 revealed that it was expressed only in glial cells and not in neurons [9]. High resolution immunogold electron microscopy has demonstrated that AQP4 is mostly restricted to the astrocytic foot processes of glial membranes in direct contact with brain capillaries [10]. Thus the expression pattern of AQP4 coincides with the known areas of glial-specific swelling.

Decreased water movement caused by AQP4 deletion provides an explanation for the improved outcome and reduced brain water accumulation in response to acute water intoxication and stroke. The regulation of water flux and fluid volume in the brain is critical because of the brain's enclosure in a rigid cranium. Much of the acute morbidity and mortality associated with head injury and stroke is a result of cerebral edema [1]. If not controlled, cerebral edema can lead to mechanical injury from displacement of brain tissue and metabolic injury from compromised blood flow as a result of increased intracranial pressure [2]. Previous studies have shown that the magnitude of cerebral edema and clinical symptoms is proportional to the quantity of the water retained [25]. Thus decreased tissue water content and astrocytic swelling in the AQP4$^{-/-}$ mice probably account for the improved neurological deficit scores and improved survival as compared with the AQP4$^{+/+}$ mice. Brain edema is also known to be a significant factor in the rapid decline and early progression to death of patients with significant ischemic infarcts. In a previous study of MCAO in mice, brain swelling, as measured by hemispheric enlargement, correlated with the neurological deficit [13]. From our studies it appears that deletion of the AQP4 water channel also reduces edema and improves neurological outcome after permanent focal cerebral ischemia. Future studies examining the effects of AQP4 deletion on infarct volume and cellular outcome after permanent and transient ischemia are warranted.

Current interventions to treat acute brain swelling include neurosurgical decompression, which permits unimpeded expansion of edematous brain matter, and hyperosmolar agents, which transiently reduce brain swelling by osmotic extraction of brain water. Although improved diagnostic and monitoring methods such as magnetic resonance imaging and intracranial pressure transducers have been introduced, there has been little change for many years in the treatment of acute brain swelling. Reduced brain edema in AQP4-deficient mice indicates that the AQP4 water channel is a potential target for drug discovery. AQP4 inhibitors might slow the accumulation of edema fluid in the brain, thereby reducing the morbidity and death associated with many common neurological disorders.

Acknowledgments

This work was supported by National Institutes of Health grants DK35124, HL58198, HL60288, HL51854 and DK43840, and grant R613 from the National Cystic Fibrosis Foundation.

REFERENCES

1 Klatzo I (1994) Evolution of brain edema concepts. *Acta Neurochirurgica Supplementum*, **60**, 3–6.

2 Fishman RA (1975) Brain edema. *New England Journal of Medicine*, **273**, 706–11.

3 Weed LH & McKibben PS (1919) Experimental alteration of brain bulk. *American Journal of Physiology*, **48**, 531–58.

4 Verkman AS, van Hoek AN, Ma T, Frigeri A, Skach WR, Mitra A, Tamarappoo BK & Farinas J (1996) Water transport across mammalian cell membranes. *American Journal of Physiology*, **270**, C12–C30.

5 King LS & Agre P (1996) Pathophysiology of the aquaporin water channels. *Annual Review of Physiology*, **58**, 619–48.

6 Nielsen S, Smith BL, Christensen EI & Agre P (1993) Distribution of the aquaporin CHIP in secretory and resorptive epithelia and capillary endothelia. *Proceedings of the National Academy of Sciences, USA*, **90**, 7275–9.

7 Hasegawa H, Zhang R, Dohrman A & Verkman AS (1993) Tissue-specific expression of mRNA encoding rat kidney water channel CHIP28k by in situ hybridization. *American Journal of Physiology*, **264**, C237–C245.

8 Ma T, Yang B, Gillespie A, Carlson EJ, Epstein CJ & Verkman AS (1997) Generation and phenotype of a transgenic knockout mouse lacking the mercurial-insensitive water channel aquaporin-4. *Journal of Clinical Investigation*, **100**, 957–62.

9 Frigeri A, Gropper MA, Turck CW & Verkman AS (1995) Immunolocalization of the mercurial-insensitive water channel and glycerol intrinsic protein in epithelial cell plasma membranes. *Proceedings of the National Academy of Sciences, USA*, **92**, 4328–31.

10 Nielsen S, Nagelhus EA, Amiry-Moghaddam M, Bourque C, Agre P & Ottersen OP (1997) Specialized membrane domains for water transport in glial cells: high-resolution immunogold cytochemistry of aquaporin-4 in rat brain. *Journal of Neuroscience*, **17**, 171–80.

11 Trachtman H (1992) Cell volume regulation: a review of cerebral adaptive mechanisms and implications for clinical treatment of osmolal disturbances: II. *Pediatric Nephrology*, **6**, 104–12.

12 Hossmann K-A (1998) Experimental models for the investigation of brain ischemia. *Cardiovascular Research*, **39**, 106–20.

13 Kondo T, Reaume AG, Huang T-T, Carlson E, Murakami K, Chen SF, Hoffman EK, Scott RW, Epstein CJ & Chan PH (1997) Reduction of CuZn-superoxide dismutase activity exacerbates neuronal cell injury and edema formation after transient focal cerebral ischemia. *Journal of Neuroscience*, **17**, 4180–9.

14 Manley GT, Fujimura M, Ma T, Noshita N, Filiz F, Bollen AW, Chan P & Verkman AS (2000) Aquaporin-4 deletion in mice reduces brain edema after acute water intoxication and ischemic stroke. *Nature Medicine*, **6**, 159–63.

15 Carrillo P, Takasu A, Safar P, Tisherman S, Stezoski SW, Stolz G, Dixon CE & Radovsky A (1998) Prolonged severe hemorrhagic shock and resuscitation in rats does not cause subtle brain damage. *Journal of Trauma-Injury Infection & Critical Care*, **45**, 239–48.

16 Marmarou A, Poll W, Shulman K & Bhagavan H (1978) A simple gravimetric technique for measurement of cerebral edema. *Journal of Neurosurgery*, **49**, 530–7.

17 Nelson SR, Mantz ML & Maxwell JA (1971) Use of specific gravity in the measurement of cerebral edema. *Journal of Applied Physiology*, **30**, 268–71.

18 Fujimura M, Morita-Fujimura Y, Kawase M, Copin J-C, Calagui B, Epstein CJ & Chan PH (1999) Manganese superoxide dismutase mediates the early release of mitochondrial cytochrome *c* and subsequent DNA fragmentation after permanent focal cerebral ischemia in mice. *Journal of Neuroscience*, **19**, 3414–22.

19 Yang G, Chan PH, Chen J, Carlson E, Chen SF, Weinstein P, Epstein CJ & Kamii H (1994) Human copper-zinc superoxide dismutase transgenic mice are highly resistant to reperfusion injury after focal cerebral ischemia. *Stroke*, **25**, 165–70.

20 Swanson RA, Morton MT, Tsao-Wu G, Savalos RA, Davidson C & Sharp FR (1990) A semiautomated method for measuring brain infarct volume. *Journal of Cerebral Blood Flow & Metabolism*, **10**, 290–3.

21 Gullans SR & Verbalis JG (1993) Control of brain volume during hyperosmolar and hypoosmolar conditions. *Annual Review of Medicine*, **44**, 289–301.

22 Wasterlain CG & Torack RM (1968) Cerebral edema in water intoxication. II. An ultrastructural study. *Archives of Neurology*, **19**, 79–87.

23 Kimelberg HK (1995) Current concepts of brain edema. Review of laboratory investigations. *Journal of Neurosurgery*, **83**, 1051–9.

24 Bullock R, Maxwell WL, Graham DI, Teasdale GM & Adams JH (1991) Glial swelling following human cerebral contusion: an ultrastructural study. *Journal of Neurology, Neurosurgery & Psychiatry*, **54**, 427–34.

25 Wasterlain CG & Posner JB (1968) Cerebral edema in water intoxication. I. Clinical and chemical observations. *Archives of Neurology*, **19**, 71–8.

12

Neuroprotection with tetracyclines in brain ischemia models

Jari Koistinaho

A.I. Virtanen Institute for Molecular Sciences, University of Kuopio, Kuopio, Finland

Introduction

Several studies have indicated that inflammation, which involves non-neuronal cells, has an important role in the pathogenesis of acute and chronic brain diseases, including stroke [1–5]. In global ischemia, delayed hippocampal damage is observed 3 to 5 days after the insult to CA1 pyramidal neurons [6], suggesting that mechanisms that develop slowly after ischemia have a role in hippocampal ischemic cell death. Furthermore, clinically common focal ischemia caused by occlusion of the middle cerebral artery involves secondary inflammation that significantly contributes to the outcome after ischemic insult [1,2,5,7–9]. Several pro-inflammatory genes or mediators, such as inducible nitric oxide synthase (iNOS), cyclooxygenase-2 (COX-2) and cytokines, are strongly expressed in the ischemic brain [2,5,9]. Inflammation is now considered an attractive pharmacological target because it progresses over several days after acute brain injury, and interference with inflammatory mechanisms, which are not fundamental for physiological brain functions, may not result in intolerable side effects [1], as the wide clinical use of non-steroidal anti-inflammatory drugs demonstrates.

Tetracyclines are well-known bacteriostatic antibiotics with broad-spectrum antimicrobial activity [10]. In the late 1960s the so-called long-acting, second-generation tetracyclines, doxycycline and minocycline, were synthesized. These semisynthetic antibiotics are rapidly and completely absorbed, even in an aged population [11–14], and, compared to many other antibiotics, they have an excellent tissue penetration into the brain and cerebrospinal fluid [10,15]. Doxycycline and minocycline are exceptional tetracycline derivatives in that they exert biological effects that are completely separate and distinct from their antimicrobial action. These effects include modulation of COX-2 activity [16], inhibition of matrix metalloproteinases [17], tumor-induced angiogenesis [18], malignant cell growth [19], bone resorption [20], depression of oxygen radical release from polymorphonuclear neutrophils [21,22], inhibition of iNOS [23,24], and inhibition of protein tyrosine nitration by scavenging peroxynitrite [25]. Experimental and clinical studies indicate that minocycline and doxycycline may be beneficial in the treatment of peripheral inflammatory diseases [26–28]. The drugs are clinically well tolerated and minocycline is currently considered for treatment of rheumatoid arthritis, a severe inflammatory human disease [26].

Protection in a global ischemia model

Because tetracyclines have anti-inflammatory properties and are clinically well tolerated, we studied whether doxycycline and minocycline could serve as neuroprotective compounds against brain ischemia [29,30]. Using a gerbil global ischemia model, we first screened the effects of the following antibiotics: erythromycin, tetracycline, doxycycline, minocycline and ceftriaxone, a third-generation cephalosporine. The antibiotics were administered intraperitoneally (ip) twice a day, starting 1 day prior to ischemia, and the treatment was continued until the day the animals were sacrificed. The screening studies indicated the neuroprotective potential of doxycycline and minocycline, which together with tetracycline, were taken to more complete studies in the same gerbil model. We used the dose of 180 to 90 mg/kg per day because the treatment did not result in severe side effects and maximal penetration of the drugs to the brain cerebrospinal fluid was desired. Twelve hours before ischemia, gerbils were injected ip with 45 mg/kg of minocycline, doxycycline or tetracycline hydrochloride. Thereafter, the animals were injected twice a day, at a dose of 90 mg/kg during the first day after ischemia and 45 mg/kg starting 36 hours after ischemia. The postischemic treatment was started 30 minutes after ischemia with 90 mg/kg. Both minocycline and doxycycline treatments significantly increased the number of surviving neurons. Six days after ischemia the minocycline-pretreated gerbils had 76.7% of the neuron profiles left in the CA1 pyramidal cell layer, the minocycline-post-treated gerbils had 71.4%, the doxycycline-pretreated gerbils had 57.2%, and the doxycycline-post-treated gerbils had 47.1%, whereas in the untreated gerbils 10.5% of the CA1 neurons were left. The neuroprotection was statistically significant in every animal group. Treatment with the same dose of tetracycline did not provide any protection. Minocycline and doxycycline did not reduce the postoperative body temperatures.

To determine whether neuroprotection by minocycline is associated with activation of non-neuronal cells, we studied glial fibrillary acidic protein (GFAP) expression, a marker of astrogliosis, and phosphotyrosine immunoreactivity and isolectin B4 binding, which are markers of activated microglia. The results showed that expression of GFAP mRNA in the hippocampus was increased to the same extent in saline- and minocycline-treated gerbils and that immunoreactivity for GFAP was

similar in these two groups. Instead, microglial activation appeared to be significantly reduced in minocycline-treated gerbils. We therefore next studied whether
induction of interleukin-1β (IL-β)converting enzyme (ICE), an apoptosis-pro-
moting gene that is strongly induced in microglia after global ischemia, or iNOS,
an enzyme that is suggested to produce toxic concentrations of nitric oxide in non-
neuronal cells after ischemia [31], are affected by neuroprotective minocycline
treatment. The semiquantitative reverse transcriptase–polymerase chain reaction
showed that 4 days after ischemia, expression of ICE mRNA was attenuated by
approximately 70% and expression of iNOS mRNA by 30% in the hippocampus of
minocycline-treated gerbils. In addition, 6 days after ischemia, NADPH-
diaphorase-reactive cells were seen in the hippocampi of saline-treated, but not
minocycline-treated, ischemic gerbils. Most of the NADPH-diaphorase-reactive
cells resembling microglia were located in the pyramidal cell layer of the CA1 subfield and some NADPH-diaphorase-reactive cells with a morphology typical of
astrocytes were detected in the stratum radiatum. Therefore, minocycline also
inhibited NOS activity in astrocytes, even though it did not block astrogliosis.

Protection in a focal brain ischemia model

Because minocycline was more neuroprotective than doxycycline in global brain
ischemia, we decided to continue with minocycline in a focal brain ischemia model
of the rat. Treatment with minocycline (45 mg/kg ip twice a day for the first day;
22.5 mg/kg for the subsequent 2 days) did not affect rectal temperature, arterial
blood pressure, plasma glucose or arterial blood gases. However, treatment started
12 hours before ischemia reduced the size of the infarct in the cerebral cortex by
76% and in the striatum by 39%. Starting the minocycline treatment 2 hours after
the onset of ischemia resulted in a reduction in the size of cortical (by 65%) and
striatal (by 42%) infarct, a reduction similar to the one obtained with pretreatment.
The cortical infarct size was reduced by 63% even when the treatment was started
4 hours after the onset of ischemia.

Because cortical spreading depression (SD), an energy-consuming wave of transient depolarizations of astrocytes and neurons, contributes to the evolution of
ischemia to infarction in focal ischemia [32–35], we tested whether minocycline
provides protection by inhibiting cortical SD. In a separate set of rats that were not
subjected to middle cerebral artery occlusion, minocycline did not alter the
number, duration or amplitude of direct current potentials induced by 60 minutes
of exposure to topical 3 M KCl, whereas MK-801, an NMDA receptor antagonist
known to reduce partial ischemic damage by blocking cortical SD, completely prevented KCl-induced direct current potentials.

As non-neuronal cells are characteristically activated in the brain in response to ischemic injury [36–38], and minocycline was found to reduce microglial activation in a global ischemia model, we studied astrogliosis and microglial activation in a focal ischemia model. Twenty-four hours after 90 minutes of ischemia, a strong induction of CD11b immunoreactivity was observed around and inside the infarction core in untreated rats. The immunoreactive cells had an amoeboid shape in the penumbra zone. Minocycline treatment started 12 hours before ischemia decreased the number of CD11b-immunoreactive cells and prevented the appearance of the amoeboid-shaped microglia adjacent to the infarction core. Instead, GFAP-immunoreactivity in the ischemic hemispheres of untreated and minocycline-treated animals was similarly increased. Similar to global ischemia studies, pretreatment with minocycline also decreased the induced ICE mRNA levels by 83% in the penumbra, indicating that minocycline treatment inhibits expression of the enzyme needed for IL-1β activation in microglia.

COX-2 is highly expressed in the brain after global and focal brain ischemia and produces superoxides and proinflammatory prostaglandins (PG) such as PGE_2 [7,9,39,40]. In general, expression of COX-2 is reduced by anti-inflammatories and can be induced by cytokines, including IL-1β (25). Because minocycline treatment inhibited microglial activation, we studied whether the treatment also affects COX-2. In gerbil global brain ischemia, we studied the hippocampal expression of COX-2 mRNA and found that minocycline downregulated the expression by 30% to 40%. The protein levels and activity of COX-2 were studied in a focal brain ischemia model. In untreated rats, the PGE_2 concentration was increased five-fold in the ischemic penumbra and was preceded by the induction of COX-2 immunoreactive neurons. Pretreatment with minocycline reduced the PGE_2 concentration in the penumbra by 55% and almost completely prevented the appearance of COX-2 immunoreactivity at 24 hours.

Protection in a cell culture model

Tetracyclines, including minocycline, efficiently reduce inflammation in the peripheral system, for example, by inhibiting the function of polymorphonuclear neutrophils [21,22]. To find out whether minocycline has a direct effect on brain cells, we studied minocycline in primary neuronal cultures. Mixed spinal cord cultures that consist of neurons (70%), astrocytes (24%) and microglia (6%) and that are devoid of endothelial cells and peripheral cells were used. When the cultures were pretreated with 0.02 mM minocycline, the neurotoxicity of 500 mM glutamate, a major mediator of neuronal death in the brain, was decreased by 85%. Therefore, we concluded that minocycline provides major neuroprotection against excitotoxicity in mixed brain cell cultures by a mechanism that is independent of peripheral systems.

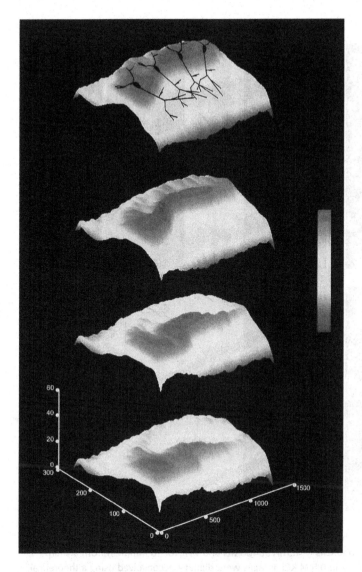

Plate 13.1 Propagating Ca^{2+} waves from SD in an HOTC. Two Ca^{2+} waves precede the electrophysiological changes of SD. The first (top image) travels rapidly at >100 μm/second along the basilar dendritic layer, and occurs shortly after an electrical stimulus in the hilus that triggers SD. The second wave subsequently travels mostly perpendicular to the pyramidal cell layer from a focus in CA3 (or less often, CA1) and spreads with the interstitial DC change of SD at millimeters/minute but always ahead of it by 6 to 16 seconds.

The images were created using a 12 bit digital camera (CH250; Photometrics, Tucson, AZ). Images were "background corrected" using a reference image consisting of an average of three images obtained immediately before SD initiation. Corrected images were enhanced using linear equalization and converted to an 8 bit format. Line profile analyses were done on images and the resultant data stored as an ASCII file. The latter were imported into Matlab (version 5.0; The Mathworks, Inc., Natick, MA) and a gaussian filter (at 10% of data standard deviation that excluded the lowest and highest 5% of the distribution along with redistribution of the resultant data over a 0 to 255 range) to extend intensity values into the z-axis. Images were pseudocolored using a 24 bit color palette that extended over the dynamic range of fluorescence intensity. Calibration bars (faint gray in bottom image) show that HOTC sectioned images are 300 pixels by 1500 pixels (or 330 μm by 1650 μm) and showed fluorescence intensity changes from 0 to 60 on an arbitrary scale.

The plates in this section are available for download in colour from www.cambridge.org/9780521187534

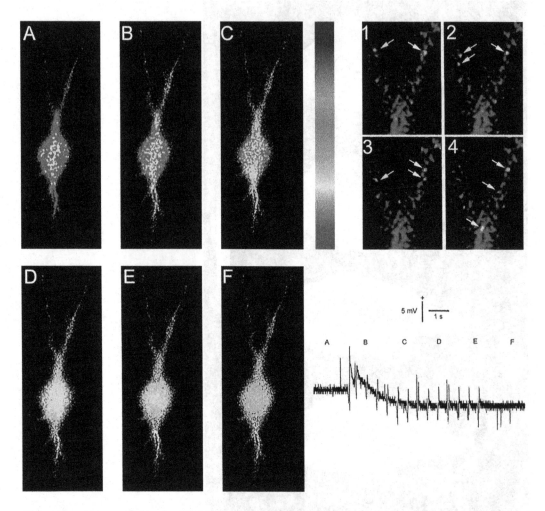

Plate 13.2 CA3 pyramidal cell Ca_i^{2+} changes to bipolar electrical stimulation in the dentate gyrus of an HOTC. Cell shown was filled via iontophoresis ($-1.5\,nA$ at 400 ms and 2 Hz for 10 minutes) from a sharp microelectrode containing 10 mM fura-2 in 0.5 M KCl. Images were digitally deconvolved using a theoretical point spread function with data containing images merged into the hue component. Furthermore, an isosbestic image was merged as the saturation component of an HSV (hue, saturation and value) color model to relay intensity information lost with ratiometric imaging. This image processing strategy improves image resolution, accuracy and the three-dimensional aspect to Ca_i^{2+} measurements [95]. A simultaneous electrophysiological record from an interstitial DC microelectrode is shown to lower right. Deflections in record represent individually evoked population spikes at the rate of 2 Hz. Images on the left side (A–F) show the propagation of Ca_i^{2+} transients beginning from the dendritic tree, progressing proximally and engulfing the soma. The color bar (middle) indicates relative Ca_i^{2+} change. Images to right (1–4) were taken before evoked stimulation and show small, spontaneous Ca_i^{2+} changes that presumably are occurring within dendritic spines (arrows).

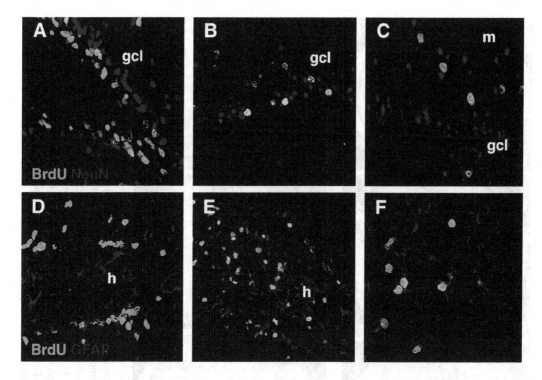

Plate 26.1 Phenotypes of proliferating cells in the dentate gyrus at various intervals after 10 minutes of global ischemia. Ten minutes of bilateral occlusion of the common carotid artery was performed on day 1, multiple doses of BrdU (twice daily) were injected from days 9 to 12, and the brains were extracted on day 14 (A, D), day 40 (B, E) or 3 months later (C). Confocal laser microscopy shows double staining images for BrdU in green and cell-type specific markers in red including NeuN (A, B, C) and glial fibrillary acidic protein (D, E, F). Fourteen days after global ischemia and 2 days after multiple injections of BrdU, the majority of BrdU-positive cells were located at the SGZ still in an undifferentiated state, expressing neither neuronal (A) nor glial (D) markers. Forty days after ischemia, the proliferating cells migrated from the SGZ to either the granule cell layer (gcl) (B) or to the dentate hilus (h) (E, F). F is a high magnification image of E. The newly divided cells survived after 3 months in the granule cell layer (C), a few of them appeared to migrate a short distance from the gcl toward the molecular layer (m).

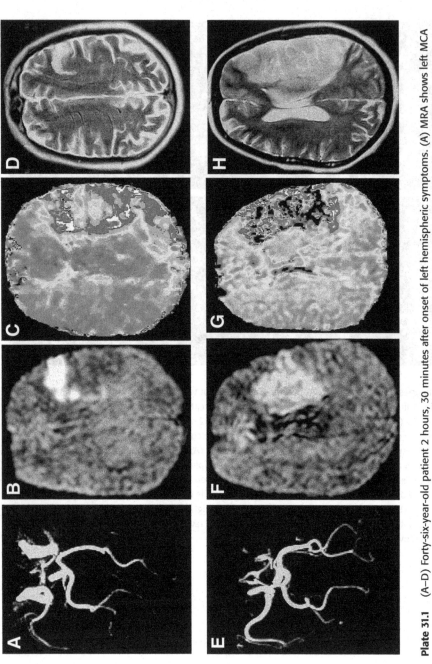

Plate 31.1 (A–D) Forty-six-year-old patient 2 hours, 30 minutes after onset of left hemispheric symptoms. (A) MRA shows left MCA occlusion. DWI (B) shows a small area of ischemically injured tissue in the left frontal lobe, while PWI (C) shows a disturbed perfusion in most of the MCA territory. After early recanalization T$_2$-weighted image on day 5 (D) reveals only a small left frontal infarct. The patient had an NIHSS score of 1 at day 90. (E–H) Forty-nine-year-old patient 2 hours after onset of left hemispheric symptoms. (E) MRA shows left MCA occlusion. DWI (F) shows medium-sized area of injury in left basal ganglia, while PWI (G) again shows a disturbed perfusion of most of the MCA territory. Early thrombolysis failed in MCA recanalization. T$_2$-weighted image (H) on day 5 shows an infarct that involves nearly the entire left MCA territory. The patient had an NIHSS of 7 at day 90.

Conclusion

In light of the present results, minocycline or synthetic tetracycline derivatives might serve as new therapeutic strategies for the treatment of stroke. The exact mechanism that mediates the salvage of ischemic tissue by minocycline is unclear, but inhibition of microglial activation may play a crucial role.

REFERENCES

1 Barone FC & Feuerstein GZ (1999) Inflammatory mediators and stroke: new opportunities for novel therapeutics. *Journal of Cerebral Blood Flow & Metabolism*, 19, 819–34.

2 Dirnagl U, Iadecola C, & Moskowitz MA (1999) Pathobiology of ischaemic stroke: an integrated view. *Trends in Neurosciences*, 22, 391–7.

3 Lee JM, Zipfel GJ & Choi DW (1999) The changing landscape of ischaemic brain injury mechanisms. *Nature*, 399 Suppl, A7–A14.

4 Rothwell NJ, Loddick SA & Stroemer P (1997) Interleukins and cerebral ischaemia. *International Review of Neurobiology*, 40, 281–98.

5 del Zoppo G, Ginis I, Hallenbeck JM, Iadecola C, Wang X & Feuerstein GZ (2000) Inflammation and stroke: putative role for cytokines, adhesion molecules and iNOS in brain response to ischemia. *Brain Pathology*, 10, 95–112.

6 Siesjö BK (1978) *Brain Energy Metabolism*. New York: Wiley.

7 Sairanen T, Ristimaki A, Karjalainen-Lindsberg ML, Paetau A, Kaste M & Lindsberg PJ (1998) Cyclooxygenase-2 is induced globally in infarcted human brain. *Annals of Neurology*, 43, 738–47.

8 DeGraba TJ (1998) The role of inflammation after acute stroke: utility of pursuing anti-adhesion molecule therapy. *Neurology*, 51 Suppl 3, S62–S68.

9 Nogawa S, Zhang F, Ross ME & Iadecola C (1997) Cyclo-oxygenase-2 gene expression in neurons contributes to ischemic brain damage. *Journal of Neuroscience*, 17, 2746–55.

10 Klein NC & Cunha BA (1995) Tetracyclines. *Medical Clinics of North America*, 79, 789–801.

11 Cunha BA, Sibley C & Ristuccia PA (1982) Doxycycline. *Therapeutic Drug Monitoring*, 4, 115–35.

12 Sande MA & Mandell GL (1990) Tetracylines, chloramphenicol, erythromycin and miscellaneous antibacterial agents. In *The Pharmacological Basis of Therapeutics*, eds. A Goodman Gilman, TW Rall, AS Nies & P Taylor, pp. 1117–45. New York: Macmillan.

13 Kramer PA, Chapron DJ, Benson J & Mercik SA (1978) Tetracycline absorption in elderly patients with achlorhydria. *Clinical Pharmacology and Therapeutics*, 23, 467–72.

14 Barza M, Brown RB, Shanks C, Gamble C & Weinstein L (1975) Relation between lipophilicity and pharmacological behavior of minocycline, doxycycline, tetracycline, and oxytetracycline in dogs. *Antimicrobial Agents and Chemotherapy*, 8, 713–20.

15 Aronson AL (1980) Pharmacotherapeutics of the newer tetracyclines. *Journal of the American Veterinary Medical Association*, 176, 1061–8.

16 Patel RN, Attur MG, Dave MN, Patel IV, Stuchin SA, Abramson SB & Amin AR (1999) A novel mechanism of action of chemically modified tetracyclines: inhibition of COX-2-mediated prostaglandin E2 production. *Journal of Immunology*, 163, 3459–67.

17 Golub LM, Ramamurthy NS, McNamara TF, Greenwald RA & Rifkin BR (1991) Tetracyclines inhibit connective tissue breakdown: new therapeutic implications for an old family of drugs. *Critical Review in Oral Biology and Medicine*, 2, 297–322.

18 Maragoudakis ME, Peristeris P, Missirlis E, Aletras A, Andriopoulou P & Haralabopoulos G (1994) Inhibition of angiogenesis by anthracyclines and titanocene dichloride. *Annals of the New York Academy of Sciences*, 732, 280–93.

19 Masumori N, Tsukamoto T, Miyao N, Kumamoto Y, Saiki I & Yoneda J (1994) Inhibitory effect of minocycline on in vitro invasion and experimental metastasis of mouse renal adenocarcinoma. *Journal of Urology*, 151, 1400–4.

20 Rifkin BR, Vernillo AT, Golub LM & Ramamurthy NS (1994) Modulation of bone resorption by tetracyclines. *Annals of the New York Academy of Sciences*, 732, 165–80.

21 Gabler WL & Creamer HR (1991) Suppression of human neutrophil functions by tetracyclines *Journal of Periodontal Research*, 26, 52–8.

22 Gabler WL, Smith J & Tsukuda N (1992) Comparison of doxycycline and a chemically modified tetracycline inhibition of leukocyte functions. *Research Communications in Chemical Pathology & Pharmacology*, 78, 151–60.

23 Amin AR, Attur MG, Thakker GD, Patel PD, Vyas PR, Patel RN, Patel IR & Abramson SB (1996) A novel mechanism of action of tetracyclines: effects on nitric oxide synthases. *Proceedings of the National Academy of Sciences, USA*, 93, 14014–19.

24 Amin AR, Patel RN, Thakker GD, Lowenstein CJ, Attur MG & Abramson SB (1997) Post-transcriptional regulation of inducible nitric oxide synthase mRNA in murine macrophages by doxycycline and chemically modified tetracyclines. *FEBS Letters*, 410, 259–64.

25 Whiteman M & Halliwell B (1997) Prevention of peroxynitrite-dependent tyrosine nitration and inactivation of α1-antiproteinase by antibiotics. *Free Radical Research*, 26, 49–56.

26 Furst DE (1998) Update on clinical trials in the rheumatic diseases. *Current Opinion in Rheumatology*, 10, 123–8.

27 Nordstrom D, Lindy O, Lauhio A, Sorsa T, Santavirta S & Konttinen YT (1998) Anti-collagenolytic mechanism of action of doxycycline treatment in rheumatoid arthritis. *Rheumatology International*, 17, 175–80.

28 Greenwald RA, Moak SA, Ramamurthy NS & Golub LM (1992) Tetracyclines suppress matrix metalloproteinase activity in adjuvant arthritis and in combination with flurbiprofen, ameliorate bone damage. *Journal of Rheumatology*, 19, 927–38.

29 Yrjänheikki J, Keinänen R, Pellikka M, Hökfelt T & Koistinaho J (1998) Tetracyclines inhibit microglial activation and are neuroprotective in global brain ischemia. *Proceedings of the National Academy of Sciences, USA*, 95, 15769–74.

30 Yrjänheikki J, Tikka T, Keinänen R, Goldsteins G, Chan PH & Koistinaho J (1999) A tetracycline derivative, minocycline, reduces inflammation and protects against focal cerebral ischemia with a wide therapeutic window. *Proceedings of the National Academy of Sciences, USA*, 96, 13496–500.

31 Endoh M, Maiese K & Wagner J (1994) Expression of the inducible form of nitric oxide synthase by reactive astrocytes after transient global ischemia. *Brain Research,* **651**, 92–100.

32 Rawanduzy A, Hansen A, Hansen TW & Nedergaard M (1997) Effective reduction of infarct volume by gap junction blockade in a rodent model of stroke. *Journal of Neurosurgery,* **87**, 916–20.

33 Mies G, Iijima T & Hossmann K-A (1993) Correlation between peri-infarct DC shifts and ischaemic neuronal damage in rat. *Neuroreport,* **4**, 709–11.

34 Busch E, Gyngell ML, Eis M, Hoehn-Berlage M & Hossmann K-A (1996) Potassium-induced cortical spreading depressions during focal cerebral ischemia in rats: contribution to lesion growth assessed by diffusion-weighted NMR and biochemical imaging. *Journal of Cerebral Blood Flow & Metabolism,* **16**, 1090–9.

35 Back T, Ginsberg MD, Dietrich WD & Watson BD (1996) Induction of spreading depression in the ischemic hemisphere following experimental middle cerebral artery occlusion: effect on infarct morphology. *Journal of Cerebral Blood Flow & Metabolism,* **16**, 202–13.

36 McGeer PL & McGeer EG (1995) The inflammatory response system of brain: implications for therapy of Alzheimer and other neurodegenerative diseases. *Brain Research Reviews,* **21**, 195–218.

37 Banati RB, Gehrmann J, Schubert P & Kreutzberg GW (1993) Cytotoxicity of microglia. *Glia,* **7**, 111–18.

38 Giulian D & Corpuz M (1993) Microglial secretion products and their impact on the nervous system. *Advances in Neurology,* **59**, 315–20.

39 Miettinen S, Fusco FR, Yrjänheikki J, Keinänen R, Hirvonen T, Roivainen R, Närhi M, Hökfelt T & Koistinaho J (1997) Spreading depression and focal brain ischemia induce cyclooxygenase-2 in cortical neurons through N-methyl-D-aspartic acid-receptors and phospholipase A2. *Proceedings of the National Academy of Sciences, USA,* **94**, 6500–5.

40 Koistinaho J, Kaponen S & Chan PH (1999) Expression of cyclooxygenase-2 mRNA after global ischemia is regulated by AMPA receptors and glucocorticoids. *Stroke,* **30**, 1900–5.

13

Spreading depression: a teleological means for self-protection from brain ischemia

Richard P. Kraig[1] & Phillip E. Kunkler[2]

[1] Departments of Neurology and Neurobiology, Pharmacology & Physiology, University of Chicago, Chicago, IL
[2] Department of Neurology, University of Chicago, Chicago, IL

Introduction

Ischemic brain injury is a leading cause of death and disability [1], with few effective treatments. Brain tissue can be "preconditioned" so that a subsequent period of ischemia either worsens or lessens the injury than otherwise would be seen [2]. Thus neural cells and tissues have an endogenous capacity to modulate the extent of their own injury. Examination of the mechanisms for these dual effects may lead to more selective cellular and molecular targets for development of new therapeutic strategies against ischemic brain injury. This conclusion follows from the fact that these dual effects reflect the teleological and composite cellular and molecular responses of brain tissue. Furthermore, successful treatments derived from their study seem most likely to be in concert with natural biological capacities and therefore have the fewest negative sequelae.

Spreading depression (SD) may be a particularly opportune perturbation for the study of mechanisms by which the brain can affect its own susceptibility to ischemic injury. SD itself is non-injurious [3] and almost completely stereotypic [4]. Thus SD may activate key processes more selectively or specifically than those begun by ischemia. Also, more detailed biophysical, biochemical and molecular biological information is available about SD than is available for ischemia.

Intracellular calcium (Ca_i^{2+}) changes within neurons are likely to be an important initial focus for understanding the mechanisms that initiate not only SD but also the cellular and tissue-based changes associated with the modulation of ischemic brain injury. First, neuronal Ca_i^{2+} changes are necessary for the initiation of SD [5]. Second, changes in Ca_i^{2+} have ubiquitous signaling capacities in eukaryotic cells [6]. Third, Ca_i^{2+} and mitochondrial Ca^{2+} changes are recognized to be of particular importance to selective neuronal vulnerability from excitotoxic injury [7–15]. Accordingly, we have begun studying the role of Ca^{2+} in SD and

SD-induced modulation of ischemic injury for the first time using a novel, in vitro preparation, the hippocampal organ culture (HOTC).

Ischemic tolerance

Brief episodes of brain ischemia make neural tissue more resistant to subsequent injury than otherwise would occur. For example, 2 minutes of global ischemia induces tolerance at 24 hours that persists for 2 days against selective neuronal destruction of CA1 pyramidal cells from a subsequent period of global ischemia [16]. Furthermore, 20 minutes of focal ischemia followed 24 hours later by global ischemia reduces injury within the zone of the previous focal reduction in flow [17] and beyond it in the ipsilateral hippocampus [18]. Brief episodes of global ischemia also reduce subsequent damage from focal ischemia [19], and tolerance to focal ischemia can be induced by preconditioning with brief episodes of focal ischemia [20]. Finally, recent work has shown bidirectional cross-tolerance between global ischemia and kainic acid excitotoxicity [21], suggesting that diverse perturbations to the brain, possibly acting through common mechanisms, can also induce ischemic preconditioning.

Mechanisms for ischemic tolerance in the brain are beginning to be defined. Potential processes include glutamate homeostasis [22], and A1 receptors [23] and adenosine triphosphate-sensitive K^+ channel activation [24]. Other evidence suggests that expression of gene products including heat shock proteins (HSPs) [25], manganese superoxide dismutase [26], interleukin-1 [27] and apoptotic-suppressor proteins may be involved in tolerance [2]. The time needed for tolerance to develop in the brain (>24 hours) and the duration of tolerance support new protein synthesis as a key element of ischemia-induced tolerance [2]. Much work has focused on potential "final" mechanisms; however, the initial specific triggers and subsequent general pathways that can induce tolerance have not been systematically examined and remain unknown.

Spreading depression

SD, which has biophysical changes similar to those of ischemia, can modulate ischemic injury. When SD precedes ischemia by less than a day, injury is greater than otherwise would be seen [28–30]. However, when SD occurs more than a day before ischemia, injury is reduced [31–33]. The mechanisms by which SD confers this dual effect are unknown but may involve anabolic processes since SD induces expression of HSP27 in astrocytes [34]. HSP27 can increase cell resistance to oxidative injury [35] but, again, the cellular signals that trigger this protein expression are unknown.

SD is a widely activating yet benign perturbation of the brain first described more than 50 years ago. It is classically defined by electrophysiological criteria as a propagating wave (in millimeters/minute) of evoked or spontaneous silence in neuronal activity associated with a large negative DC potential [4]. SD is seen in many gray matter brain regions including the hippocampus of both lower animals [4] and humans [35] in response to electrical, chemical or mechanical stimuli [4]. Near total depolarization of both neurons and glia occurs during the 30 to 60 seconds of electrical silence seen with SD. This depolarization is associated with a dramatic shift in interstitial ion concentrations ($[\text{"X"}]_o$). $[K^+]_o$ rises from 3 to about 40 mM. $[Na^+]_o$ falls from 150 to 57 mM. $[Ca^{2+}]_o$ drops from 1.2 to 0.01 mM and $[Cl^-]_o$ falls from 137 mM to 47 mM [36,37]. $[H^+]_o$ also changes dramatically, showing first an alkaline transient, followed by a more long-lasting acid shift [37]. Simultaneously, carbon dioxide tension rises and $[HCO_3^-]_o$ rises and then falls [38]. Finally, levels of glutamate, lactate [39,40] and arachidonic acid [41] also rise in the interstitial space during SD. These changes are similar to those seen in ischemia [42]. Unlike ischemia, SD is never sufficient to cause irreversible injury of brain cells [3]. However, SD does cause microgliosis and astrogliosis that peak at times associated with SD-induced worsening or lessening of excitotoxic injury, respectively [43].

Similarly dramatic intracellular changes also occur with SD. K^+ released from neurons [44] enters the interstitial space and is taken up by astrocytes [45,46]. Astrocytic K^+ rises by 50 mM during SD. This rise occurs with an equally large (i.e., electroneutral) rise in astrocytic HCO_3^- [46]. The latter stems from a rise in tissue carbon dioxide tension [38] and intracellular pH (pH_i) [47,48]. This astrocytic rise in pH_i reaches a peak during maximal depolarization from SD, a time when neuronal pH_i is invariant or swings slightly in the more acidic direction [49]. Mechanisms for these pH_i changes remain incompletely defined. The decline in neuronal pH_i may be due to proton flux into the cells [50], while the rise in astrocytic pH_i may be due to depolarization-induced electrogenic HCO_3^- transport [51,52]. Acid produced during SD is likely to be the result of energy expenditure directed at ion transport needed to restore normal gradients across plasma membranes [53]. Nonetheless, energy stores are maintained during SD. Phosphocreatine falls slightly and briefly to maintain adenosine triphosphate [4,54]. Thus, although ion concentration and passive membrane electrical properties of SD resemble those of ischemia, energy failure is never seen with SD [4]. Lack of energy failure may be a key to why SD does not injure the brain [55]. What is more important, yet-unknown aspects of these dramatic interstitial and intracellular SD-induced changes are likely to be important triggers, not only of SD but of SD-induced changes associated with altering the severity of ischemic brain injury. This conclusion stems from the realization that voltage [46], pH_i [56], or Ca_i^{2+} [6] changes are often used by eukaryotic cells as initial signals for the induction of enhanced anabolic activity.

SD and gap junctions

Despite the wealth of data generated about SD over the last 50 years, the underlying biophysical events of SD remain essentially unknown. Two theories initially proposed by Grafstein and Van Harreveld, respectively, attributed both the initiation and propagation of SD to excessive release of either K^+ [57] or glutamate [58,59]. Others believe the process is more complex and consists of a cascade of events that includes the generalized release of neurotransmitters and neuromodulators [4,60]. Each of these theories is supported by data. For example, it is well known that both K^+ and glutamate are released during SD. Furthermore, at least part of their build up in the interstitial space is due to release from neurons. However, these theories do not adequately account for the basic electrophysiological properties of SD. On the other hand, work by Somjen and co-workers begins to suggest mechanisms that might account for the basic electrophysiological changes of SD.

Recently, Somjen and co-workers [61–63] have proposed that the opening of gap junctions between hippocampal pyramidal cells is essential for SD. Their suggestion is based on observations generated from extracellular potential measurements, current source density analyses and patch clamp recordings [62]. First, they showed that a large current sink occurs in the basal dendrites of hippocampal pyramidal cells with the onset of SD [62]. The source for this sink is unknown but was suggested to lie ahead of the propagating SD wave [62]. Second, Somjen and co-workers proposed the novel idea that the opening of previously closed neuronal gap junctions occurs with SD [62,64]. The notion of synchronous electrical interaction among pyramidal neurons in SD is supported by the finding of such interactions during seizures [65,66]. Third, Somjen and co-workers produced the first patch clamp recordings during SD [61,64]. While preliminary, this work reveals no changes in astrocytic conductance during SD. Astrocytes simply depolarize, probably due to elevated $[K^+]_o$. Pyramidal cells, on the other hand, show a large inward current that is due neither to K^+ nor to Na^+ but may be due to Ca^{2+} [5]. We have begun to extend these observations from acute brain slices with SD to SD in HOTCs, where studies can be designed to test the mechanisms by which changes associated with SD trigger the modulation of subsequent excitotoxic injury.

Gap junctions between pyramidal cells and between astrocytes are known to exist in the hippocampus [67]. However, direct evidence for the opening of previously closed neuronal or astrocytic gap junctions during SD is lacking. Changes in gap junctional connections associated with SD are likely to be labile since their conductance can be influenced by pH_i, Ca_i^{2+}, and possibly voltage, each of which change dramatically in SD. Thus, while gap junctions between pyramidal cells and between astrocytes are expected, the characterization of dynamic changes in these connections with SD will begin to define the potential for an immensely powerful means of non-synaptic communication between neurons and between astrocytes [66].

The spatiotemporal characteristics of current sources and sinks of SD are unknown. They are also potentially important signaling mechanisms for SD and SD-induced modulation of ischemic injury that is under investigation in our laboratory. We are using optical current source density analysis techniques on whole HOTCs or single cells filled with a voltage-sensitive dye [68,69]. This work confirms that SD occurs with a massive current sink in the distal dendrites of hippocampal pyramidal neurons that may at least in part be due to Ca^{2+} flux. Furthermore, for the first time, it identifies a large current source. Current flows out of CA1 pyramidal cells at their basilar somata, axons and probably axon terminals. At least some aspect of this current source appears to be due to chloride flux into the involved neurons. Finally, as expected, aspects of a current source do indeed lie ahead of the propagating wave of SD.

HOTCs, SD and Ca_i^{2+}

Neural cells do not normally exist in isolation. Instead, they interact with other brain cells, with the vasculature and with products from still other organ systems. The notion that interactions necessarily occur between individual brain cell types and their local environment is likely also to apply to how these cells respond to degeneration, modulation and possibly the lack of regeneration that follows from ischemic brain injury. The notion of interaction may be applied equally well to how ions, molecules, cells and even tissues influence the behavior of neural cells associated with, for example, SD and SD-induced ischemic tolerance [70].

Given the high capacity of neural cells to influence, and be influenced by, their environment, one must decide how best to study SD and its effects. Of course, SD occurs only within susceptible neural tissues. Animal preparations that include multiple cell types are essential for interactive cellular phenomena. Whole animals are indispensable for the definition of the size and extent of changes that occur in experimental variables during and after SD or ischemia. However, whole animal studies are limited by their relative inability to manipulate experimental conditions as compared with in vitro preparations. Brain slices are well suited for acute studies that examine plasma membrane-based issues of cellular interaction, while mixed and cocultures are well suited for more long-term studies.

Slice cultures (e.g., HOTCs) may be the most advantageous tissue culture preparations for study of SD and SD-related phenomena, since they possess several distinct advantages over other biological preparations. First, the HOTC is an intact area of brain tissue that maintains most cell-to-cell interrelationships found in vivo, yet HOTCs survive in vitro for months [71–73]. Thus individual cells within the HOTC can be followed in space and time over a period that allows measurements of SD-induced modulation of excitotoxic injury. Also, the gap junctional coupling ratios for pyramidal cell neurons from CA3 or CA1 areas are analogous in HOTCs to those found in vivo (Figure 13.1). Second, HOTCs possess functional capacities that parallel their in vivo counterparts. For example, HOTCs support SD [74], SD-induced gliosis [75] and SD-induced modulation of excitotoxic injury [76]. Third, neural cell differentiation in HOTCs is comparable to that seen in vivo. For example in addition to SD, neurons within HOTCs show typical trisynaptic (e.g., dentate gyrus to CA3 to CA1) neuronal activity [74], electrographic seizures [74], and long-term potentiation and long-term synaptic depression [72,77].

Astrocytes in vivo show immunopositive staining only for the cytoskeletal element vimentin during development or when they become reactive in association with irreversible neuronal injury [78]. Under such a circumstance, these astrocytes also undergo cellular division [79]. Injury without neuronal death [79] and physiological phenomena such as SD [80] are associated with a lesser degree of astrocytic gliosis that consists of a transient increase in cell size and increased immunostaining for glial fibrillary acidic protein. In contrast, astrocytes in primary culture are always vimentin positive and continue to divide [78]. However, astrocytes within HOTCs show little evidence for vimentin staining or cell division after 21 days in culture [75], suggesting that these cells are more like astrocytes in vivo than cells found in primary cultures. Similarly, microglia, though easily activated by a host of physiological and pathophysiological stimuli [81], are quiescent in HOTCs to a degree consistent with that seen in vivo [82].

Despite the increased use of HOTCs, SD has never been reported before in these cultures. This lack is due to at least two facts. First, while acute brain slices easily support SD [83,84], HOTCs typically do not. A sufficient volume of tissue must be synchronously depolarized to initiate SD [4]. Perhaps the CA3 volume of cells activated by bipolar DG stimulation to evoke SD is simply too low in HOTCs, since they are much thinner (e.g., 50 to 150 μm thick) compared to acute slices (e.g., 200 to 400 μm thick). The second potential reason that SD has never been reported in HOTCs, may be that brief exposure to low-Cl^- Ringer's is often needed to evoke SD [74]. Exposure to reduced Cl^- Ringer's is a well-recognized means to increase the susceptibility of brain tissue to SD [4].

Brief exposure to sodium acetate-based Ringer's solution, coupled with a single bipolar electrical stimulus in the dentate gyrus used to evoke a field potential in CA3, triggers SD in HOTCs [74]. SD in HOTCs occurs with the classic electrophysiological changes of a slowly propagating interstitial DC potential change associated with a transient loss of spontaneous and evoked synaptic activity.

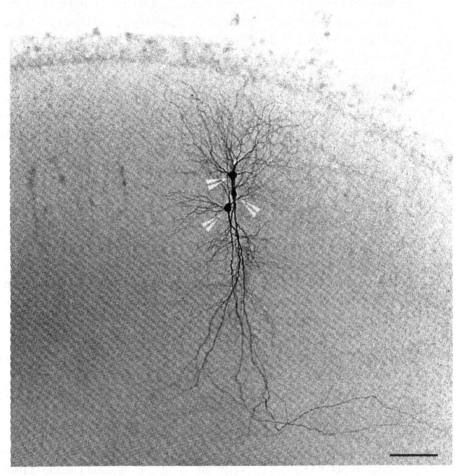

Figure 13.1   Gap junctional connectivity of CA pyramidal cells in HOTCs. Intracellular staining with
Biocytin was used to detect the degree of gap junctional connectivity between CA3
pyramidal neurons and between CA1 pyramidal neurons. An example of the degree of
gap junctional connectivity is shown. Arrows show cell bodies of three pyramidal cell
neurons in the CA region filled from a single intracellular injection. Microelectrodes for
dye injections were filled with 3% Biocytin and 1% Texas Red in 1 M potassium acetate.
Dye was iontophoresed into cells using 0.7 to 0.9 nA with a duty cycle of 400 ms at 2 Hz
for 5 to 20 minutes. Texas Red confirmed the original cell injected and Biocytin confirmed
the number of cells connected via gap junctions. Results were consistent with those
found in acute brain slices, namely a coupling ratio of 1.71 per injection [94]. Here CA3
pyramidal cell injections ($n = 90$) showed 53% at 1 : 1, 31% at 1 : 2, 10% at 1 : 3 and 6% at
1 : 4–7 coupling ratios. CA1 pyramidal cell injections ($n = 28$) showed 68% at 1 : 1, 28% at
1 : 2 and 4% at 13. Bar = 100 μm.

Slowly propagating intracellular and intercellular Ca^{2+} waves are a recently recognized phenomenon of neurons [85], astrocytes [86] and brain tissues [87], and may be a concomitant of SD [77]. Although Ca^{2+} waves resemble SD and occur in HOTCs [87], SD has not been reported in these cultures before our recently completed study [74]. Furthermore, Ca^{2+} waves occur within astrocytes and between astrocytes for distances that extend up to 200 μm [88–90]. However, SD can propagate for tens of millimeters [4], so astrocytic Ca^{2+} waves alone cannot explain SD. Similarly, the Ca^{2+} waves that occur between neurons travel ten times faster than SD [85], so they too alone cannot explain SD. Results using HOTCs show for the first time that HOTCs support SD and how these two distinct Ca^{2+} waves relate to SD. Both Ca^{2+} waves precede SD by seconds. Plate 13.1 illustrates the propagation of these two waves. The first travels >100 μm/second along the stratum radiatum (top image). The second, slower wave spreads with the interstitial DC change at millimeters/minute but always ahead of it by 6 to 16 seconds (second to fourth images). Heptanol, which uncouples gap junctions, blocked both types of Ca^{2+} waves and SD. Thus two types of Ca^{2+} wave occur with the initiation and propagation of SD. The first might reflect interneuronal changes linked by gap junctions. This conclusion stems from the fact that Ca^{2+} waves among neurons travel as rapidly as this first Ca^{2+} wave [85]. Furthermore this more rapid wave travels along the stratum radiatum, where dendritic gap junctions are found [65,67]. The second wave might be due to intercellular spread among astrocytes, since it does not follow a cytoarchitectural pattern and moves at a speed reminiscent of those seen among astrocytes [86–90].

Figure 13.2 summarizes three major Ca^{2+} changes (and associated waves) that may be essential for SD and SD-associated changes in brain function. These changes can be summarized as follows. With initiation of SD, (i) an influx of Ca^{2+} occurs across neuronal plasma membranes, and neurons become synchronized via the opening of gap junctional connections from stimulus-induced depolarization. Neuronal synchronization is associated with a rapidly propagating (i.e., ~100 μm/second) interneuronal Ca^{2+} wave. This influx leads (ii) to a drop in $[Ca^{2+}]_o$, that (iii) may be one trigger associated with initiation of interastrocytic Ca^{2+} waves that propagate at the speed of SD (~3 mm/minute), but 3 to 4 seconds ahead of it.

The bases for these Ca^{2+} changes, their role in SD and in SD-induced modulation of excitotoxic injury are now a major focus of inquiry in our laboratories. Our most recent efforts in this regard involve injection of a fluorescent Ca^{2+}-sensitive dye into single, identified CA pyramidal neurons within HOTCs. An illustration of its capacities is shown in Plate 13.2. The images show the propagation of Ca^{2+}_i transients within a single CA3 pyramidal cell from dentate gyrus-evoked synaptic activity. Ca^{2+}_i changes begin from the dendritic tree, progress proximally and eventually engulf the soma. Images to the right (1 to 4) were taken before evoked

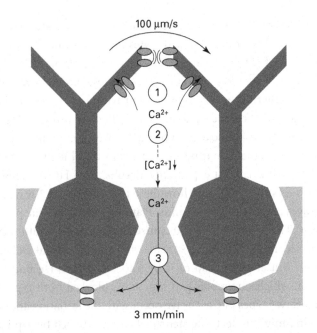

Figure 13.2 Schematic of the proposed three major Ca^{2+} changes of SD. With initiation of SD, (1) an influx of Ca^{2+} occurs across neuronal plasma membranes and neurons become synchronized via the opening of gap junctional connections from stimulus-induced depolarization. Neuronal synchronization is associated with a rapidly propagating (i.e., ~100 μm/second) interneuronal Ca^{2+} wave. This influx leads (2) to a drop in interstitial $[Ca^{2+}]$, which (3) may be one trigger associated with initiation of interastrocytic Ca^{2+} waves that propagate at the speed of SD (~3 mm/minute) but 3 to 4 seconds ahead of it.

stimulation and show small, spontaneous Ca_i^{2+} changes that presumably were occurring within dendritic spines (arrows). Such measurements illustrate that highly circumscribed and rapid changes in subregional cellular Ca_i^{2+} can be measured in a functioning area of brain tissue. These are reminiscent of similar Ca_i^{2+} changes originally shown in cerebellar Purkinje cells within acute brain slices [91].

Our goal, to study in detail these Ca_i^{2+} changes associated with SD-induced modulation of ischemic injury, requires use of HOTCs. In recently completed work we have shown that SD induces a robust bimodal rise in pyramidal cell Ca_i^{2+} [92]. Furthermore, this Ca_i^{2+} change is essential for SD since a blockade of plasma-membrane Ca^{2+} flux blocks the initiation and propagation of SD [5].

Conclusion

The predominant approach to scientific inquiry for at least the past century has been reductionist. However, shortcomings to this approach to deciphering "mechanisms" of brain function in health and disease are increasingly apparent [93]. A special recent section published in *Science* entitled, "Beyond Reductionism" suggests that "something may be gained from supplementing the predominant reductionist approach (i.e., study of isolated cells) with an integrative agenda (i.e., study of an isolated tissue where cell-to-cell relationships are maintained)" [93]. The latter is supported by use of HOTCs as outlined here.

SD, SD-induced gliosis and SD-induced tolerance that require days to evolve can now be examined for the first time in vitro using a novel and highly advantageous preparation, the HOTC. Thus the experimental advantages of easy access and microenvironmental control of in vitro preparations can be applied to answer "mechanistic" questions at the cellular and molecular levels about events that occur within tissue. Initial support for this contention is evident from studies of Ca_i^{2+} in HOTCs that show sufficient neuronal Ca_i^{2+} changes must occur to induce SD. Further support should come from work recently initiated and designed to explore how neural Ca_i^{2+} changes trigger alterations in inflammatory mediators involved in the modulation of ischemic brain injury such as cyclooxygenase-2 (i.e., worsening of injury) and interleukin-1 (i.e., lessening of ischemic injury).

Acknowledgments

This work was supported by grant NS-19108 from the National Institute of Neurological Disorders and Stroke. We thank Raymond Hulse for assistance in figure preparation and Marcia P. Kraig for hippocampal organ culture maintenance.

REFERENCES

1 Lyden PD (1996) Magnitude of the problem of stroke and the significance of acute intervention. In *Rapid Identification and Treatment of Acute Stroke*, eds. J. R. Marler, P. W. Jones & M. Emr, pp. 1–4. Bethesda, MD: Office of Scientific and Health Reports, National Institute of Neurological Disorders and Stroke.

2 Chen J & Simon R (1997) Ischemic tolerance in the brain. *Neurology*, **48**, 306–11.

3 Nedergaard M & Hansen AK (1988) Spreading depression is not associated with neuronal injury in the normal brain. *Brain Research*, **449**, 395–8.

4 Bureš J, Burešova O & Krivánek J (1974) *The Mechanisms and Applications of Leão's Spreading Depression of Electroencephalographic Activity*. New York: Academic Press.

5 Kunkler PE & Kraig RP (2000) Transmembrane calcium flux is essential for spreading depression in hippocampal organ cultures. *Society for Neuroscience Abstracts*, **26**, 762.

6 Whitfield JF (1990) *Calcium, Cell Cycles, and Cancer*. Boca Raton, FL: CRC Press.

7 Dykens JA (1994) Isolated cerebral and cerebellar mitochondria produce free radicals when exposed to elevated Ca^{2+} and Na^+: implications for neurodegeneration. *Journal of Neurochemistry*, **63**, 584–91.

8 White RJ & Reynolds IJ (1996) Mitochondrial depolarization in glutamate-stimulated neurons: an early signal specific to excitotoxin exposure. *Journal of Neuroscience*, **16**, 5688–97.

9 Schinder AF, Olson EC, Spitzer NC & Montal M (1996) Mitochondrial dysfunction is a primary event in glutamate neurotoxicity. *Journal of Neuroscience*, **16**, 6125–33.

10 Choi D (1997) The excitotoxic concept. In *Primer on Cerebrovascular Diseases*, eds. K.M.A. Welch, L.R. Caplan, D.J. Reis, B.K. Siesjö & B. Weir, pp. 187–90. New York: Academic Press.

11 Tymianski MM & Sattler RG (1997) Is calcium involved in excitotoxic or ischemic neuronal damage? In *Primer on Cerebrovascular Diseases*, eds. K.M.A. Welch, L.R. Caplan, D.J. Reis, B.K. Siesjö & B. Weir, pp. 190–2. New York: Academic Press.

12 Sims NR (1997) Mitochondrial function and calcium sequestration during reperfusion. In *Primer on Cerebrovascular Diseases*, eds. K.M.A. Welch, L.R. Caplan, D.J. Reis, B.K. Siesjö & B. Weir, pp. 1184–7. New York: Academic Press.

13 Siesjö BK, Hu B & Kristian T (1999) Is the cell death pathway triggered by the mitochondrion or the endoplasmic reticulum? *Journal of Cerebral Blood Flow & Metabolism*, **19**, 19–26.

14 Nicholls DG & Budd SL (1998) Mitochondria and neuronal glutamate excitotoxicity. *Biochimica et Biophysica Acta*, **1366**, 97–112.

15 Stout AK, Raphael HM, Kanterewicz BI, Klann E & Reynolds IJ (1998) Glutamate-induced neuron death requires mitochondrial calcium uptake. *Nature Neuroscience*, **1**, 366–73.

16 Kitagawa K, Matsumoto M, Tagaya M, Hata R, Ueda H, Niinobe M, Handa N, Fukunaga R, Kimura K, Mikoshiba K & Kamada T (1990) "Ischemic tolerance" phenomenon found in the brain. *Brain Research*, **528**, 21–4.

17 Glazier SS, O'Rourke DM, Graham DI & Welsh FA (1994) Induction of ischemic tolerance following brief focal ischemia in rat brain. *Journal of Cerebral Blood Flow & Metabolism*, **14**, 545–53.

18 Miyashita K, Abe H, Nakajima T, Ishikawa A, Nishiura M, Sawada T & Naritomi H (1994) Induction of ischaemic tolerance in gerbil hippocampus by pretreatment with focal ischaemia. *Neuroreport*, **6**, 46–8.

19 Simon RP, Niiro M & Gwinn R (1993) Prior ischemic stress protects against experimental stroke. *Neuroscience Letters*, **163**, 135–7.

20 Chen J, Graham SH, Zhu RL & Simon RP (1996) Stress proteins and tolerance to focal cerebral ischemia. *Journal of Cerebral Blood Flow & Metabolism*, **16**, 566–77.

21 Plamondon H, Blondeau N, Heurteaux C & Lazdunski M (1999) Mutually protective actions of kainic acid epileptic preconditioning and sublethal global ischemia on hippocampal neuronal death: involvement of adenosine A_1 receptors and K_{ATP} channels. *Journal of Cerebral Blood Flow & Metabolism*, **19**, 1296–308.

22 Marini AM & Paul SM (1992) *N*-methyl-D-aspartate receptor-mediated neuroprotection in cerebellar granule cells requires new RNA and protein synthesis. *Proceedings of the National Academy of Sciences, USA*, **89**, 6555–9.

23 Abele AE & Miller RJ (1990) Potassium channel activators abolish excitotoxicity in cultured hippocampal pyramidal neurons. *Neuroscience Letters*, **115**, 195–200.

24 Reshef A, Sperling O & Zoref-Shani E (2000) Opening of K(ATP) channels is mandatory for acquisition of ischemic tolerance by adenosine. *Neuroreport*, **11**, 463–5.

25 Nakata N, Kato H & Kogure K (1993) Inhibition of ischaemic tolerance in the gerbil hippocampus by quercetin and anti-heat shock protein-70 antibody. *Neuroreport*, **4**, 695–8.

26 Kato H, Kogure K, Araki T, Liu XH, Kato K & Itoyama Y (1995) Immunohistochemical localization of superoxide dismutase in the hippocampus following ischemia in a gerbil model of ischemic tolerance. *Journal of Cerebral Blood Flow & Metabolism*, **15**, 60–70.

27 Ohtsuki T, Ruetzler CA, Tasaki K & Hallenbeck JM (1996) Interleukin-1 mediates induction of tolerance to global ischemia in gerbil hippocampal CA1 neurons. *Journal of Cerebral Blood Flow & Metabolism*, **16**, 1137–42.

28 Takano K, Latour LL, Formato JE, Carano RA, Helmer KG, Hasegawa Y, Sotak CH & Fisher M (1996) The role of spreading depression in focal ischemia evaluated by diffusion mapping. *Annals of Neurology*, **39**, 308–18.

29 Busch E, Gyngell ML, Eis M, Hoehn-Berlage M & Hossmann KA (1996) Potassium- induced cortical spreading depressions during focal cerebral ischemia in rats: contribution to lesion growth assessed by diffusion-weighted NMR and biochemical imaging. *Journal of Cerebral Blood Flow & Metabolism*, **16**, 1090–9.

30 Mies G, Iijima T & Hossmann KA (1993) Correlation between peri-infarct DC shifts and ischaemic neuronal damage in rat. *Neuroreport*, **4**, 709–11.

31 Kobayashi S, Harris VA & Welsh FA (1995) Spreading depression induces tolerance of cortical neurons to ischemia in rat brain. *Journal of Cerebral Blood Flow & Metabolism*, **15**, 721–7.

32 Kawahara N, Ruetzler CA & Klatzo I (1995) Protective effect of spreading depression against neuronal damage following cardiac arrest cerebral ischaemia. *Neurological Research*, **17**, 9–16.

33 Matsushima K, Hogan MJ & Hakim AM (1996) Cortical spreading depression protects against subsequent focal cerebral ischemia in rats. *Journal of Cerebral Blood Flow & Metabolism*, **16**, 221–6.

34 Plumier J-CL, David J-C, Robertson HA & Currie RW (1997) Cortical application of potassium chloride induces the low-molecular weight heat shock protein (Hsp27) in astrocytes. *Journal of Cerebral Blood Flow & Metabolism*, **17**, 781–90.

35 Avoli M, Drapeau C, Louvel J, Pumain R, Olivier A & Villemure J-G (1991) Epileptiform activity induced by low extracellular magnesium in the human cortex maintained in vitro. *Annals of Neurology*, **30**, 589–96.

36 Kraig RP & Nicholson C (1978) Extracellular ionic variations during spreading depression. *Neuroscience*, **3**, 1045–59.

37 Kraig RP, Ferreira-Filho CR & Nicholson C (1983) Alkaline and acid transients in cerebellar microenvironment. *Journal of Neurophysiology*, **49**, 831–50.

38 Kraig RP & Cooper AJL (1987) Bicarbonate and ammonia changes in brain during spreading depression. *Canadian Journal of Physiology & Pharmacology*, **65**, 1099–104.

39 Krivanek J (1961) Some metabolic changes accompanying Leão's spreading cortical depression in the rat. *Journal of Neurochemistry*, **6**, 183–9.

40 Mutch WAC & Hansen AJ (1984) Extracellular pH changes during spreading depression and cerebral ischemia: mechanisms of brain pH regulation. *Journal of Cerebral Blood Flow & Metabolism*, **4**, 17–27.

41 Lauritzen M, Hansen AJ, Kronborg D & Wieloch T (1990) Cortical spreading depression is associated with arachidonic acid accumulation and preservation of energy charge. *Journal of Cerebral Blood Flow & Metabolism*, **10**, 115–22.

42 Hansen AJ (1985) Effect of anoxia on ion distribution in the brain. *Physiological Reviews*, **65**, 101–48.

43 Caggiano AO & Kraig RP (1996) Eicosanoids and nitric oxide influence induction of reactive gliosis from spreading depression in microglia but not astrocytes. *Journal of Comparative Neurology*, **369**, 93–108.

44 Grafe P & Ballanyi K (1987) Cellular mechanisms of potassium homeostasis in the mammalian nervous system. *Canadian Journal of Physiology & Pharmacology*, **65**, 1038–42.

45 Kraig RP & Iadecola C (1989) Reduction of astroglial K$^+$ accumulation enhances elevation in cerebral blood flow from neuronal activation. *Journal of Cerebral Blood Flow & Metabolism*, **9** (Suppl. 1), S207.

46 Kraig RP & Jaeger CB (1990) Ionic concomitants of astroglial transformation to reactive species. *Stroke*, **21** (Suppl.), III-184–III-187.

47 Chesler M & Kraig RP (1987) Intracellular pH of astrocytes increases rapidly with cortical stimulation. *American Journal of Physiology*, **253**, 666–70.

48 Chesler M & Kraig RP (1989) Intracellular pH transients of mammalian astrocytes. *Journal of Neuroscience*, **9**, 2011–19.

49 Kraig RP & Chesler M (1988) Dynamics of volatile buffers in brain cells during spreading depression. In *Mechanisms of Cerebral Hypoxia and Stroke*, ed. G.G. Somjen, pp. 279–89. New York: Plenum Press.

50 Smith SE, Gottfried JA, Chen JC & Chesler M (1994) Calcium dependence of glutamate receptor-evoked alkaline shifts in hippocampus. *Neuroreport*, **5**, 2441–5.

51 Bevensee MO, Weed RA & Boron WF (1997) Intracellular pH regulation in cultured astrocytes from rat hippocampus. I. Role of HCO$_3^-$. *Journal of General Physiology*, **110**, 453–65.

52 Bevensee MO, Apkon M & Boron WF (1997) Intracellular pH regulation in cultured astrocytes from rat hippocampus. II. Electrogenic Na/HCO$_3^-$ cotransport. *Journal of General Physiology*, **110**, 467–83.

53 Erecinska M & Silver IA (1989) ATP and brain function. *Journal of Cerebral Blood Flow & Metabolism*, **9**, 2–19.

54 Mies G & Paschen W (1984) Regional changes of blood flow, glucose, and ATP content determined on brain sections during a single passage of spreading depression in rat brain cortex. *Experimental Neurology*, **84**, 249–58.

55 Siesjö BK & Bengtsson F (1989) Calcium fluxes, calcium antagonists, and calcium-related pathology in brain ischemia, hypoglycemia, and spreading depression: a unifying hypothesis. *Journal of Cerebral Blood Flow & Metabolism*, **9**, 127–40.

56 Busa WB (1986) The proton as an integrating effector in metabolic activation. *Current Topics in Membrane Transport*, **26**, 291–310.

57 Van Harreveld A (1959) Compounds in brain extracts causing spreading depression of cerebral cortical activity and contraction of crustacean muscle. *Journal of Neurochemistry*, **3**, 300–15.

58 Van Harreveld A (1978) Two mechanisms for spreading depression in the chicken retina. *Journal of Neurobiology*, **9**, 419–31.

59 Grafstein B (1956) Mechanism of spreading cortical depression. *Journal of Neurophysiology*, **19**, 154–71.

60 Nicholson C & Kraig RP (1981) The behavior of extracellular ions during spreading depression. In *The Application of Ion-Selective Microelectrodes*, ed. T Zeuthen, pp. 217–38. Amsterdam: Elsevier/North-Holland.

61 Somjen GG, Aitken PG, Czeh GL, Herreras O, Jing J & Young JN (1992) Mechanism of spreading depression: a review of recent findings and a hypothesis. *Canadian Journal of Physiology & Pharmacology*, **70**, S248–S254.

62 Herreras O, Largo C, Ibarz JM, Somjen GG & Martin del Rio R (1994) Role of neuronal synchronizing mechanisms in the propagation of spreading depression in the in vivo hippocampus. *Journal of Neuroscience*, **14**, 7087–98.

63 Largo C, Tombaugh GC, Aitken PG, Herreras O & Somjen GG (1997) Heptanol but not fluoroacetate prevents the propagation of spreading depression in rat hippocampal slices. *Journal of Neurophysiology*, **77**, 9–16.

64 Czeh G, Aitken PG & Somjen GG (1992) Whole-cell membrane current and membrane resistance during hypoxic spreading depression. *Neuroreport*, **3**, 197–200.

65 Perez-Velazquez JL, Valiante TA & Carlen PL (1994) Modulation of gap junctional mechanisms during calcium-free induced field burst activity: a possible role for electrotonic coupling in epileptogenesis. *Journal of Neuroscience*, **14**, 4308–17.

66 Jeffery JGR (1995) Nonsynaptic modulation of neuronal activity in the brain: electric currents and extracellular ions. *Physiological Reviews*, **75**, 689–723.

67 MacVicar BA & Dudek FE (1981) Electrotonic coupling between pyramidal cells: a direct demonstration in rat hippocampal slices. *Science*, **213**, 782–5.

68 Kraig RP, Hulse R, Kunkler PE & Nicholson C (1999) Optical current source densities with spreading depression in hippocampal organ cultures. *Society for Neuroscience Abstract*, **25**, 2101.

69 Kraig RP, Hulse RE, Kunkler PE & Nicholson C (2000) Optical current source density analyses show that chloride flow contributes to the somatic current source from hippocampal pyramidal cells during spreading depression. *Annals of Neurology*, **58**, 445.

70 Kraig RP, Lascola CD & Caggiano AO (1995) Glial response to brain ischemia. In *Neuroglia*, eds. H. Kettenmann & BR Ransom, pp. 964–76. New York: Oxford.

71 Buchs P-A, Stoppini L & Muller D (1993) Structural modifications associated with synaptic development in area CA1 of rat hippocampal organotypic cultures. *Developmental Brain Research*, **71**, 81–91.

72 Muller D, Buchs P-A & Stoppini L (1993) Time course of synaptic development in hippocampal organotypic cultures. *Developmental Brain Research*, **71**, 93–100.

73 Bahr BA (1995) Long-term hippocampal slices: a model system for investigating synaptic mechanisms and pathologic processes. *Journal of Neuroscience Research*, **42**, 294–305.

74 Kunkler PE & Kraig RP (1998) Calcium waves precede electrophysiological changes of spreading depression in hippocampal organ cultures. *Journal of Neuroscience*, **18**, 3416–25.

75 Kunkler PE & Kraig RP (1997) Reactive astrocytosis from excitotoxic injury in hippocampal organ culture parallels that seen in vivo. *Journal of Cerebral Blood Flow & Metabolism*, **17**, 26–43.

76 Kraig RP & Kunkler PE (1998) Spreading depression induces tolerance to excitotoxic injury in hippocampal organ cultures. *Society for Neuroscience Abstract*, **24**, 2013.

77 Muller D, Djebbara-Hannas Z, Jourdain P, Vutskits L, Durbec P, Rougon G & Kiss JZ (2000) Brain-derived neurotrophic factor restores long-term potentiation in polysialic acid- neural adhesion molecule-deficient hippocampus. *Proceedings of the National Academy of Sciences, USA*, **97**, 4315–20.

78 DeVillis J, Wu DK & Kumar S (1986) Enzyme induction and regulation of protein synthesis. In *Astrocytes*, vol. 2, eds. S Federoff & A Vernadakis, pp. 209–37. New York: Academic Press.

79 Petito CK, Morgello S, Felix JC & Lesser ML (1990) The two patterns of reactive astrocytosis in postischemic rat brain. *Journal of Cerebral Blood Flow & Metabolism*, **10**, 850–9.

80 Kraig RP, Dong LM, Thisted R & Jaeger CB (1991) Spreading depression increases immunohistochemical staining of glial fibrillary acidic protein. *Journal of Neuroscience*, **11**, 2187–98.

81 Giulian D (1995) Microglia and neuronal dysfunction. In *Neuroglia*, eds. H Kettenmann & BR Ransom, pp. 671–84. New York: Oxford.

82 Czapiga M & Colton CA (1999) Function of microglia in organotypic slice cultures. *Journal of Neuroscience Research*, **56**, 644–51.

83 Snow RW, Taylor CP & Dudek FE (1983) Electrophysiological and optical changes in slices of rat hippocampus during spreading depression. *Journal of Neurophysiology*, **50**, 561–72.

84 Psarropoulou C & Avoli M (1993) 4–Aminopyridine-induced spreading depression episodes in immature hippocampus: developmental and pharmacological characteristics. *Neuroscience*, **55**, 57–68.

85 Charles AC, Kodali SK & Tyndale RF (1996) Intercellular calcium waves in neurons. *Molecular and Cellular Neurosciences*, **7**, 337–53.

86 Cornell-Bell AH, Finkbeiner SM, Cooper MS & Smith SJ (1990) Glutamate induces calcium waves in cultured astrocytes: long-range glial signaling. *Science*, **247**, 470–3.

87 Dani JW, Chernjavsky A & Smith SJ (1992) Neuronal activity triggers calcium waves in hippocampal astrocyte networks. *Neuron*, **8**, 429–40.

88 Nedergaard M (1994) Direct signaling from astrocytes to neurons in cultures of mammalian brain cells. *Science*, **263**, 1768–71.

89 Wang Z, Tymianski M, Jones OT & Nedergaard M (1997) Impact of cytoplasmic calcium buffering on the spatial and temporal characteristics of intercellular calcium signals in astrocytes. *Journal of Neuroscience*, **17**, 7359–71.

90 Pasti L, Volterra A, Pozzan T & Carmignoto G (1997) Intracellular calcium oscillations in astrocytes: a highly plastic, bidirectional form of communication between neurons and astrocytes in situ. *Journal of Neuroscience*, **17**, 7817–30.

91 Tank DW, Sugimori M, Connor JA & Llinas RR (1988) Spatially resolved calcium dynamics of mammalian Purkinje cells in cerebellar slice. *Science*, **242**, 773–7.

92 Kunkler PE & Kraig RP (2000) Neuronal calcium changes during spreading depression in hippocampal organ cultures. *Society for Neuroscience Abstract*, **25**, 2101.

93 Gallagher R & Appenzeller T (1999) Beyond reductionism. *Science*, **284**, 79.

94 Church J & Baimbridge KG (1991) Exposure to high-pH medium increases the incidence and extent of dye coupling between rat hippocampal CA1 pyramidal neurons in vitro. *Journal of Neuroscience*, **11**, 3289–95.

95 Hinman LE & Sammak PJ (1998) Intensity modulation of pseudocolor images. *Biotechniques*, **25**, 124–8.

Part V

Hemorrhage, edema, and secondary injury

Co-Chairs: Philip R. Weinstein & Julian T. Hoff

14

The role of matrix metalloproteinases and urokinase in blood–brain barrier damage with thrombolysis

Gary A. Rosenberg[1], Susan Alexander[2], Edward Y. Estrada[2] & Mark Grostette[2]

[1] Departments of Neurology, Neuroscience and Cell Biology and Physiology, University of New Mexico, Albuquerque, NM
[2] Department of Neurology, University of New Mexico, Albuquerque, NM

Introduction

Recombinant tissue plasminogen activator (rtPA) benefits patients who have had an acute stroke, but a delay in treatment for over 3 hours raises the risk of intracerebral hemorrhage [1,2]. Reperfusion of blood into an ischemic region, while preserving metabolic function, results in the production of molecules that may damage the injured tissue [3]. The cerebral microvasculature is a major site of injury during reperfusion with a biphasic disruption of the blood–brain barrier (BBB) seen after reperfusion [4]. Multiple factors have been implicated in the damage to the microvasculature by ischemia with reperfusion, including free radicals, blood products and proteases. Matrix metalloproteinases (MMPs) are a gene family of neutral proteases. Once formed and activated, the MMPs attack the basal lamina around the cerebral blood vessels, leading to the opening of the BBB [5]. MMPs are induced in cerebral ischemia [6–10].

MMPs are secreted in a latent form that requires activation [11]. Plasminogen activators (PAs) are serine proteases involved in angiogenesis, neuronal growth and regulation of other proteases through activation processes [12,13]. Brain cells produce PAs in response to an ischemic injury [6,14]. Urokinase-type plasminogen activator (uPA) is secreted by microglial cells in culture [15]. Urokinase generates plasmin, which activates MMPs [16,17]. Latent MMP-2 (gelatinase A) is activated by a membrane-type metalloproteinase (MT-MMP), which is activated by plasmin [18,19]. Latent MMP-9 (gelatinase B) is activated by stromelysin-1 (MMP-3), which also requires plasmin for activation [20]. Because of the role of PAs in the activation of MMPs, and the induction of MMPs in reperfusion injury, we hypothesized that rtPA use in acute ischemia facilitates the activation of the MMPs, opening the BBB and increasing the risk of hemorrhage. In vivo studies were done in rats with middle cerebral artery occlusion (MCAO) by the suture method with 90 or 180 minutes of ischemia and 24 hours of reperfusion. BBB integrity was measured by radiolabeled sucrose, and MMPs and PAs by zymography. In vitro studies of the effect of plasminogen on the activation of MMPs were done in mixed glial cell cultures.

Methods

MCAO and the BBB

Twenty Wistar–Kyoto rats were anesthetized with 2% halothane with nitrous oxide and oxygen. The neck vessels were exposed and a suture was placed in the common carotid artery and advanced to occlude the MCA, using a described method [21]. The MCAO was maintained for either 90 or 180 minutes, and reperfusion was done by withdrawing the catheter. After 24 hours the rats were deeply anesthetized with pentobarbital (50 mg/kg intraperitoneally) and were given an intravenous injection of [^{14}C]sucrose (10 μCi). Ten minutes later the heart was stopped with an intracardiac injection of saturated potassium chloride and the brain was rapidly removed and frozen in isopentane cooled with liquid nitrogen.

Three coronal sections of about 5 mm were made through the region of the infarct. The most anterior sections were used to verify the existence of an infarct by staining the section for 30 minutes in 2% (v/v) 2,3,5-triphenyltetrazolium chloride. Only those rats showing an infarct were included in the analysis. The cortex and caudate from the second brain section of the infarcted and non-infarcted hemispheres were used for analysis of BBB permeability. The concentration of [^{14}C]sucrose in the brain and in a sample of blood removed at the time of death was measured by liquid scintillation counting. The ratio of sucrose in the brain to that in the blood was used to estimate the BBB permeability [22]. The third contiguous brain section was used for zymography.

Ten animals each were subjected to 90 or 180 minutes of MCAO and half of each of the two groups received an intravenous infusion of 10 mg rtPA/kg (Alteplase; Genentech, Inc., South San Francisco, CA). The rtPA was infused for 30 seconds with reperfusion.

Zymography

Tissue samples were prepared for gelatin-substrate and casein zymography to measure for the presence of gelatinases A and B (MMP-2 and -9, respectively) and for PAs as described elsewhere [23]. In brief, tissue was taken from the ischemic and non-ischemic hemispheres in a region posterior to that used for isotopic measurements. Tissue samples were extracted in 0.2% (w/v) Triton X-100 in 20 mM phosphate buffer at pH 7.2 for 24 hours at 4 °C. The tissue was centrifuged and the supernatant removed for zymography in 10% (w/v) polyacrylamide/sodium dodecyl sulfate-gels with gelatin or casein added. After electrophoresis at 150 V, gels were rinsed in 2.5% Triton X-100 followed by water and incubated for 70 hours for gelatinases and overnight for PAs. Proteolytic bands were visualized by staining with Coomassie G-250 dye. To determine the type of PA, casein gels were incubated with amiloride (Sigma), an inhibitor of uPA. Relative molecular masses were determined from protein standards and MMP-2 and -9 standards (Calbiochem). Protein content in the samples was determined by the Micro BCA assay (Pierce Co., Rockford, IL) and read on a microtiter plate reader. Zymograms were scanned with an Agfa Duo Scanner using the transparency mode and an image analysis software program designed for electrophoresis gels was used to quantify the images (AlphaImage; Alpha Innotech Corp.). Electrophoresis data were expressed as relative lysis units per microgram protein.

Cell cultures

Glial cultures were established from the cortex of newborn Sprague–Dawley rats using methods previously described [24]. Briefly, the cortical tissue was pooled from 12 to 15 rat pups on the day of birth and mechanically dissociated by syringe needles and a mesh sieve. The cells were pelleted and plated into $75\,cm^2$ tissue culture flasks at a density of approximately 15×10^6 cells/flask in Hepes-buffered Dulbecco's modified Eagle's medium/F12 medium (Gibco BRL) with 10% (v/v) fetal calf serum and gentamicin, and grown to confluency in 10 to 14 days. Confluent mixed glial cultures were subcultured into six-well plates (Falcon) at a plating density of 5×10^5 cells/well. Cell cultures were maintained at a viability greater than 92% as assessed by the trypan blue exclusion method and used for experiments 3 days after subculturing.

To determine the composition of mixed glial cultures, a portion of the cells were subcultured onto 12 mm round glass coverslips and grown for 3 days. The cells were fixed with 4% (v/v) paraformaldehyde and stored in phosphate-buffered saline for immunostaining. Primary antibodies used to identify cell phenotypes included rabbit anti-bovine glial fibrillary acidic protein (Accurate Labs) to identify astrocytes, mouse monoclonal anti-rat OX-42 (Harlan Sera-Lab) to identify microglia and A2B5 (Boehringer Mannheim). Cell counts were performed on immunocytochemically stained specimens. An estimate of culture cell types indicated that 67% were astrocytes, 26% were microglia and 5% to 7% were of the O2–A or neuronal lineage.

For plasminogen cell stimulation studies, confluent cells were changed to serum-free media and grown either in the presence or absence of plasminogen (2 μg/ml;

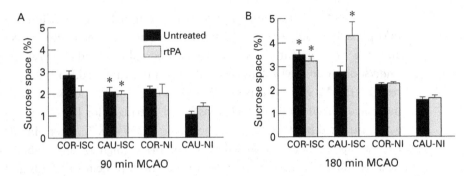

Figure 14.1   Blood–brain barrier permeability estimated by the percentage of sucrose space after either 90 or 180 minutes of MCAO with reperfusion for 24 hours. (A) Values for the cortex (COR) and caudate (CAU) for the ischemic (ISC) and the non-ischemic (NI) hemispheres in untreated rats (black bars) and in those treated with rtPA (shaded bars). Both ischemic hemispheres were compared statistically with the untreated non-ischemic hemispheres by ANOVA. The caudate of the ischemic rats showed increased sucrose space. (B) Values for the 180 minute group. Sucrose uptake in the cortex was increased in both the untreated and treated rats, but the caudate lost the significance seen at 90 minutes in the untreated group, and showed a large increase with rtPA treatment. Asterisks indicate significant differences by ANOVA ($P < 0.05$).

Sigma) for 24 hours with or without aprotinin (100 μg/ml, Sigma). After 24 hours the conditioned media were collected and frozen. Enzyme activity was determined by zymography as described above. Data were expressed in relative lysis units per number of cells per well.

Statistical analysis

Statistical analysis was done between experimental groups, using a one-way analysis of variance (ANOVA) with the Bonferroni correction for multiple t tests. Results were expressed as mean ± standard error of the mean. The significance level was set at $P < 0.05$.

Results

Sucrose space

In the rats undergoing 90 minutes of MCAO with 24 hours of reperfusion, the cortical tissue sucrose spaces were similar on the ischemic and non-ischemic sides in the rtPA-treated and untreated rats. Caudate tissue showed a significant increase in the sucrose spaces in both the treated and untreated rats (Figure 14.1A). The uptake of sucrose was higher in the cortical tissue than in the caudate in both the ischemic and non-ischemic hemispheres.

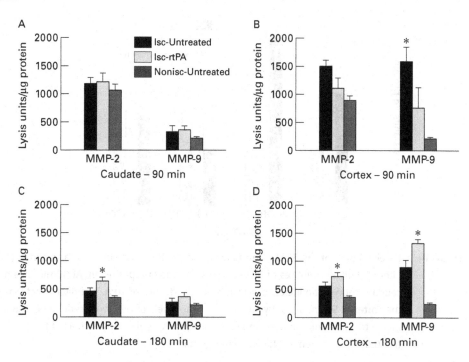

Figure 14.2 Quantitative zymography for the gelatinases in the regions and times shown. (A) The caudate at 90 minutes showed no increase in either MMP-2 or MMP-9. (B) MMP-9 was increased in the cortex at 90 minutes. (C) rtPA-treated rats showed an increase in MMP-2 in the caudate, but no effect of either ischemia (Isc) alone or rtPA treatment for MMP-9. (D) In the cortex the rtPA treatment increased both the MMP-2 and MMP-9 levels. Note that the MMPs are reduced at 180 minutes as compared with the 90 minute values, which are shown on the same scale. Asterisks indicate a statistically significant difference compared to the non-ischemic (Nonisc) side ($P < 0.05$).

After 3 hours of MCAO, the cortical tissue showed a significantly increased sucrose uptake that was similar in the treated and untreated rats. In the caudate, the untreated rats lost the statistically significant increase, and the rtPA-treated rats showed the highest level of sucrose uptake seen in any region (Figure 14.1B). The difference between the rtPA-treated and the untreated hemispheres was statistically significant using Student's unpaired t test ($P < 0.05$).

MMPs

Caudate tissue from the animals that were subjected to 90 minutes of MCAO had similar levels of MMP-2 in the ischemic and non-ischemic tissue (Figure 14.2A). Cortical tissue showed a marked rise in the levels of MMP-9 in the untreated ischemic hemisphere, approaching those of MMP-2. Treatment with rtPA reduced the MMP-9 levels, resulting in a loss of significance compared to the non-ischemic

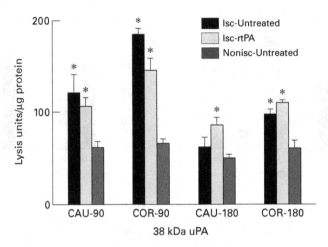

Figure 14.3   Levels of uPA for the 38 kDa form are shown for the caudate (CAU) and cortex (COR) after either 90 or 180 minutes of MCAO with 24 hours of reperfusion. At 90 minutes the caudate showed an increase, which was not affected by rtPA. A similar effect was seen in the cortex at 90 minutes. By 180 minutes the levels of uPA were reduced in the untreated rats in the ischemic caudate and cortex, and rtPA significantly increased the levels ($P<0.05$). Isc, ischemic; Nonisc, non-ischemic.

side (Figure 14.2B). Cortical levels at 90 minutes for MMP-2 were statistically similar in the treated and untreated rats. The levels of MMP-9 in the cortex approached those of MMP-2.

By 3 hours the levels of MMP-2 were similar on the ischemic and non-ischemic sides in the caudate and cortex tissue. Treatment with rtPA caused a statistically significant increase in the levels of MMP-2 in both areas (Figure 14.2C). MMP-9 in the caudate was unaffected by the prolonged ischemia, but in the cortex an increase in the levels of MMP-9 reached statistical significance (Figure 14.2D).

PAs were measured in the casein gels, which showed two bands. The higher relative molecular mass band appeared at 58 kDa, while the lower one appeared at 39 kDa. Amiloride, which blocks uPA, abolished the lower band, but only partially depleted the upper one. Since the lower band was uPA and the upper band contained both uPA and tPA, measurements were made from the lower band.

In the rats that underwent 90 minutes of MCAO, a significant increase in uPA was seen in both the ischemic caudate and the cortex (Figure 14.3). Treatment with rtPA slightly lowered the increase, but the tissue levels remained significantly higher than those found on the non-ischemic side. At 3 hours the levels of uPA were similar in the caudate of the ischemic and non-ischemic hemispheres, and the rtPA caused a significant increase in the levels. In the cortex at 3 hours there was a significant increase in uPA in the ischemic, untreated rats, which was unaltered by treatment with rtPA.

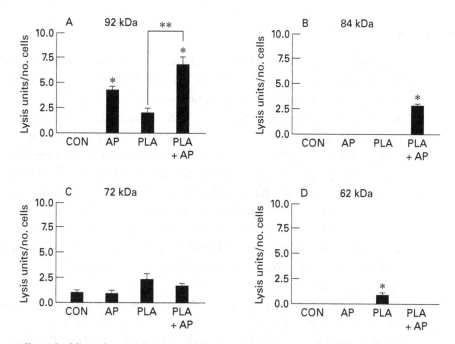

Figure 14.4   Effect of adding plasminogen to mixed astrocyte and microglial cell cultures. (A) MMP-9 (92 kDa) without plasminogen (CON), with the plasmin inhibitor aprotinin (AP), with plasminogen (PLA) and both plasminogen and aprotinin (PLA+AP). The aprotinin alone significantly increased the 92 kDa. Plasminogen alone also raised the 92 kDa, but not significantly. The combination had the greatest effect. The single asterisks indicate significant differences compared with the control, and the double asterisks indicate differences between the two by a *t* test ($P < 0.05$). (B) Activated MMP-9 (84 kDa) was seen only with plasminogen plus aprotinin. (C) No effect was seen on 72 kDa. (D) Plasminogen alone caused a significant rise in the levels of active MMP-2 (62 kDa), which was completely blocked by aprotinin.

Cell cultures

Mixed glial cell cultures derived from rat cortex were grown in the presence and absence of plasminogen (2 μg/ml). Levels of 92 kDa latent MMP-9 were undetectable in the cultures grown in the absence of plasminogen. When plasminogen was added a small increase that was statistically insignificant was observed. Addition of aprotinin resulted in increased production of latent MMP-9, which was further increased in the presence of plasminogen. An active 84 kDa form of MMP-9 was seen only in the cells treated with both aprotinin and plasminogen (Figure 14.4B). Control cells grown without plasminogen or aprotinin showed a small production of latent 72 kDa MMP-2, which was slightly increased by plasminogen (Figure 14.4C). Addition of plasminogen to the cell cultures resulted in the production of the active 62 kDa form of MMP-2, which was blocked by the addition of aprotinin (Figure 14.4D).

Discussion

We found that 90 minutes of MCAO selectively opened the BBB in the caudate and that the opening was unaffected by the infusion of rtPA. However, when the time of MCAO was extended to 3 hours, disruption of the BBB took place in the cortex and rtPA caused a selective increase in BBB permeability in the ischemic caudate. At 90 minutes, despite a rise in the levels of MMP-9 and uPA in the cortex, the BBB remained intact, suggesting that the enzymes were in a latent form. Extension of the ischemic period to 3 hours caused an increase in MMP-2 and uPA in the caudate of the rtPA-treated rats that corresponded to the selective opening of the BBB by rtPA at that site. At 3 hours there was also an increase in MMP-2, MMP-9 and uPA in the cortex of rtPA-treated rats, but the BBB, which was already opened, failed to show any further opening. The vulnerability of the caudate to rtPA after prolonged occlusion of the MCA occurs in association with a combination of factors, including the production of MMPs and uPA.

MMPs are secreted in a latent form that requires activation. Studies of activation mechanisms, which were done in vitro using cell cultures, suggest that plasminogen is required to generate plasmin for the activation of MMP-2. The increased BBB permeability seen at 90 minutes in the caudate without rtPA treatment, allowed extravasation of serum components, including plasminogen. Infusion of rtPA after the BBB was open, may have exaggerated the injury by the plasmin formed from the extravasated plasminogen. The reason for the selective vulnerability of the caudate to the action of rtPA is unclear. Other toxic substrates formed in the reperfused areas, such as free radicals, lipid peroxidation products and injury to mitochondria, may have also contributed to the damage to the microvasculature in the caudate. Cortical tissue had increases in MMP-2, MMP-9 and uPA, and the opening of the BBB at 3 hours in the rtPA-treated rats. However, the BBB was already affected in the cortex in the untreated rats and the infusion of rtPA did not cause a further increase in the permeability to sucrose.

Regulation of MMPs is tightly controlled at transcription, activation and inhibition [25]. Transcription of MMP-2 and MMP-9 occurs through different gene promoters. MMP-2 has an activator protein-2 site that is consistent with its role in the constitutive expression of the enzyme. On the contrary, MMP-9 is produced under inflammatory conditions, and has activator protein-1 and nuclear factor-κB sites that respond to immediate early gene products, c-Fos and c-Jun, and to cytokines, such as tumor necrosis factor-α and interleukin-1β. They are produced as latent enzymes by astrocytes, endothelial cells, microglia and neurons [26]. Activation is done by other enzymes and by self-activation [27]. MMP-2 is activated by MT-MMP, which is activated by plasmin. MMP-9 is activated by MMP-3, which also requires plasmin for activation [20]. This interplay between the MMPs and PAs is an important feature of extracellular matrix disruption in normal and pathological processes [28].

The cell cultures showed that plasminogen participates in the activation of MMP-2 and in the production of latent MMP-9. Aprotinin, which inhibits uPA, was able to inhibit the activation of MMP-2, implicating plasmin in the activation of MMP-2. Aprotinin also enhanced the expression of MMP-9 for reasons that remain to be elucidated.

Conclusion

In summary, an ischemic episode of 90 minutes prior to reperfusion opened the BBB in the caudate and increased MMP-9 and uPA in the caudate and cortex. Since MMP-2 was already high in both regions and uPA was increased in both, we would have expected the increase in BBB permeability to be seen in both regions unless the MMPs were inactive. The changes in the caudate at 90 minutes reached statistical significance, although the absolute increases in permeability were small. At 3 hours the rtPA selectively increased the sucrose space in the caudate and raised the levels of MMP-2 and uPA. We propose that plasmin generated from rtPA and uPA activated MMP-2 and increased BBB damage. Other factors appear to be involved in the process and further studies will be needed to identify these factors and to understand their relationship to the MMPs.

Acknowledgments

The study was supported by grants from the National Institutes of Health (RO1 NS21169). The rtPA was a generous gift from Dr. N. van Bruggen (Genentech Corp.). Dr. L. Cunningham provided helpful advice and reviewed the manuscript.

REFERENCES

1 The National Institute of Neurological Disorders; Stroke rtPA Stroke Study Group (1995) Tissue plasminogen activator for acute ischemic stroke. *New England Journal of Medicine*, 333, 1581–7.

2 Hacke W, Kaste M, Fieschi C, Toni D, Lesaffre E, von Kummer R, Boysen G, Bluhmki E, Hoxter G, Mahagne MH & Hennerici M (1995) Intravenous thrombolysis with recombinant tissue plasminogen activator for acute hemispheric stroke: the European Cooperative Acute Stroke Study (ECASS). *Journal of the American Medical Association*, 274, 1017–25.

3 Siesjö BK (1978) In *Brain Energy Metabolism*, pp. 255–6. Chichester: John Wiley.

4 Kuroiwa T, Ting P, Martinez H & Klatzo I (1985) The biphasic opening of the blood–brain barrier to proteins following temporary middle cerebral artery occlusion. *Acta Neuropathologica*, **68**, 122–9.

5 Rosenberg GA, Kornfeld M, Estrada E, Kelley RO, Liotta LA & Stetler-Stevenson WG (1992) TIMP-2 reduces proteolytic opening of blood-brain barrier by type IV collagenase. *Brain Research*, **576**, 203–7.

6 Rosenberg GA, Navratil M, Barone F & Feuerstein G (1996) Proteolytic cascade enzymes increase in focal cerebral ischemia in rat. *Journal of Cerebral Blood Flow & Metabolism*, **16**, 360–6.

7 Romanic AM, White RF, Arleth AJ, Ohlstein EH & Barone FC (1998) Matrix metalloproteinase expression increases after cerebral focal ischemia in rats: inhibition of matrix metalloproteinase-9 reduces infarct size. *Stroke*, **29**, 1020–30.

8 Rosenberg GA, Estrada EY & Dencoff JE (1998) Matrix metalloproteinases and TIMPs are associated with blood–brain barrier opening after reperfusion in rat brain. *Stroke*, **29**, 2189–95.

9 Gasche Y, Fujimura M, Morita-Fujimura Y, Copin J-C, Kawase M, Massengale J & Chan PH (1999) Early appearance of activated matrix metalloproteinase-9 after focal cerebral ischemia in mice: a possible role in blood–brain barrier dysfunction. *Journal of Cerebral Blood Flow & Metabolism*, **19**, 1020–8.

10 Heo JH, Lucero J, Abumiya T, Koziol JA, Copeland BR & del Zoppo GJ (1999) Matrix metalloproteinases increase very early during experimental focal cerebral ischemia. *Journal of Cerebral Blood Flow & Metabolism*, **19**, 624–33.

11 Nagase H (1997) Activation mechanisms of matrix metalloproteinases. *Biological Chemistry*, **378**, 151–60.

12 Reich R, Thompson EW, Iwamoto Y, Martin GR, Deason JR, Fuller GC & Miskin R (1988) Effects of inhibitors of plasminogen activator, serine proteinases, and collagenase IV on the invasion of basement membranes by metastatic cells. *Cancer Research*, **48**, 3307–12.

13 Mignatti P & Rifkin DB (1996) Plasminogen activators and matrix metalloproteinases in angiogenesis. *Enzyme & Protein*, **49**, 117–37.

14 Ahn MY, Zhang ZG, Tsang W & Chopp M (1999) Endogenous plasminogen activator expression after embolic focal cerebral ischemia in mice. *Brain Research*, **837**, 169–76.

15 Nakajima K, Tsuzaki N, Shimojo M, Hamanoue M & Kohsaka S (1992) Microglia isolated from rat brain secrete a urokinase-type plasminogen activator. *Brain Research*, **577**, 285–92.

16 Carmeliet P, Moons L, Lijnen R, Baes M, Lemaitre V, Tipping P, Drew A, Eeckhout Y, Shapiro S, Lupu F & Collen D (1997) Urokinase-generated plasmin activates matrix metalloproteinases during aneurysm formation. *Nature Genetics*, **17**, 439–44.

17 Mazzieri R, Masiero L, Zanetta L, Monea S, Onisto M, Garbisa S & Mignatti P (1997) Control of type IV collagenase activity by components of the urokinase-plasmin system: a regulatory mechanism with cell-bound reactants. *EMBO Journal*, **16**, 2319–32.

18 Sato H, Takino T, Okada Y, Cao J, Shinagawa A, Yamamoto E & Seiki M (1994) A matrix metalloproteinase expressed on the surface of invasive tumour cells. *Nature*, **370**, 61–5.

19 Okumura Y, Sato H, Seiki M & Kido H (1997) Proteolytic activation of the precursor of membrane type 1 matrix metalloproteinase by human plasmin. A possible cell surface activator. *FEBS Letters*, **402**, 181–4.

20 Ramos-DeSimone N, Hahn-Dantona E, Sipley J, Nagase H, French DL & Quigley JP (1999) Activation of matrix metalloproteinase-9 (MMP-9) via a converging plasmin/stromelysin-1 cascade enhances tumor cell invasion. *Journal of Biological Chemistry*, **274**, 13066–76.

21 Longa EZ, Weinstein PR, Carlson S & Cummins R (1989) Reversible middle cerebral artery occlusion without craniectomy in rats. *Stroke*, **20**, 84–91.

22 Ohno K, Pettigrew KD & Rapoport SI (1978) Lower limits of cerebrovascular permeability to nonelectrolytes in the conscious rat. *American Journal of Physiology*, **235**, H299–H307.

23 Rosenberg GA, Dencoff JE, McGuire PG, Liotta LA & Stetler-Stevenson WG (1994) Injury-induced 92-kilodalton gelatinase and urokinase expression in rat brain. *Laboratory Investigation*, **71**, 417–22.

24 McCarthy KK & de Vellis J (1980) Preparation of separate astroglial and oligodendroglial cell cultures from rat cerebral tissue. *Journal of Cell Biology*, **85**, 890–902.

25 Birkedal-Hansen H (1995) Proteolytic remodeling of extracellular matrix. *Current Opinion in Cell Biology*, **7**, 728–35.

26 Gottschall PE & Deb S (1996) Regulation of matrix metalloproteinase expressions in astrocytes, microglia and neurons. *Neuroimmunomodulation*, **3**, 69–75.

27 Nagase H & Woessner JF Jr (1999) Matrix metalloproteinases. *Journal of Biological Chemistry*, **274**, 21491–4.

28 Yong VW, Krekoski CA, Forsyth PA, Bell R & Edwards DR (1998) Matrix metalloproteinases and diseases of the CNS. *Trends in Neurosciences*, **21**, 75–80.

15

Does brain nitric oxide generation influence tissue oxygenation after severe human subarachnoid hemorrhage?

Ahmad Khaldi[1], Alois Zauner[1], Michael Reinert[1], Itaf Fakhry[2],
Domenic A. Sica[2] & Ross Bullock[1]

[1] Division of Neurosurgery, Medical College of Virginia, VCU, Richmond, VA
[2] Department of Internal Medicine–Clinical Pharmacology, Medical College of Virginia, VCU, Richmond, VA

Introduction

Nitric oxide (NO) is now believed to be involved in many physiological events, especially vasoregulation. In the brain, NO has been implicated in retrograde neurotransmission, synaptic plasticity and vasomotor control [1–3]. NO leads to vasodilation by diffusing across all membranes, and interrelates with guanylate cyclase in the smooth muscle, as its primary receptor target, thus regulating cerebral perfusion and cerebral blood flow (CBF) [3–5]. NO is rapidly synthesized on demand by nitric oxide synthase (NOS), which is present in a wide variety of tissues, including endothelial cells. Three isoforms of NOS are described, and all of them are expressed in the brain. The constitutive, endothelial and neuronal NOSs are believed to be primarily responsible for cerebral perfusion [6].

In neurons, NO release is stimulated by the excitatory amino acid glutamate via N-methyl-D-aspartate receptors. The NO then acts as a retrograde or orthodox neurotransmitter. Endothelial cells may supply tonically released NO that influences cerebral resistance vessels; however, the presence of NOS in glial and neuronal cells makes it likely that the coupling of CBF and neuronal activity is achieved via NO activity. The vasodilatory function of NO may be reduced after subarachnoid hemorrhage (SAH), due to reduced NO production or a disturbance of the basal vasomotor balance. Endothelial NO is profoundly reduced in some forms of experimental ischemia, leading to compensatory induction of NOS [7]. Hemoglobin derived from the blood and oxyhemoglobin in the subarachnoid space (after SAH) binds to NO, thereby reducing its vasodilating effect.

NO, a free radical with an extremely short half-life of only few seconds, is difficult to study [8]. Therefore, NO breakdown products or metabolites are studied routinely instead in plasma and cerebrospinal fluid (CSF) [9], or in brain tissue using direct tissue analysis or microdialysis. In two animal studies, vasospasm could be reversed after experimental SAH by infusing NO donors [10,11]. In this pilot study, we used microdialysis to test the relationship between NO metabolites, endothelin-1, and brain tissue oxygenation measured in the same brain region in patients after severe SAH.

Patients and methods

Patients

The studies were approved by the Committee for Conduct of Human Research at Virginia Commonwealth University. Patients were selected for this study when their Hunt and Hess (H & H) grade was 3 or greater or when they developed clinically significant vasospasm. All patients were treated according to a standardized protocol and underwent cerebral arteriography prior to occlusion of the ruptured aneurysm. All patients had a ventriculostomy catheter placed for intracranial pressure monitoring and for CSF drainage. Middle cerebral artery blood flow velocities were studied as needed using transcranial Doppler. Xenon CBF studies were done after treatment of the aneurysm and whenever vasospasm was suspected. Significant vasospasm was diagnosed by deterioration of the neurological exam, by xenon CBF studies and by cerebral arteriography.

Neurochemical monitoring

A triple lumen transcranial bolt tapped into the skull under local anesthesia was used to grip and immobilize the ventricular catheter, a microdialysis probe (CMA Microdialysis, Acton, MA), and a "neurotrend" or "paratrend" oxygen sensor (Codman, Randolph, MA) [12]. The neurotrend (paratrend) sensor was used for continuous measurements of ptiO$_2$, ptiCO$_2$, pHti and brain temperature.

A custom-built 10 mm flexible, microdialysis probe, 0.5 mm in diameter (molecular weight cut-off of 20 000 daltons), was used for measuring extracellular NO metabolites. It was perfused at 2 μl/minute using sterile 0.9% (w/v) saline, allowing 60 μl dialysates to be collected every half hour using a refrigerated (4°C), automated collector system (CMA 170, CMA Microdialysis). When possible, placement of the microdialysis probe and oxygen sensor system was in the vascular territory, which had the highest probability of developing ischemia and/or vasospasm. This was usually in the ipsilateral middle cerebral artery distribution, or in the territory of the anterior cerebral artery.

Nitrite and nitrate measurements

For total NO (nitrite and nitrate) measurements, a dialysate fraction (25 μl) was incubated with 5 μl nitrite reductase (10 U/ml), 1 μl NADP (4 mM), 5 μl phosphate-buffered saline and 14 μl 0.9% saline for 1 hour at room temperature. Thereafter, 15 μl sulfanilamide (1 mg/ml with 60 μl phosphoric acid) and 15 μl N-naphthylenediamine (10 mg/ml) were added to the samples for 10 minutes. The total volume (80 μl) was then measured for absorbance at 545 nm. For measuring nitrite alone, the Griess reagent was added to a 50 μl dialysate sample, instead of a 25 μl sample [13].

Endothelin-1 measurements

Endothelin-1 was measured by radioimmunoassay using an endothelin-1 radioimmunoassay (RIA) kit (Peninsula Laboratories, Belmont, CA). To increase the level of sensitivity of the assay, samples were lyophilized and reconstituted in 100 μl of the assay buffer.

Data collection and statistical analysis

The neurotrend data were collected every 5 minutes into a Macintosh computer (Apple Computers, Cupertino, CA). The mean $ptiO_2$ values over a period of 2 hours before and 2 hours after each nitrite/nitrate measurement were used for comparison. To calculate the relationship between NO and oxygen, the percentage change in NO production and $ptiO_2$ was used. The average $ptiO_2$ was calculated and the percentage change from the average $ptiO_2$ was calculated. Similarly, the percentage change in NO production from the average level of NO production for each patient was calculated and StatView 4.1 (Abacus Concepts, Berkeley, CA) was used for statistical analysis.

Results

Ten patients were selected who had a poor H & H grade (≥ 3), and two other patients with an initial H & H grade of 2, who later developed new neurological deficits and deteriorated to a grade 3, were included. Seven patients developed clinically significant vasospasms as diagnosed by xenon computed tomography CBF studies. Ten patients received full or partial "triple H" therapy to treat the vasospasms. Using the Glasgow Outcome Score to assess outcome at 3 months, the patients had made a good recovery; three patients had become moderately disabled, one patient remained vegetative and five patients had died.

Dialysate NO measurements

Nitrite and nitrate in the cerebral dialysate was used as an indirect indicator for NO production in these patients and there were significant fluctuations in microdialysis NO production during each patient's clinical course (Figure 15.1).

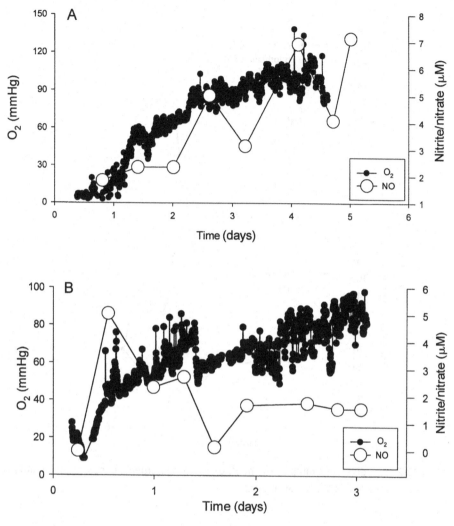

Figure 15.1   Close and linear relationship between dialysate NO (microdialysis NO) and oxygen tension (ptiO$_2$) in a patient (A) without vasospasm and (B) with vasospasm and ischemia.

Endothelin-1 in CSF and microdialysate

Endothelin-1 was measured in microdialysis as well as in CSF. On average, two CSF samples were taken from each patient every day and the corresponding microdialysis was used for endothelin-1 measurements. Figure 15.2 shows examples of two different patients' CSF and microdialysis changes of endothelin-1 over time.

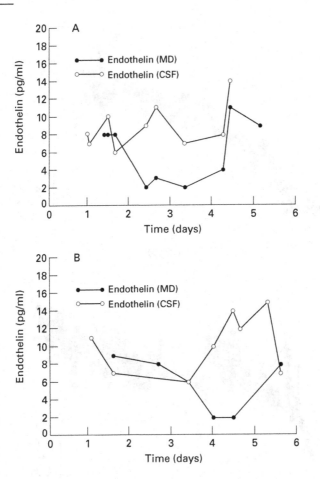

Figure 15.2. Two different examples of endothelin-1 measurements in cerebrospinal fluid (CSF) and microdialysis (MD) over time.

Correlation between NO metabolites, brain tissue oxygen and metabolism

A linear relationship was seen between brain tissue oxygen and NO metabolites in all patients, independent of whether the patient had a vasospasm. Single patient examples with and without vasospasm are shown in Figure 15.1. Figure 15.3 shows the relationship between percentage change in $ptiO_2$ and percentage change in NO production. A decrease in NO was significantly associated with a decline in $ptiO_2$ levels ($r^2 = 0.326$; $P < 0.001$). $ptiCO_2$, a possible indicator of the magnitude of aerobic metabolism and/or substrate clearance, did not change significantly and did not correlate with the changes in nitrite/nitrate.

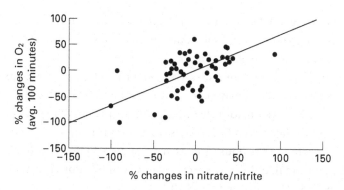

Figure 15.3 Percentage of changes in dialysate nitrate/nitrite and oxygen tension (ptiO$_2$) of all patients are shown ($r^2 = 0.326$; $P < 001$).

Discussion

NO is a highly reactive molecule that plays an important role in cerebral circulation in neurotransmission, platelet aggregation and in other peripheral physiological functions [5]. Because NO has a half-life of only seconds, clinical researchers have had great difficulty with its measurement in human tissue. Hence, its metabolites, such as nitrite and nitrate, are often measured in vivo as a surrogate indicator of its activity [14]. Unfortunately, the results obtained with nitrate measurements in plasma, CSF and urine have been highly inconsistent [15]. More recent studies have therefore focused on measuring extracellular NO metabolites in brain tissue using microdialysis. In this way, the systemic effects that overshadow central nervous system NO production are eliminated, and the measurements may be more accurate indicators of true cerebral NO events [16–18].

Previous studies have shown that endothelin-1 might be a good indicator of vasospasm when measured in the CSF of SAH patients [19–21]. However, we were unable to confirm that changes in CSF endothelin-1 or in microdialysate endothelin-1 correlate with changes in either brain tissue oxygen or NO metabolites (data not shown). Moreover, elevation in CSF endothelin-1 measurements (range: 3 to 20 pg/ml) was consistent with previous studies and seems to be closely related to microdialysis endothelin-1 (Figure 15.2).

In our small series, dialysate nitrite and nitrate ranged widely over time after SAH, and was not accompanied by changes in the production of NO in CSF (data not shown). The mean "NO metabolite" level over the entire monitoring period ranged from 1.8 to 5.8 μM in different patients. However, an increase in NO metabolites was significantly related to changes in brain tissue oxygen tension (Figure 15.3). Interestingly, brain tissue CO$_2$, which may be an indicator of cerebral substrate clearance, was unrelated to NO metabolites. A simultaneous increase in tissue NO and oxygen tension may reflect cerebral vasodilation and thus oxygen delivery, without changing cerebral oxidative metabolism and oxygen consumption, so that net tissue oxygen tension increases.

In animal models, there is an increase in NO production after ischemia, but its role is not understood [9]. It may be neurotoxic or neuroprotective in different situations. The known vasodilator role of NO, with its primary target being smooth muscle cells of regulatory cerebral vessels, makes its role in SAH-induced vasospasm intriguing [4,6]. Previous studies have shown that cerebral perfusion is increased by NO and that the intra-arterial delivery of NO donors actually reverses vasospasm in an SAH animal model [5,10,11].

These findings are supported by our data that show an increase in NO correlates with increased brain oxygen tension, suggestive of vasodilation. However, if severe vasospasm and tissue ischemia are present, extracellular NO decreases along with tissue oxygen tension. It is unknown whether this increase in NO production is due to stimulation of the constitutive NOS by glutamate-induced increases in intracellular calcium, or due to an upregulation of the inducible NOS. Furthermore, the source and significance of NO generated in neurons and glial cells vs. NO production in smooth muscles of cerebral vessels themselves remains unknown. The fact that CSF-NO was unrelated to dialysate NO and tissue oxygen tension in our study, may suggest that cerebral ischemia is related to NO generated from neurons and glial cells rather than from arterial wall cells alone. CSF may also fail to show dynamic changes in the NO metabolites, acting rather as a "sump" or storage reservoir, for these metabolites and thus, "averaging out" any fluctuations. Further studies, in which microdialysis probes are placed adjacent to the large cerebral vessels after aneurysm surgery and NO metabolite levels are compared with those from probes placed opposite, could provide more information in this area.

Conclusion

In summary, our study showed a decline in tissue NO production, accompanied by low brain tissue oxygen tension, during periods of ischemia, brain infarction and severe clinical vasospasm. Patients with normal or high ptiO$_2$ had a simultaneous increase in dialysate NO levels. CSF-NO was not related to extracellular NO production nor to oxygen tension. This study does provide evidence to support the hypothesis that NO donors may prevent or reverse post-SAH vasospasm and thus improve tissue oxygenation if administered early enough after SAH.

Acknowledgments

We are grateful for support from the Reynolds Foundation, the Lind Lawrence Foundation and National Institutes of Health grant no. NS 12587.

REFERENCES

1 Bredt DS, Hwang PM & Snyder SH (1990) Localization of NOS indicating a neural role of NO. *Nature,* **347,** 768–70.

2 Bredt DS & Snyder SH (1992) Nitric oxide, a novel neuronal messenger. *Neuron,* **8,** 3–11.

3 Garthwaite J & Boulton CL (1995) NO signaling in the CNS. *Annual Review of Physiology,* **57,** 683–706.

4 Furchgott RF & Zawadzki JV (1980) The obligatory role of endothelial cells in the relaxation of arterial smooth muscle by acetylcholine. *Nature,* **288,** 373–6.

5 Faraci FM & Brian JE (1994) NO and cerebral circulation. *Stroke,* **25,** 692–703.

6 Paakkari I & Lindsberg P (1995) NO in CNS. *Annals of Medicine,* **27,** 369–77.

7 Pluta RM, Thompson BG, Dawson TM, Snyder SH, Boock RJ & Oldfield EH (1996) Loss of nitric oxide synthase immunoreactivity in cerebral vasospasm. *Journal of Neurosurgery,* **84,** 648–54.

8 Wink DA, Hanbauer I, Grisham MB, Laval F, Nims RW, Laval J, Cook J, Pacelli R, Liebmann J, Krishna M, Ford PC & Mitchell JB (1996) Chemical biology of nitric oxide: regulation and protective and toxic mechanisms. *Current Topics in Cellular Regulation,* **34,** 159–87.

9 Suzuki Y, Osuka K, Noda A, Tanazawa T, Takayasu M, Shibuya M & Yoshida J (1997) Nitric oxide metabolites in the cisternal cerebral spinal fluid of patients with subarachnoid hemorrhage. *Neurosurgery,* **41,** 807–12.

10 Pluta RM, Oldfield EH & Boock RJ (1997) Reversal and prevention of cerebral vasospasm by intracarotid infusion of nitric oxide donors in a primate model of subarachnoid hemorrhage. *Journal of Neurosurgery,* **87,** 746–51.

11 Wolf EW, Banerjee A, Soble-Smith J, Dohan FC Jr, White RP & Robertson JT (1998) Reversal of cerebral vasospasm using an intrathecally administered nitric oxide donor. *Journal of Neurosurgery,* **89,** 279–88.

12 Zauner A, Bullock R, Di X & Young HF (1995) Brain oxygen, CO_2, pH and temperature monitoring: evaluation in the feline brain. *Neurosurgery,* **37,** 1168–76.

13 Green LC, Wagner DA, Glogowski J, Skipper PL, Wishnok JS & Tannenbaum SR (1982) Analysis of nitrate, nitrite, and [^{15}N]nitrate in biological fluids. *Analytical Biochemistry,* **126,** 131–8.

14 Grisham M, Johnson GG & Lancaster JR (1996) Quantification of nitrate and nitrite in extracellular fluids. *Methods in Enzymology,* **268,** 237–46.

15 Moshage H (1997) Nitric oxide determination: much ado about NO-thing? *Clinical Chemistry,* **43,** 553–6.

16 Luo D, Knezevich S & Vincent SR (1993) NMDA induced nitric oxide release: an in vivo microdialysis study. *Neuroscience,* **57,** 897–900.

17 Shintani F, Kanba S, Nakaki T, Sato K, Yagi G, Kato R & Asai M (1994) Measurement by in vivo brain microdialysis of nitric oxide release in the rat cerebellum. *Journal of Psychiatry & Neuroscience,* **19,** 217–21.

18 Yamada K & Nabeshima T (1997) Simultaneous measurement of nitrite and nitrate levels as indices of nitric oxide release in the cerebellum of conscious rats. *Journal of Neurochemistry,* **68,** 1234–43.

19 Suzuki R, Masaoka H, Hirata Y, Marumo F, Isotani E & Hirakawa K (1992) The role of endothelin-1 in the origin of cerebral vasospasm in patients with aneurysmal subarachnoid hemorrhage. *Journal of Neurosurgery,* 77, 96–100.

20 Zimmermann M (1997) Endothelin in cerebral vasospasm. Clinical and experimental results. *Journal of Neurosurgical Sciences,* 41, 139–51.

21 Suzuki K, Meguro K, Sakurai T, Saitoh Y, Takeuchi S & Nose T (2000) Endothelin-1 concentration increases in the cerebrospinal fluid in cerebral vasospasm caused by subarachnoid hemorrhage. *Surgical Neurology,* 53, 131–5.

16

Tissue plasminogen activator and hemorrhagic brain injury

Minoru Asahi[1], Rick M. Dijkhuizen[2], Xiaoying Wang[3], Bruce R. Rosen[4] & Eng H. Lo[5]

[1,2,3,5] Neuroprotection Research Laboratory, Departments of Neurology and Radiology, Massachusetts General Hospital, and Program in Neuroscience, Harvard Medical School, Boston, MA
[2,4] NMR Center, Massachusetts General Hospital, Harvard Medical School, Boston, MA

Effects of tissue-type plasminogen activator in acute clinical stroke

A rational approach to cerebral ischemia involves reperfusion of occluded arteries. Recent clinical trials have shown that thrombolytic therapy with tissue-type plasminogen activator (tPA) may be effective for acute ischemic stroke [1,2]. However, there is also an elevated risk of cerebral hemorrhage and further brain injury [3,4]. In all three of the major clinical trials (National Institute of Neurological Disorders and Stroke, European Cooperative Acute Stroke Study I and II), the odds ratio for intracerebral hemorrhage after tPA therapy was increased by about three-fold compared with placebo [5]. The precise mechanisms that underlie these negative effects of tPA remain unclear, but are clearly related to severity of the ischemic insult as well as to the timing of tPA-induced reperfusion. In this chapter, the literature on the neurotoxic effects of tPA will be briefly discussed, and data from our own laboratory will be provided with which we examine some of these mechanisms.

Effects of tPA in experimental cerebral ischemia

Although tPA-induced reperfusion of ischemic brain tissue is expected to salvage tissue, recent reports from the experimental literature have suggested that tPA may have neurotoxic effects as well. Wang and colleagues [6] have shown that infusion of tPA increased infarct size in a mouse model of focal cerebral ischemia. Potentially negative effects of tPA may be based on its ability to activate plasminogen and induce damaging extracellular proteolytic pathways [7,8]. Specifically, non-fibrin substrates for plasmin, such as laminin, may be degraded [9]. Proteolysis of laminin and other proteins in the extracellular matrix may amplify excitotoxicity.

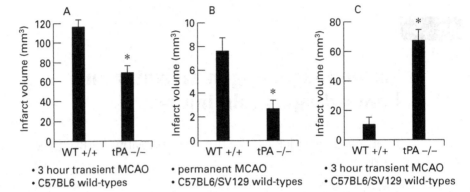

Figure 16.1 Ischemic infarct volumes (mean ± SEM) in tPA-deficient knockout mice. Variable results were obtained depending on the precise arterial occlusion conditions and background mouse strains used. * $P<0.05$. (A) Data from ref. 6; (B) data from ref. 17; (C) data from ref. 18. MCAO, middle cerebral artery occlusion.

It has been shown that knockout mice deficient in tPA or plasminogen were resistant to excitotoxic injury after intracerebral injections of kainate, N-methyl-D-aspartate and α-amino-3-hydroxy-5-methyl-4-isoxazole propionic acid [7,10,11]. Since excitotoxicity plays a central role in ischemic pathophysiology [12,13], it is conceivable that tPA can have detrimental effects on neuronal survival after stroke. Fundamentally, extracellular proteolysis can disrupt cell–matrix and cell–cell interactions leading to cell death [14–16].

The responses to cerebral ischemia in the knockout mouse models have been examined. The data in this area have been somewhat controversial. In the first study, knockout mice deficient in endogenous tPA expression showed reduced infarct size as compared with their wild-type littermates [6]. Since this first seminal paper, other groups have also examined these tPA knockouts, with variable results (Figure 16.1). One group confirmed that tPA knockouts were more resistant to focal ischemia [17], whereas another found that tPA knockouts actually had larger infarcts as compared with wild-type littermates [18]. This variability in ischemic outcomes is probably related to complex issues regarding genetic backgrounds of the contributing strains [19,20].

In an effort to further dissect these variable effects of tPA, several other groups [21,22], including our own [23], have attempted to detect negative effects of tPA in normal rat and mouse models of cerebral ischemia. In these three reports where cerebral ischemia was achieved by mechanically occluding arteries, no negative effects of exogenously administered tPA were discerned. These data suggest that while mechanisms for tPA-induced neurotoxicity certainly exist, the precise outcomes may depend critically on the model systems used.

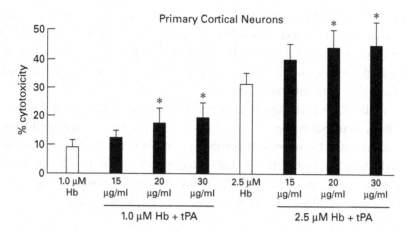

Figure 16.2   tPA amplifies hemoglobin-induced neurotoxicity in primary neuronal cultures. Hemoglobin (Hb) doses associated with low levels of cytotoxicity were combined with non-toxic low doses of tPA. Percentage cytotoxicity (mean ± SD) was calculated on the basis of maximal lactate dehydrogenase release. * $P < 0.05$ between cultures treated with hemoglobin alone vs. cultures treated with a combination of hemoglobin plus various doses of tPA.

tPA amplifies neuronal damage in vitro

As discussed above, the beneficial effects of tPA thrombolysis and cerebral reperfusion may sometimes be negated by hemorrhage. Obviously, any involvement of tPA in the pathophysiology of hemorrhagic injury would be of considerable clinical importance. Hemoglobin is a major component of blood, and one of the likely mediators of neurotoxicity after hemorrhagic injury [24]. Hemoglobin, via heme or Fe^{2+}, can induce oxidative damage and may also potentiate excitotoxic injury in neuronal cells [25]. Therefore, we sought to determine whether tPA could amplify hemoglobin-induced neurotoxicity in vitro [26].

In both PC12 cells and rat primary cortical cultures, hemoglobin induced a dose-dependent cytotoxic response, as expected. The highest dose examined (30 μM) resulted in over 80% cell death. On the other hand, 24 hours of exposure to tPA alone at low to medium concentrations (5 to 20 μg/ml, 580 IU/μg) did not induce significant lactate dehydrogenase release as compared with untreated control cultures. However, when cells were exposed to a combination of hemoglobin plus tPA, cytotoxicity was amplified. Whereas 1 or 2.5 μM hemoglobin alone resulted in low levels of cell damage, the combination of hemoglobin plus non-toxic doses of tPA significantly increased levels of cell death in both PC12 cells and primary cortical neurons (Figure 16.2). The possible relevance of our results is underlined by the fact that the doses of tPA used here are within the range of plasma concentrations (approximately 10 to 20 μg/ml) achieved after intravenous infusion of tPA in ischemic stroke [2]. Local concentrations of tPA can be even higher after intra-arterial applications or when used for clot lysis during surgical procedures for removal of intracerebral hematomas.

While tPA is being used as a form of thrombolytic therapy for acute ischemic stroke, some patients are exposed to elevated risks of intracerebral hemorrhage. Our data raise the important possibility that tPA may worsen outcomes after hemorrhage. When hemorrhage occurs as a complication of tPA therapy, further deterioration of the patient may be due to both the effects of hemorrhage per se as well as the additional toxicity of tPA-amplified hemoglobin effects.

tPA induces hemorrhage in a rat model of embolic focal ischemia

Traditional animal models of cerebral ischemia have involved occlusion of cerebral arteries by mechanical means, via external ligation with a suture, clamping with aneurysm clips or permanent vascular occlusion via cautery. While these models have provided a wealth of data on the pathophysiology of cerebral ischemia, they are not suitable for investigating tPA thrombolysis and its associated effects in vivo. More recently, models of embolic focal cerebral ischemia have been developed [27–31]. In these rodent models that use homologous blood clots, delayed treatment with tPA resulted in hemorrhagic transformations [32–34]. In our laboratory, we have used a quantitative model of tPA-induced hemorrhage in rats to investigate the pathophysiology of tPA-induced reperfusion and possible secondary tissue injury related to cerebral hemorrhage [35]. Focal cerebral ischemia was induced by selectively placing homologous blood clots within the proximal trunk of the middle cerebral artery in rats, and delayed administration of 10 mg tPA/kg was performed intravenously at 6 hours after ischemic onset.

Clinical data suggest that high systemic blood pressure may increase the risk of cerebral hemorrhage [36]. Therefore, experiments were conducted to compare normotensive Wistar–Kyoto (WK) rats with spontaneously hypertensive (SH) rats. Overall, hemorrhage severity was much lower in the normotensive WK rats compared with the SH rats, and tPA did not significantly increase cerebral hemorrhage (Figure 16.3). Indeed, 24 hour infarct volumes and neurological deficits were significantly improved by tPA in the normotensive WK rats. In contrast, tPA significantly increased the severity of hemorrhage in the SH rats (Figure 16.3). Concomitantly, infarct volumes and neurological deficits in SH rats were also worsened by tPA, and the severity of hemorrhage was positively correlated with infarct volumes ($r=0.611$, $P<0.01$). Although we cannot unequivocally exclude a role for

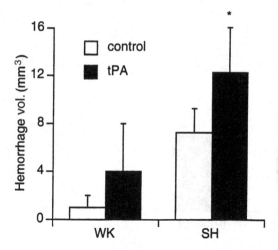

Figure 16.3 In spontaneously hypertensive (SH) rats subjected to clot-induced embolic stroke, tPA significantly increased hemorrhage volumes (mean ± SD) compared with untreated rats. Although tPA appeared to slightly increase hemorrhage in normotensive Wistar–Kyoto (WK) rats, the difference was not statistically significant. * $P < 0.05$.

other genetic differences in the hypertensive SH rats, it is likely that increased blood pressure may be the most parsimonious explanation here.

Alpha-phenyl-tert-butyl-nitrone reduces tPA-induced hemorrhage and brain injury

Reperfusion injury after ischemia involves mechanisms of oxidative stress and injury [37–39]. Oxidative injury may play a role in mediating cerebrovascular damage after tPA thrombolytic stroke therapy, thus predisposing brain tissue to hemorrhage [40,41]. Based on this supposition, we sought to determine whether combining some form of free radical scavenging therapy with tPA would decrease risks and severity of tPA-induced hemorrhage and enhance positive outcomes [35]. Hypertensive SH rats were subjected to embolic focal ischemia as before. Rats treated with 10 mg tPA/kg 6 hours postischemia were compared with rats treated with tPA plus 20 mg of the free radical spin trap alpha-phenyl-tert-butyl-nitrone (α-PBN) per kilogram.

Delayed tPA administration induced hemorrhage as expected (Figure 16.4). Combination treatment with α-PBN significantly reduced hemorrhage severity (6.7 ± 4.2 mm³ in rats treated with α-PBN plus tPA vs. 11.1 ± 3.8 mm³ in rats given tPA

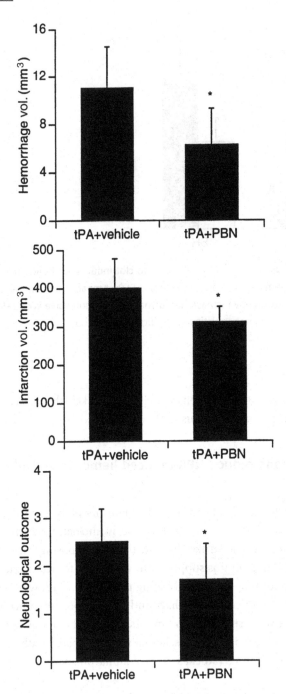

Figure 16.4 In SH rats subjected to clot-induced embolic stroke, tPA-associated hemorrhage was significantly reduced by cotreatment with the free radical spin trap α-PBN. Concomitantly, infarct volumes were reduced and neurological deficits were improved.
Mean ± SD. * $P < 0.05$. PBN, alpha-phenyl-tert-butyl-nitrone.

alone; $P = 0.004$) (Figure 16.4). Concomitantly, infarct volumes and neurological outcomes were significantly improved as well (Figure 16.4).

These findings suggest that compounds targeted against oxidative injury may prove valuable when used in combination treatments for ameliorating hemorrhage risks associated with thrombolytic stroke therapy. Clearly, the underlying molecular mechanisms involved remain to be fully established. Additional studies utilizing this model are warranted to explore the mechanisms involved, test therapeutic windows and translate these findings into potential clinical applications.

Magnetic resonance markers of tPA-induced hemorrhage

In recent years, magnetic resonance imaging (MRI) has become an important tool in the diagnosis of both clinical and experimental stroke. Conventional T_1- and T_2-weighted imaging, and newly developed diffusion- and perfusion-weighted MRI techniques enable comprehensive and non-invasive assessments of acute ischemic tissue damage and perfusion deficits. Recently, these techniques have been applied to assess the efficacy of tPA treatment in rat embolic stroke models. It was demonstrated that tPA administration within 1 hour after stroke improves cerebral blood flow and reduces ischemic tissue damage [42,43]. However, delayed tPA treatment (4 hours after ischemic onset) did not significantly alter MRI parameters [44].

In our laboratory, we have applied MRI after embolic stroke in hypertensive SH rats to correlate ischemic brain damage, before and after late tPA therapy (6 hours after stroke), with development of intracerebral hemorrhage. Perfusion-weighted dynamic susceptibility contrast-enhanced MRI, using GdDTPA (gadolinium diethylene triamine penta-acetic acid) as a contrast agent, demonstrated incomplete and variable reperfusion after tPA injection. Administration of tPA led to an increase in the apparent diffusion coefficient and T_2 of tissue water, suggestive of development of vasogenic edema. As expected, intracerebral hemorrhage developed in all animals. In order to assess the blood–brain barrier status, we performed pre- and post-GdDTPA T_1-weighted MRI. GdDTPA tissue enhancement reflects blood–brain barrier breakdown, which has been shown to occur early after reperfusion. A previous study demonstrated that GdDTPA leakage matched areas of hemorrhage in the intraluminal filament model of transient focal cerebral ischemia in rats [45]. In the present model of embolic focal ischemia, clear post-GdDTPA T_1-weighted signal intensity enhancement was evident prior to tPA administration in areas where hemorrhage emerged at later stages after tPA (Figure 16.5). Additionally, areas with tPA-induced intracerebral hemorrhage had significantly lower relative cerebral blood flow levels as compared with areas in which there was no hemorrhagic transformation. These results suggest that intracerebral hemorrhage emerges in areas with relatively low perfusion levels and early blood–brain

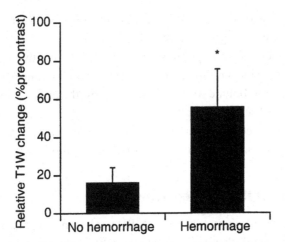

Figure 16.5 MRI predictors of hemorrhage. SH rats were subjected to embolic focal ischemia, and tPA was administered 6 hours later. Relative post-GdDTPA T_1-weighted (T1W) signal intensity change (percentage of precontrast) obtained 1 hour before tPA administration was significantly higher in the ischemic areas, with subsequent intracerebral hemorrhage. Mean ± SD. * $P<0.05$ vs. areas with no hemorrhage.

barrier perturbations. Hence, MRI may be used to quantify the effects of thrombolytic therapy and possibly predict the risk of hemorrhagic transformation.

Conclusion

Thrombolysis with tPA has been shown to be effective in acute ischemic stroke if administered within the proper therapeutic window. However, there are emerging reports that, aside from its beneficial clot lysis properties, tPA may also have complex neurotoxic effects in the cerebral parenchyma. These effects may critically depend on the model systems used, and warrant further investigation. One clear negative with tPA is the increased risk of hemorrhage. Here, we described a rat model of tPA-induced hemorrhage and showed that combination therapy with free-radical spin traps may be a potentially important way of ameliorating these risks. Finally, MRI markers of stroke and hemorrhagic risks are now being elucidated by our laboratory and others. The use of in vivo MRI correlates and predictors, together with combination therapies, may significantly optimize the efficacy and safety of thrombolytic therapy for acute ischemic stroke.

Acknowledgments

This work was supported in part by National Institutes of Health grants R01–NS37074, R01–NS38731, R01–NS40529, R01–HL39810, and P50–NS10828.

Dr. Dijkhuizen was supported by the Netherlands Organization for Scientific Research (NWO) and currently holds a fellowship from the American Heart Association. The authors thank Drs. Michael Moskowitz and Stella Tsirka for helpful discussions.

REFERENCES

1 Hacke W, Kaste M, Fieschi C, Toni D, Lesaffre E, von Kummer R, Boysen G, Bluhmki E, Höxter G, Mahagne M-H & Hennerici M, for the ECASS Study Group (1995) Intravenous thrombolysis with recombinant tissue plasminogen activator for acute hemispheric stroke. The European Cooperative Acute Stroke Study (ECASS). *Journal of the American Medical Association*, **274**, 1017–25.

2 The National Institute of Neurological Disorders and Stroke rtPA Stroke Study Group (1995) Tissue plasminogen activator for acute ischemic stroke. *New England Journal of Medicine*, **333**, 1581–7.

3 Larrue V, von Kummer R, del Zoppo G & Bluhmki, E. (1997) Hemorrhagic transformation in acute ischemic stroke. Potential contributing factors in the European Cooperative Acute Stroke Study. *Stroke*, **28**, 957–60.

4 The NINDS t-PA Stroke Study Group (1997) Intracerebral hemorrhage after intravenous t-PA therapy for ischemic stroke. *Stroke*, **28**, 2109–18.

5 Hacke W, Brott T, Caplan L, Meier D, Fieschi C, von Kummer R, Donnan G, Heiss WD, Wahlgren NG, Spranger M, Boysen G & Marler JR (1999) Thrombolysis in acute ischemic stroke: controlled trials and clinical experience. *Neurology*, **53** (Suppl 4), S3–S15.

6 Wang YF, Tsirka SE, Strickland S, Stieg PE, Soriano SG & Lipton SA (1998) Tissue plasminogen activator (tPA) increases neuronal damage after focal cerebral ischemia in wild-type and tPA-deficient mice. *Nature Medicine*, **4**, 228–31.

7 Tsirka SE, Rogove AD, Bugge TH, Degen JL & Strickland S (1997) An extracellular proteolytic cascade promotes neuronal degeneration in the mouse hippocampus. *Journal of Neuroscience*, **17**, 543–52.

8 Tsirka SE, Bugge TH, Degen JL & Strickland S (1997) Neuronal death in the central nervous system demonstrates a non-fibrin substrate for plasmin. *Proceedings of the National Academy of Sciences, USA*, **94**, 9779–81.

9 Chen ZL & Strickland S (1997) Neuronal death in the hippocampus is promoted by plasmin-catalyzed degradation of laminin. *Cell*, **91**, 917–25.

10 Tsirka SE, Gualandris A, Amaral DG & Strickland S (1995) Excitotoxin-induced neuronal degeneration and seizure are mediated by tissue plasminogen activator. *Nature*, **377**, 340–4.

11 Tsirka SE, Rogove AD & Strickland S (1996) Neuronal cell death and tPA. *Nature*, **384**, 123–4.

12 Choi DW & Rothman SM (1990) The role of glutamate neurotoxicity in hypoxic-ischemic neuronal death. *Annual Review of Neuroscience*, **13**, 171–82.

13 Lipton SA & Rosenberg PA (1994) Mechanisms of disease: excitatory amino acids as a final common pathway for neurologic disorders. *New England Journal of Medicine*, **330**, 613–22.

14 Frisch SM & Francis H (1994) Disruption of epithelial cell-matrix interactions induces apoptosis. *Journal of Cell Biology*, **124**, 619–26.

15 Meredith JE Jr, Fazeli B & Schwartz MA (1993) The extracellular matrix as a cell survival factor. *Molecular Biology of the Cell*, **4**, 953–61.

16 Shi YB, Damjanowski S, Amano T & Ishizuya A (1998) Regulation of apoptosis during development: input from the extracellular matrix. *International Journal of Molecular Medicine*, **2**, 273–82.

17 Nagai N, De Mol M, Lijnen HR, Carmeliet P & Collen D (1999) Role of plasminogen system components in focal cerebral ischemic infarction. A gene targeting and gene transfer study in mice. *Circulation*, **99**, 2440–4.

18 Tabrizi P, Wang L, Seeds N, McComb JG, Yamada S, Griffin JH, Carmeliet P, Weiss MH & Zlokovic BV (1999) Tissue plasminogen activator (tPA) deficiency exacerbates cerebrovascular fibrin deposition and brain injury in a murine stroke model: studies in tPA-deficient mice and wild-type mice on a matched genetic background. *Arteriosclerosis, Thrombosis, and Vascular Biology*, **19**, 2801–6.

19 Ginsberg MD (1999) On ischemic brain injury in genetically altered mice. *Arteriosclerosis, Thrombosis, and Vascular Biology*, **19**, 2581–3.

20 Schauwecker PE & Steward O (1997) Genetic determinants of susceptibility to excitotoxic cell death: implications for gene targeting approaches. *Proceedings of the National Academy of Sciences, USA*, **94**, 4103–8.

21 Klein GM, Li H, Sun P & Buchan AM (1999) Tissue plasminogen activator does not increase neuronal damage in rat models of global and focal ischemia. *Neurology*, **52**, 1381–4.

22 Kilic E, Hermann DM & Hossmann KA (1999) Recombinant tissue plasminogen activator reduces infarct size after reversible thread occlusion of middle cerebral artery in mice. *Neuroreport*, **10**, 107–11.

23 Meng W, Wang X, Asahi M, Kano T, Asahi K, Ackerman RH & Lo EH (1999) Effects of tissue type plasminogen activator in embolic versus mechanical models of focal cerebral ischemia in rats. *Journal of Cerebral Blood Flow & Metabolism*, **19**, 1316–21.

24 Regan RF & Panter SS (1993) Neurotoxicity of hemoglobin in cortical cell culture. *Neuroscience Letters*, **153**, 219–22.

25 Regan RF & Panter SS (1996) Hemoglobin potentiates excitotoxic injury in cortical cell culture. *Journal of Neurotrauma*, **13**, 223–31.

26 Wang X, Asahi M & Lo EH (1999) Tissue type plasminogen activator amplifies hemoglobin-induced neurotoxicity in rat neuronal cultures. *Neuroscience Letters*, **274**, 79–82.

27 Busch E, Krüger K & Hossmann K-A (1997) Improved model of thromboembolic stroke and rtPA induced reperfusion in the rat. *Brain Research*, **778**, 16–24.

28 Kudo M, Aoyama A, Ichimori S & Fukunaga N (1982) An animal model of cerebral infarction. Homologous blood clot emboli in rats. *Stroke*, **13**, 505–8.

29 Overgaard K, Sereghy T, Boysen G, Pedersen H, Hoyer S & Diemer NH (1992) A rat model of reproducible cerebral infarction using thrombotic blood clot emboli. *Journal of Cerebral Blood Flow & Metabolism*, **12**, 484–90.

30 Sakurama T, Kitamura R & Kaneko M (1994) Tissue-type plasminogen activator improves neurological functions in a rat model of thromboembolic stroke. *Stroke*, **25**, 451–6.

31 Zhang Z, Zhang RL, Jiang Q, Raman SBK, Cantwell L & Chopp M (1997) A new rat model of thrombotic focal cerebral ischemia. *Journal of Cerebral Blood Flow & Metabolism,* **17,** 123–35.

32 Chopp M, Zhang RL, Zhang ZG & Jiang Q (1999) The clot thickens – thrombolysis and combination therapies. *Acta Neurochirurgica Supplementum,* **73,** 67–71.

33 Brinker G, Pillekamp F & Hossmann KA (1999) Brain hemorrhages after rtPA treatment of embolic stroke in spontaneously hypertensive rats. *Neuroreport,* **10,** 1943–6.

34 Kano T, Katayama Y, Tejima E & Lo EH (2000) Hemorrhagic transformation after fibrinolytic therapy with tissue plasminogen activator in a rat thromboembolic model of stroke. *Brain Research,* **854,** 245–8.

35 Asahi M, Asahi K, Wang X & Lo EH (2000) Reduction of tissue plasminogen activator-induced hemorrhage and brain injury by free radical spin trapping after embolic focal cerebral ischemia in rats. *Journal of Cerebral Blood Flow & Metabolism,* **20,** 452–7.

36 Levy DE, Brott TG, Haley EC Jr, Marler JR, Sheppard GL, Barsan W & Broderick JP (1994) Factors related to intracranial hematoma formation in patients receiving tissue-type plasminogen activator for acute ischemic stroke. *Stroke,* **25,** 291–7.

37 Akins PT, Liu PK & Hsu CY (1996) Immediate early gene expression in response to cerebral ischemia. Friend or foe? *Stroke,* **27,** 1682–7.

38 Chan PH (1996) Role of oxidants in ischemic brain damage. *Stroke,* **27,** 1124–9.

39 Hallenbeck JM & Dutka AJ (1990) Background review and current concepts of reperfusion injury. *Archives of Neurology,* **47,** 1245–54.

40 del Zoppo GJ, Zeumer H & Harker LA (1986) Thrombolytic therapy in stroke: possibilities and hazards. *Stroke,* **7,** 595–607.

41 Lyden PD & Zivin JA (1993) Hemorrhagic transformation after cerebral ischemia: mechanisms and incidence. *Cerebrovascular & Brain Metabolism Reviews,* **5,** 1–16.

42 Busch E, Krüger K, Allegrini PR, Kerskens CM, Gyngell ML, Hoehn-Berlage M & Hossmann K-A (1998) Reperfusion after thrombolytic therapy of embolic stroke in the rat: magnetic resonance and biochemical imaging. *Journal of Cerebral Blood Flow & Metabolism,* **18,** 407–18.

43 Jiang Q, Zhang RL, Zhang ZG, Ewing JR, Divine GW & Chopp M (1998) Diffusion-, T_2-, and perfusion-weighted nuclear magnetic resonance imaging of middle cerebral artery embolic stroke and recombinant tissue plasminogen activator intervention in the rat. *Journal of Cerebral Blood Flow & Metabolism,* **18,** 758–67.

44 Jiang Q, Zhang RL, Zhang ZG, Ewing JR, Jiang P, Divine GW, Knight RA & Chopp M (2000) Magnetic resonance imaging indexes of therapeutic efficacy of recombinant tissue plasminogen activator treatment of rat at 1 and 4 hours after embolic stroke. *Journal of Cerebral Blood Flow & Metabolism,* **20,** 21–7.

45 Knight RA, Barker PB, Fagan SC, Li Y, Jacobs MA, Welch KMA & Fisher M (1998) Prediction of impending hemorrhagic transformation in ischemic stroke using magnetic resonance imaging in rats. *Stroke,* **29,** 144–51.

17

Dynamics of infarct evolution after permanent and transient focal brain ischemia in mice

Konstantin-Alexander Hossmann[1], Ryuji Hata[2] & Takayuki Hara[3]

[1-3] Max-Planck-Institute for Neurological Research, Department of Experimental Neurology, Cologne, Germany

Introduction

Acute occlusion of a large brain artery causes focal ischemia with a flow gradient that decreases from the peripheral to the more central parts of the occluded vascular territory. According to the threshold concept of brain ischemia, tissue viability is immediately endangered in the core of the ischemic territory in which blood flow declines below the critical level required to support energy metabolism [1,2]. The surrounding penumbra is only functionally impaired, but with increasing time of vascular occlusion, tissue viability deteriorates until, within 6 to 12 hours, both the core and penumbra undergo ischemic infarction [3]. If vascular occlusion is reversed, part of the ischemic territory may recover, depending on the duration and severity of the flow impairment. However, after a delay that can be as long as several weeks, a secondary type of brain injury may evolve, which leads to delayed infarction within the territory of the formerly occluded brain vessel [4,5]. Finally, a spontaneous or drug-induced recirculation may occur, which differs from transient surgical occlusion by the slow restitution of flow, and which may aggravate rather than reverse ischemic injury [6,7].

Obviously, each of these ischemic conditions presents a different pathophysiology, with different requirements for therapeutic interventions. To analyze the underlying mechanisms it is necessary to describe, in a first step, the detailed regional and temporal evolution of tissue injury. A straightforward way to achieve this goal is the application of multiparametric imaging techniques to the various focal ischemia models. This approach includes bioluminescence imaging of adenosine triphosphate (ATP) to detect energy failure, amino acid autoradiography to image cerebral protein synthesis (CPS), terminal deoxynucleotidyl transferase-mediated uridine 5'-triphosphate-biotin nick end labeling (TUNEL) histochemistry to detect DNA fragmentation and in situ hybridization autoradiograms to image specific genomic expression patterns. In a series of experimental investigations, which are described in more detail elsewhere, this approach was used in three models of murine focal ischemia, i.e., permanent thread occlusion to study the expansion of the infarct core into the penumbra [3], transient thread occlusion to investigate the evolution of secondary infarction under conditions of undisturbed recirculation [8] and reversible clot embolism to replicate the clinically more relevant gradual restoration of blood flow after thrombolytic therapy [9].

Material and methods

Production of focal brain ischemia

Experiments were carried out in halothane-anesthetized adult male C57 Black/6J mice weighing 20 to 30 g. Transient or permanent middle cerebral artery (MCA) thread occlusion was done by a modification of the technique described by Koizumi et al. [10], using threads with silicon-coated tips the diameter of which (0.05 to 0.20 mm) was matched to the body weight of the animals [3]. MCA clot embolism was performed by a method developed in our laboratory [11]. Cylindrical blood clots were prepared in PE10 catheters by mixing fresh arterial blood with thrombin, and four fibrin-rich segments 4 mm in length (corresponding to 0.284 μl clot material) were flushed retrogradely through the external into the internal carotid artery. Thrombolysis of clots was carried out by intracarotid infusion of 10 mg recombinant tissue plasminogen activator (rtPA)/kg (Alteplas, Boehringer-Ingelheim, Germany). In both thread- and clot-occluded animals, blood flow was monitored by laser Doppler flowmetry.

Brain imaging in animals with permanent thread occlusion was performed 1, 3 and 6 hours and 3 days after thread insertion, respectively. In experiments with reversible thread occlusion, the thread was withdrawn after 1 hour and the brains were investigated after 1, 3, 6 and 24 hours and 3 days of reperfusion. Thrombolysis of the MCA clot embolism was started 1 hour after injection of the clots, and the animals were investigated before and after 1, 3, 6 and 24 hours of treatment. Embolized animals selected for 3 day survival died between the first and second days, and therefore could not be submitted to the brain imaging protocol.

Brain imaging

Forty-five minutes before termination of experiments, the animals received an intraperitoneal injection of L-[4, 5-³H]leucine (150 μCi, Amersham, Braunschweig, Germany) for autoradiographic measurement of global protein synthesis [12]. The brains were frozen in situ with liquid nitrogen and cut into 20 μm thick coronal cryostat sections. Pictorial ATP measurements were prepared using an ATP-specific bioluminescence assay [13]. For measurement of CPS, brain slices were incubated in 10% (v/v) trichloroacetic acid to remove labeled free leucine and metabolites other than proteins. Subsequently, slices were exposed for 14 days with ^{3}H standards to tritium-sensitive X-ray film (Hyperfilm ^{3}H; Amersham) for autoradiography of ^{3}H-labeled proteins.

Pictorial assays of c-Fos, JunB and HSP70 mRNAs were performed by in situ hybridization using appropriate ^{35}S-labeled oligonucleotide probes [3]. Brain sections were fixed for 15 minutes in 4% (v/v) paraformaldehyde/phosphate-buffered saline, pH 7.4, and after overnight hybridization at 42 °C, were exposed to autoradiographic film (Hyperfilm β-max; Amersham).

TUNEL was performed by incubating paraformaldehyde/phosphate-buffered saline-fixed cryostat sections in a terminal deoxynucleotidyl transferase mix (150 U/ml; Life Technologies, Eggenstein, Germany, and 10 pmol/l biotin-16-deoxyuridine 5′-triphosphate; Boehringer-Mannheim, Germany) [3]. Incorporated biotin was visualized with the avidin-biotin peroxidase complex method (Vector Laboratories, Burlingame, CA).

For image analysis, the National Institutes of Health image software (version 1.61) was used. Images were digitized with a closed-circuit digital camera and the volumes of ATP depletion and CPS inhibition were measured using a semiautomated method [14]. ATP depletion was defined as a decline to less than 30% of the value of the contralateral side. The threshold for CPS was set to the lowest CPS value of the non-ischemic hemisphere, excluding fiber tracts. The areas of ATP depletion and CPS inhibition were measured on each section by subtracting the area of the non-lesioned ipsilateral hemisphere from that of the contralateral hemisphere. The areas of preserved ATP and protein synthesis were outlined and superimposed to demarcate penumbral tissue in which protein synthesis was suppressed but ATP was preserved [3].

To evaluate the regional reproducibility of measurements, regional incidence maps were constructed [3]. The areas of biochemical disturbances were outlined on representative brain sections from each individual experiment and superimposed at two coronal levels at the caudate putamen and the dorsal hippocampus. Using the image analysis software, the incidence of the metabolic alterations was calculated for each pixel and expressed as percentage of the number of animals per group.

Statistics

All values are given as means ± standard deviation (SD). Differences in metabolic parameters and relative in situ hybridization radioactivity of mRNAs were compared using one-way analysis of variance.

Permanent MCA thread occlusion

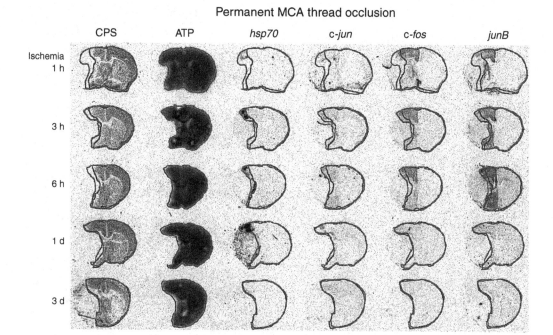

Figure 17.1   Coronal sections of the mouse brain at the level of the caudate putamen at various intervals after the onset of permanent middle cerebral artery occlusion. Multiparametric imaging of CPS, ATP content and the expression of Hsp70, c-Jun, c-Fos and JunB mRNA. The outlines of preserved ATP and CPS have been superimposed to demarcate the core from the penumbra of the evolving infarct. Note gradual expansion of infarct core (defined as the ATP-depleted tissue) into the penumbra (defined as the tissue with suppressed CPS but preserved ATP) and differential expression of *hsp*70 and immediate early genes in the penumbra and the peri-infarct normal brain tissue.

Results

Permanent MCA thread occlusion

Brain metabolism

In the sham-operated controls, regional ATP content and regional CPS did not differ between hemispheres. After MCA occlusion (MCAO), both ATP and CPS were severely reduced in the ipsilateral hemisphere, but the regional distribution of the changes differed between ATP and CPS, on the one hand, and with the duration of ischemia on the other (Figures 17.1 and 17.2).

After 1 hour of vascular occlusion, ATP was depleted in the frontoparietal cortex, the lateral part of the caudate putamen and the piriform cortex. Suppression of protein synthesis was present in the same areas, but the changes extended distinctly

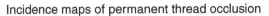

Incidence maps of permanent thread occlusion

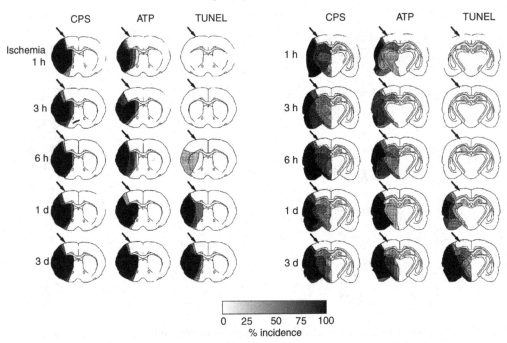

Figure 17.2 Incidence maps of suppressed CPS, ATP depletion and neurons positive for TUNEL on coronal sections of the mouse brain at various times after the onset of permanent MCAO. Areas of disturbed metabolism were outlined in five animals per time point at the level of the caudate putamen (left) and dorsal hippocampus (right) and superimposed to calculate the incidence of alterations as the percentage of the number of animals per group. The demarcation between normal and disturbed protein synthesis in the parietal cortex visible at 1 hour of MCAO was marked by the arrows to estimate the evolution of the metabolic disturbances at later time points. Notice the gradual expansion of the ATP-depleted area into, but not beyond, the area of disturbed CPS visible after 1 hour, and the delayed appearance of TUNEL within, but not outside, the ATP-depleted region. These findings demonstrate that early inhibition of protein synthesis heralds the final manifestation of infarction and that DNA fragmentation occurs in the core, but not in the penumbra of evolving infarcts.

more into the frontal, medial and temporooccipital parts of the MCA territory. With increasing ischemia time, the ATP-depleted tissue mass, but not the volume of tissue with inhibition of CPS, gradually expanded until within 1 day, ATP- and CPS-impaired regions merged (Figure 17.1). On coronal brain sections at the level of the caudate putamen, the ATP-depleted area thus increased from $40.1 \pm 11\%$ (means $\pm$ SD) of the hemispheric cross-sectional area at 1 hour of MCAO to $47.4 \pm 11.9\%$ after 3 hours, $49.0 \pm 13.6\%$ after 6 hours, $56.2 \pm 4.7\%$ after 1 day and 58.2

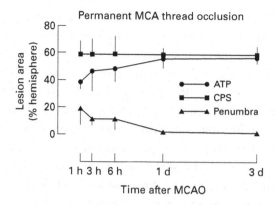

Figure 17.3   Dynamics of infarct evolution in the mouse brain during permanent MCAO. The areas of suppressed CPS, ATP depletion and penumbral tissue (defined as the area of suppressed CPS but preserved ATP) were measured at the level of the caudate putamen and expressed as percentage of the opposite non-ischemic hemisphere. Note the gradual expansion of the ATP-depleted brain tissue into the region of suppressed protein synthesis, indicating growth of the infarct core into the peri-infarct penumbra.

± 3.9% after 3 days, respectively (Figure 17.3). The area of CPS inhibition remained almost constant during this time and amounted to 58.9 ± 5.5% after 1 hour, 59.3 ± 14.9% after 3 hours, 59.6 ± 9.4% after 6 hours, 59.0 ± 5.4% after 1 day and 60.2 ± 3.8% after 3 days of MCAO. Accordingly, the penumbra, defined as the area of disturbed protein synthesis but preserved energy state, gradually declined from close to 20% after 1 hour of ischemia to less than 3% after 1 day.

Quantitative evaluations of ATP and CPS in different anatomical structures confirmed the progression of metabolic disturbances and revealed that 3 days after MCAO ATP reduction was most pronounced in the somatosensory, temporal and piriform cortex, as well as in the lateral and medial caudate putamen. Reductions were also seen in the hippocampus, thalamus and hypothalamus, but these changes did not reach a level of significance.

To evaluate the consistency of the regional extent of metabolic alterations, injury incidence maps were prepared by superposition of the areas of reduced ATP and CPS observed in each individual experiment (Figure 17.2). These incidence maps revealed a remarkable reproducibility of the metabolic alterations and confirmed the robustness of early CPS inhibition for predicting the final size of brain infarcts.

Genomic expressions

Representative examples of in situ hybridization autoradiograms of the mRNAs of HSP70 and the products of the immediate early genes c-*fos*, c-*jun* and *junB* are shown in Figure 17.1. Transcription of the stress gene HSP70 was confined mainly to the penumbra, whereas transcription of the immediate early genes c-*jun*, c-*fos* and *JunB* extended into the normal brain tissue of the ipsilateral hemisphere.

The dynamics of gene expression were studied by measuring the optical densities of the in situ hybridization signals in the infarct core, in the penumbral cortex and in the paramedian normal cortex of the ipsilateral hemisphere. HSP70 mRNA expression sharply increased in the penumbra, reaching a peak 3 hours after vascular occlusion. Expression of the immediate early genes increased from 1 to 6 hours after MCAO, both in the penumbra and the peri-ischemic normal cortex, but the relative distributions were different: the concentrations of c-Fos and JunB mRNAs were highest in the non-ischemic normal cortex of the ipsilateral hemisphere, whereas c-Jun mRNA was increased more in the penumbra. Interestingly, c-Jun mRNA expression remained elevated throughout the observation time of 3 days, whereas all the other mRNAs returned to normal during this time.

TUNEL

After MCAO, DNA fragmentation as visualized by TUNEL was clearly confined to neurons and appeared much later than the changes in ATP and CPS (Figure 17.2). The number of TUNEL-positive neurons was highest in the central parts of the ischemic territory, and at no time could TUNEL be detected in the penumbral regions. Quite to the contrary, TUNEL became prominent 1 day after MCAO, i.e., at a time at which the penumbra had disappeared and brain infarcts had already reached their final size. This excludes any significant contribution of TUNEL-visible DNA fragmentation to infarct expansion.

Transient MCA thread occlusion

Brain metabolism

When the brain was reperfused after 1 hour of MCAO, inhibition of CPS was initially little changed (Figures 17.4 and 17.5). At the level of the caudate putamen the CPS-inhibited area was $54.1 \pm 2.6\%$ at 1 hour, $56.9 \pm 6.1\%$ at 3 hours and $56.6 \pm 4.8\%$ 6 hours after the onset of reperfusion (Figure 17.6). Later, the area with suppressed CPS decreased to $48.7 \pm 4.5\%$ at 1 day ($P<0.05$) and to $37.2 \pm 7.3\%$ at 3 days ($P<0.01$) after reperfusion, but it never fully recovered.

In contrast to CPS, ATP returned transiently. After recirculation for 1 hour, ATP was almost completely restored, but with longer periods of reperfusion, ATP again deteriorated. The mean area of ATP depletion at the level of the caudate putamen thus secondarily increased from $7.2 \pm 10.9\%$ of the non-ischemic contralateral hemisphere at 3 hours to $14.2 \pm 10.4\%$ at 6 hours, $19.7 \pm 17.9\%$ at 1 day and $34.8 \pm 9.2\%$ 3 days, after the onset of reperfusion, respectively. At 3 days, ATP depletion had merged with the area of CPS inhibition, leading to the sharp demarcation of the brain infarct from the normal brain tissue.

Transient MCA thread occlusion

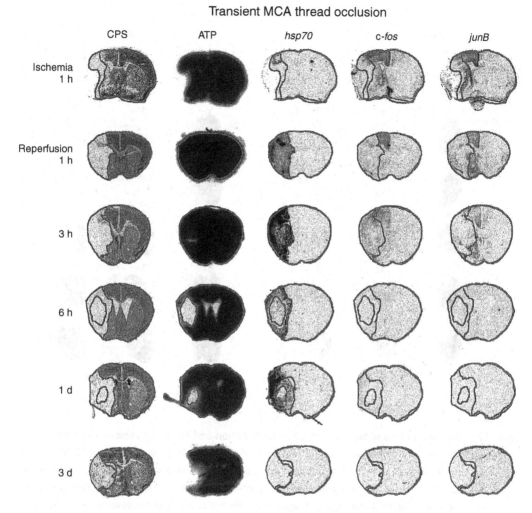

Figure 17.4   Multiparametric images of CPS, tissue ATP content and Hsp70, c-Fos and JunB mRNAs of representative brain sections of mice at the level of the caudate putamen after various reperfusion times following transient MCAO for 1 hour. The outlines of preserved ATP and CPS have been superimposed to demarcate the metabolically impaired areas from the normal brain tissue.

The reproducibility of these changes was confirmed by the injury incidence maps (Figure 17.5). These maps document clearly that CPS inhibition remained virtually constant from the end of the 1 hour ischemic period up to 6 hours after reperfusion, whereas ATP transiently recovered. However, starting 3 hours after ischemia ATP secondarily deteriorated, first in the dorsal hippocampus and the central parts of the caudate putamen and later in the more peripheral parts of the MCA-supplying territory. After 3 days of recirculation the region of ATP depletion precisely matched the region of suppressed CPS.

Incidence maps of transient thread occlusion

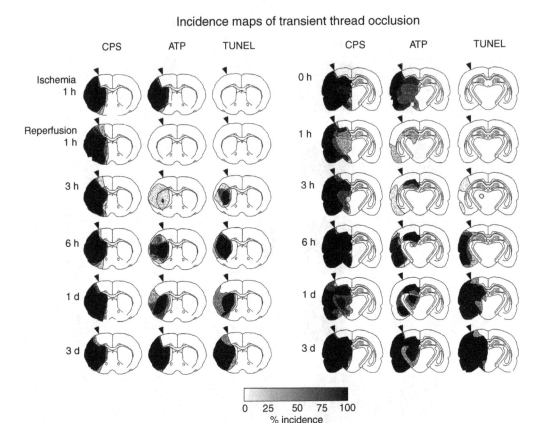

Figure 17.5   Incidence maps of suppressed CPS, ATP depletion and TUNEL-positive neurons on coronal sections of the mouse brain at various reperfusion times following transient MCAO for 1 hour. Areas of disturbed metabolism were outlined in 4 to 5 animals per time point at the level of the caudate putamen (left) and dorsal hippocampus (right) and superimposed to calculate the incidence of alterations as percentage of the number of animals per group. The demarcation between normal and disturbed protein synthesis in the parietal cortex visible at the end of 1 hour of MCAO was marked by the arrowheads to estimate the evolution or regression of the metabolic lesions at later time points. Note the transient recovery of ATP after the beginning of reperfusion and correlation of TUNEL with secondary energy failure.

Genomic expression

Representative in situ hybridization autoradiograms of HSP70, c-Fos and JunB mRNAs are demonstrated in Figure 17.4. The outlining of preserved ATP and normal CPS was superimposed on adjacent cryostat sections to facilitate the regional allocation of hybridization signals.

At the end of 1 hour of MCAO, expression of HSP70 mRNA was slightly

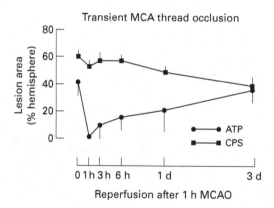

Figure 17.6   Dynamics of metabolic lesions in the mouse brain after transient MCAO for 1 hour. The areas of suppressed CPS and ATP depletion were measured at the level of the caudate putamen and expressed as percentage of the opposite hemisphere. Note the transient recovery of ATP followed by secondary deterioration.

increased in the cortical penumbra, i.e., the region of suppressed CPS but preserved ATP located in the periphery of the MCA territory. c-Fos and JunB mRNAs also increased in the lateral part of the penumbra but even more so in the normal cortex outside the area of suppressed CPS, extending up to the midline but not into the opposite hemisphere.

After reperfusion, HSP70 mRNA expression sharply increased throughout the area of suppressed CPS, peaking 3 hours after the release of vascular occlusion. With longer recirculation times it gradually declined, particularly in the areas of secondary ATP failure, and completely disappeared after 3 days, i.e., at a time when the area of secondary ATP depletion began to merge with that of CPS suppression. In contrast to HSP70 mRNA, the expression pattern of the immediate early genes changed little after reperfusion, the signal intensity declining gradually to the control value between 6 hours and 1 day after the onset of reperfusion.

TUNEL

Double-stranded DNA breaks visualized by TUNEL could first be detected between 3 and 6 hours after the beginning of reperfusion (Figure 17.5). Most of the TUNEL-positive cells appeared to be neurons but the use of cryostat sections precluded precise identification. The comparison of the distribution pattern of TUNEL-positive cells with the inhibition of CPS revealed an initially central localization, which between 1 and 3 days merged with but did not expand beyond the area of CPS suppression. On the other hand, TUNEL-positive cells were encountered mainly in areas of secondary ATP depletion, although precise colocalization was not present in all animals.

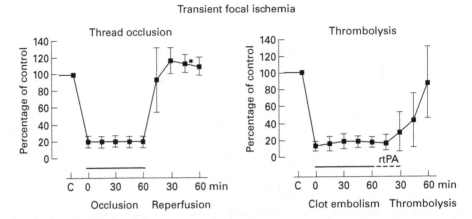

Figure 17.7   Comparison of blood reperfusion after 60 minutes of transient MCA thread occlusion (left) and after rtPA-induced thrombolysis starting 60 minutes after MCA clot embolism (right). Note the considerably longer delay of reperfusion after initiation of thrombolysis.

Thrombolysis of MCA clot embolism

Blood reperfusion

A major difference in reversible focal ischemia brought about by transient thread occlusion or by thrombolysis of clot embolism was the speed of recirculation. After retraction of the intraluminal thread, the brain was recirculated almost instantaneously in analogy to the reperfusion profile following vascular clipping in aneurysm surgery (Figure 17.7). Thrombolysis of clot embolism, in contrast, produced a slowly progressing improvement of flow that took about 1 hour to reach pre-occlusion values.

Brain metabolism

One hour after clot embolism, the regional pattern of metabolic impairment was similar to that observed after 1 hour of thread occlusion, but the volume of the metabolic lesion was slightly larger (Figure 17.8). At the level of the caudate putamen, the ATP depletion area amounted to $58 \pm 10.1\%$ and the CPS-impaired region to $68.0 \pm 6.7\%$ of the hemispheric cross-section (Figure 17.9). In untreated animals, the area of CPS suppression remained constant for the next 24 hours ($67.7 \pm 8.9\%$), whereas the ATP-depleted area gradually expanded until it merged at 24 hours with that of CPS suppression ($66.1 \pm 0.2\%$).

Intra-arterial thrombolysis with 10 mg rtPA/kg 1 hour after embolism gradually reversed these changes. ATP returned in most parts of the ischemic territory between 3 and 6 hours, and had fully recovered after 24 hours (Figures 17.8 and 17.9). Interestingly, CPS also improved, initially in the peripheral areas and after

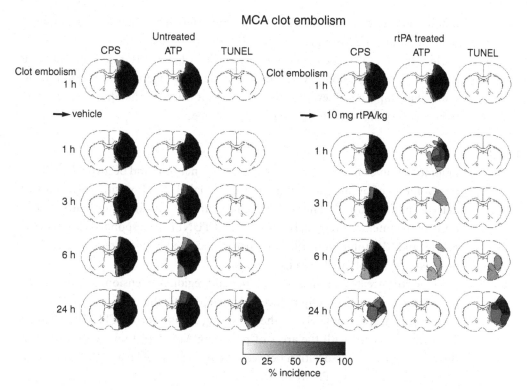

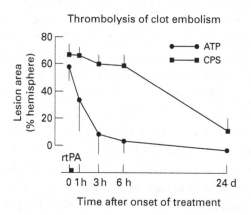

Figure 17.8   Evolution of ischemic injury after clot embolism with and without rtPA treatment.
Incidence maps of suppressed CPS, ATP depletion and double-stranded DNA
fragmentation (TUNEL; for calculations see Figure 17.2). Note the DNA fragmentation in
the rtPA-treated animals, despite a gradual return of energy metabolism and a partial
restoration of protein synthesis.

Figure 17.9   Effect of rtPA-induced thrombolysis on the evolution of ischemic injury after clot
embolism of the MCA. Hemispheric areas of suppressed ATP and CPS were measured at
the level of the caudate putamen (mean ± SD). Thrombolysis induces gradual
improvement of ATP and, after longer delays, CPS.

6 hours in the more central parts of the MCA territory, leading to a significant reduction in the CPS-suppressed area at 24 hours ($15.5 \pm 9.6\%$, $P < 0.05$).

Despite this amazing recovery compared with 1 hour of transient thread occlusion, the animals did not survive. Between 1 and 3 days all mice, treated or not, died under the symptoms of severe brain edema, demonstrating that the observed metabolic recovery did not prevent fatal brain damage.

TUNEL

Fragmentation of nuclear DNA was confined to neurons and occurred late during the evolution of brain injury. In untreated animals TUNEL-positive neurons were detected between 6 and 24 hours after vehicle infusion. Twenty-four hours after the onset of treatment the regional distribution of TUNEL corresponded clearly to that of ATP and CPS inhibition which, in turn, colocalized with the region of critically reduced cerebral blood flow (Figure 17.8).

In the rtPA-treated animals the number and regional extension of TUNEL-positive neurons were distinctly reduced compared with the untreated animals and corresponded approximately to the persisting inhibition of CPS. Interestingly, TUNEL colocalized with the areas of persisting ATP depletion after 6 hours but there was a distinct dissociation between the recovery of ATP and the progression of TUNEL at 24 hours (Figure 17.8).

Discussion

The comparison of infarct evolution in the three experimental models of this investigation clearly reveal that the manifestation of either early or late ischemic injury cannot be explained by a unified hypothesis of ischemic cell damage. In permanent focal brain ischemia, early core injury is the result of a critical reduction of glucose and oxygen supplies leading to primary energy failure [15]. The gradual progression of ischemic injury in the penumbra is more difficult to explain. A genetically controlled programmed type of cell injury is unlikely because TUNEL-associated DNA fragmentation, a hallmark of apoptosis, was never detected before the breakdown of ATP, indicating unspecific alterations. This is in line with previous electron microscopic studies that did not reveal the typical morphological features of apoptosis [16]. The expression pattern of immediate early and stress genes was also at variance with current concepts of the genetic control of programmed cell death [17]. HSP70, considered to be neuroprotective, did not prevent penumbral infarction despite its strong upregulation, and the mRNAs of the injury-promoting immediate early genes c-fos and junB were most strongly expressed in the peri-infarct healthy tissue where cell injury never evolved.

The pathophysiologically more important alteration is presumably the inhibition of protein synthesis, which heralded the final size of the infarct at an early stage of infarct evolution. It is unlikely that the inhibition of protein synthesis was responsible for cell death per se because its pharmacological suppression can survive for much longer times [18]. However, it is conceivable that the inhibition of protein synthesis is the marker of another disturbance that is the ultimate cause of secondary energy failure. Such a disturbance could be the generation of peri-infarct spreading depression-like depolarizations, with the resulting massive activation of the ion exchange pumps [19,20]. Since blood flow, and hence oxygen supply, is reduced in the peri-infarct surrounding, the increased energy requirements of spreading depression are not coupled to a parallel increase in oxidative respiration, causing repeated episodes of relative hypoxia and eventual irreversible tissue injury [21]. This interpretation is supported by magnetic resonance spectroscopic evidence of spreading depression-associated increases of tissue lactate and tissue damage visible on diffusion-weighted imaging [22], as well as by the observation that both infarct expansion and the penumbral inhibition of CPS could be prevented by inhibiting the generation of peri-infarct depolarizations [19].

This situation basically differs from reversible focal ischemia, and here again between fast and slow reperfusion, as exemplified by transient thread occlusion and thrombolysis of clot embolism. After transient thread occlusion, blood flow is restored almost instantaneously, leading to the rapid restoration of energy-producing metabolism. Recovery of the energy state, in turn, restores ion and water homeostasis, as documented among others by magnetic resonance imaging of the apparent diffusion coefficient of water [23]. Thrombolysis of clot embolism, in contrast, reverses the reduction of blood flow, hence of energy metabolism, much more slowly. In the present study in which thrombolysis was started 1 hour after embolism, blood flow returned to the control level after about 1 hour, and ATP between 3 and 6 hours. Obviously, the longer recovery delay is equivalent to a longer energy depletion time and, therefore, to a more severe ischemic impact. Slow reperfusion may also provoke additional damage, owing to the generation of cytotoxic brain edema, which progresses until the energy-dependent ion homeostasis has been restored. The aggravating effect of slow reperfusion has, in fact, been documented in reversible global ischemia, where a clear correlation existed between the initial recirculation rate and the quality of biochemical and functional recovery [24].

The present investigation shows that this may not be true in reversible focal ischemia. In the thread-occluded animals, CPS did not recover and energy metabolism secondarily failed despite fast reperfusion, whereas in the slowly thrombolysed animals ATP recovery was persistent and CPS returned.

Secondary tissue injury after reversible thread occlusion has been described before and has been related to a genetically programmed type of cell death [4,5].

However, the tempororegional evolution of injury does not support this interpretation. In the central parts of the MCA territory where secondary infarction evolved, HSP70 mRNA, but not c-Fos or JunB mRNAs, was strongly upregulated and DNA fragmentation became visible at the same time or after but not before the secondary breakdown of the energy state.

The alternative explanation is a flow–metabolism mismatch in analogy to the penumbra of permanent ischemia. Although blood flow in the recirculated territory may be in the normal range [23,25], postischemic disturbances of vascular reactivity may result in the uncoupling of flow and metabolism, which, under conditions of postischemic hypermetabolism, can provoke relative hypoxia [26].

Such a hypermetabolic situation may arise from mitochondrial injury. There is compelling evidence that postischemic recirculation generates reactive oxygen species, which interfere with mitochondrial function and which impair oxidative respiration because of increased leak currents across the inner mitochondrial membrane [27]. Mitochondrial respiration is also impaired by excessive cytosolic calcium flooding because mitochondrial calcium accumulation diverts part of the capacity of the respiratory chain to calcium transport [28]. Both events reduce the ATP yield of mitochondrial respiration and have to be compensated for by increased oxidation of glucose. The great number of interventions that have been shown to alleviate ischemic injury could, in fact, be explained by the improvement of such a mismatch: flow promoting interventions by increasing oxygen supply, free radical scavengers by reducing mitochondrial damage, calcium antagonists by reducing cytosolic calcium flooding and antiepileptics, hypothermia or anesthetics by reducing the energy requirements of the tissue (for a recent review of therapeutic interventions, see ref. 29).

Interestingly, slow reperfusion initiated 1 hour after clot embolism by thrombolysis did not cause secondary deterioration of energy metabolism during the first day after the onset of therapy. A more delayed manifestation of injury is unlikely because the duration of energy failure, which in this model is longer than after 1 hour of reversible thread occlusion, correlates inversely with the maturation interval of secondary injury [30]. We propose two putative explanations for this unexpected finding. One factor could be an improved microcirculation because rtPA treatment reduces plasma fibrinogen content and, in consequence, lowers blood viscosity [31,32]. The other factor could be amelioration of free radical injury, which has been postulated to decline when postischemic tissue reoxygenation is delayed [33]. Together, these effects may alleviate the postischemic flow/metabolism mismatch and, therefore, on the one hand promote recovery of protein synthesis and on the other prevent secondary energy failure.

A disappointing observation in our thrombolysis experiment was the fact that the metabolic improvement did not prevent DNA fragmentation and fatal brain edema between the first and third day after the onset of treatment. At the present time we do not have experimental data to analyze this pathophysiology in more detail, but it is noteworthy that DNA fragmentation occurred in the presence of both undisturbed protein synthesis and energy metabolism. They may, therefore, reflect an active type of cell death that deserves further investigation.

Conclusion

The three models of focal brain ischemia presented in this chapter exhibit basic differences in the tempororegional evolution of ischemic injury and, therefore, should be critically evaluated in respect to their clinical relevance. In particular, the widely used reversible thread occlusion model, which causes instantaneous reperfusion after a relatively short period of severe focal ischemia, does not replicate either spontaneous or thrombolysis-induced reperfusion and is probably of limited relevance for clinical stroke. This may be the reason that therapeutic interventions that succeeded in improving injury in this model failed under clinical conditions. Further studies should, therefore, be carried out in more appropriate experimental stroke models.

REFERENCES

1 Heiss W-D (1992) Experimental evidence of ischemic thresholds and functional recovery. *Stroke*, **23**, 1668–72.

2 Hossmann K-A (1994) Viability thresholds and the penumbra of focal ischemia. *Annals of Neurology*, **36**, 557–65.

3 Hata R, Maeda K, Hermann D, Mies G & Hossmann K-A (2000) Dynamics of regional brain metabolism and gene expression after middle cerebral artery occlusion in mice. *Journal of Cerebral Blood Flow & Metabolism*, **20**, 306–15.

4 Chen J, Jin K, Chen M, Pei W, Kawaguchi K, Greenberg DA & Simon RP (1997) Early detection of DNA strand breaks in the brain after transient focal ischemia: implications for the role of DNA damage in apoptosis and neuronal cell death. *Journal of Neurochemistry*, **69**, 232–45.

5 Du C, Hu R, Csernansky CA, Hsu CY & Choi DW (1996) Very delayed infarction after mild focal cerebral ischemia: a role for apoptosis? *Journal of Cerebral Blood Flow & Metabolism*, **16**, 195–201.

6 Koudstaal PJ, Stibbe J & Vermeulen M (1988) Fatal ischaemic brain oedema after early thrombolysis with tissue plasminogen activator in acute stroke. *British Medical Journal*, **297**, 1571–4.

7 Rudolf J, Grond M, Stenzel C, Neveling M & Heiss W-D (1998) Incidence of space-occupying brain edema following systemic thrombolysis of acute supratentorial ischemia. *Cerebrovascular Diseases*, **8**, 166–71.

8 Hata R, Maeda K, Hermann D, Mies G & Hossmann K-A (2000) Evolution of brain infarction after transient focal cerebral ischemia in mice. *Journal of Cerebral Blood Flow & Metabolism*, **20**, 937–46.

9 Hara T, Mies G & Hossmann K-A (2000) Effect of thrombolysis on the dynamics of infarct evolution after clot embolism of middle cerebral artery in mice. *Journal of Cerebral Blood Flow & Metabolism*, **20**, 1483–91.

10 Koizumi J, Yoshida Y, Nakazawa T & Oneda G (1986) Experimental studies of ischemic brain edema. 1. A new experimental model of cerebral embolism in rats in which recirculation can be introduced in the ischemic area. *Japanese Journal of Stroke*, **8**, 1–8.

11 Kilic E, Hermann DM & Hossmann K-A (1998) A reproducible model of thromboembolic stroke in mice. *Neuroreport*, **9**, 2967–70.

12 Mies G, Djuricic B, Paschen W & Hossmann K-A (1997) Quantitative measurement of cerebral protein synthesis in vivo: theory and methodological considerations. *Journal of Neuroscience Methods*, **76**, 35–44.

13 Kogure K & Alonso OF (1978) A pictorial representation of endogenous brain ATP by a bioluminescent method. *Brain Research*, **154**, 273–84.

14 Swanson RA & Sharp FR (1994) Infarct measurement methodology. *Journal of Cerebral Blood Flow & Metabolism*, **14**, 697–8.

15 Mies G, Ishimaru S, Xie Y, Seo K & Hossmann K-A (1991) Ischemic thresholds of cerebral protein synthesis and energy state following middle cerebral artery occlusion in rat. *Journal of Cerebral Blood Flow & Metabolism*, **11**, 753–61.

16 van Lookeren Campagne M & Gill R (1996) Ultrastructural morphological changes are not characteristic of apoptotic cell death following focal cerebral ischaemia in the rat. *Neuroscience Letters*, **213**, 111–14.

17 MacManus JP & Linnik MD (1997) Gene expression induced by cerebral ischemia: an apoptotic perspective. *Journal of Cerebral Blood Flow & Metabolism*, **17**, 815–32.

18 Kesner RP, Partlow LM, Bush LG & Berman RF (1981) A quantitative regional analysis of protein synthesis inhibition in the rat brain following localized injection of cycloheximide. *Brain Research*, **209**, 159–76.

19 Mies G, Iijima T & Hossmann K-A (1993) Correlation between peri-infarct DC shifts and ischaemic neuronal damage in rat. *Neuroreport*, **4**, 709–11.

20 Nedergaard M & Hansen AJ (1993) Characterization of cortical depolarizations evoked in focal cerebral ischemia. *Journal of Cerebral Blood Flow & Metabolism*, **13**, 568–74.

21 Back T, Ginsberg MD, Dietrich WD & Watson BD (1996) Induction of spreading depression in the ischemic hemisphere following experimental middle cerebral artery occlusion: effect on infarct morphology. *Journal of Cerebral Blood Flow & Metabolism*, **16**, 202–13.

22 Gyngell ML, Back T, Hoehn-Berlage M, Kohno K & Hossmann K-A (1994) Transient cell depolarization after permanent middle cerebral artery occlusion: an observation by diffusion-weighted MRI and localized ^{1}H-MRS. *Magnetic Resonance in Medicine*, **31**, 337–41.

23 van Dorsten FA, Hata R, Maeda K, Franke C, Eis M, Hossmann K-A & Hoehn M (1999) Diffusion- and perfusion-weighted MR imaging of transient focal cerebral ischaemia in mice. *NMR in Biomedicine*, **12**, 525–34.

24 Hossmann K-A (1988) Resuscitation potentials after prolonged global cerebral ischemia in cats. *Critical Care Medicine*, **16**, 964–71.

25 Tsuchidate R, He QP, Smith ML & Siesjö BK (1997) Regional cerebral blood flow during and after 2 hours of middle cerebral artery occlusion in the rat. *Journal of Cerebral Blood Flow & Metabolism*, **17**, 1066–73.

26 Hossmann K-A (1997) Reperfusion of the brain after global ischemia: hemodynamic disturbances. *Shock*, **8**, 95–101.

27 Kuroda S & Siesjö BK (1997) Reperfusion damage following focal ischemia: pathophysiology and therapeutic windows. *Clinical Neuroscience*, **4**, 199–212.

28 Kristian T, Gido G, Kuroda S, Schutz A & Siesjö BK (1998) Calcium metabolism of focal and penumbral tissues in rats subjected to transient middle cerebral artery occlusion. *Experimental Brain Research*, **120**, 503–9.

29 Grotta JC & Hickenbottom S (1999) Neuroprotective therapy. *Revue Neurologique*, **155**, 644–6.

30 Ito U, Kirino T, Kuroiwa T & Klatzo I (eds.) (1992) *Maturation Phenomenon in Cerebral Ischemia*. Berlin: Springer-Verlag.

31 Gulba DC, Bode C, Runge MS & Huber K (1998) Thrombolytic agents: an updated overview. *Fibrinolysis and Proteolysis*, **12** Suppl 2, 39–58.

32 Lowe G (1998) The pharmacology of thrombolytic and fibrinogen-depleting agents in the treatment of acute ischaemic stroke. *Cerebrovascular Diseases*, **8** Suppl 1, 36–42.

33 Hammerman C & Kaplan M (1998) Ischemia and reperfusion injury. The ultimate pathophysiologic paradox. *Clinics in Perinatology*, **25**, 757–77.

Part VI

Inflammation

Co-Chairs: Midori A. Yenari & Gregory J. del Zoppo

18

Inflammation and stroke: benefits or harm?

Giora Z. Feuerstein[1], Elaine E. Peters[2] & Xinkang Wang[3]

[1-3] DuPont Pharmaceuticals Company, Wilmington, DE

Introduction

Stroke is the third leading cause of death in most developed countries and the primary cardiovascular cause of death in Japan and China. The health burden of the disease is staggering, as loss of a productive life inflicts a heavy toll on patients, families and the society at large. Yet, this disease has no effective therapeutic treatment beyond a limited (about 2%) treatment with thrombolytics that has a significant adverse effect, and despite intense research efforts and numerous clinical trials to develop drugs to reduce morbidity and mortality. Over the past two decades, the focus of drug development efforts has targeted modulators of ion channels (Ca^{2+}, Na^{+}), scavengers of oxygen radicals and antagonists of excitotoxic neurotransmitters (primarily glutamate and glycine receptors). However, all phase III clinical trials with these compounds (Table 18.1), where such compounds were tested for efficacy of treatment in ischemic stroke, have failed due to lack of efficacy, adverse effects or other development difficulties. Debates on the reasons for this grim reality have sprung up in recent meetings, where "finger pointing" to possible causes of failure include wrong animal models, wrong mechanism of action, poor clinical design, inadequate timing of treatment, etc. While this debate is ongoing, the stroke research community seems to have been disenchanted by the "classic" targets for drug development (*vide supra*) as evidenced by emerging hope that other strategies such as "reconstruction", "apoptosis" and "inflammation" may yield the desired success. In this short review, we will analyze the case for a role inflammation might have in ischemic stroke. However, rather than pointing only to possible adverse effects of inflammatory cells and mediators in ischemic brain injury [extensively reviewed in refs. 1–3], this review will evaluate evidence that both beneficial and detrimental mechanisms could be promoted by inflammatory cells and mediators.

Inflammation is defined as a local reaction at the microvessel interfaces that results in fluid and cell translocation from the intravascular medium into the tissue

Table 18.1. Recent stroke trials

Drug	Mechanism	Time/route	Status phase
Lubeluzole	Blocks nitric oxide/ion channels	6–8 hours/iv	One III positive; III continues
Enlimomab	Anti-ICAM-1 antibody	6 hours/iv	III negative
Citicoline	Free radical scavenger?	24 hours/po	III negative
Fosphenytoin	Membrane stabilizer	6 hours/iv	III negative
Cerestat	N-methyl-D-aspartate antagonist	6 hours/iv	III terminated
Cervene	Opioid agonist	6 hours/iv	III terminated
Tirilazad	Free radical scavenger	6 hours/iv	III negative
Nimodipine	Calcium antagonist	24–48 hours/iv	III negative
Eliprodil	N-methyl-D-aspartate antagonist	6 hours/iv	III terminated
GM1 ganglioside	Ganglioside	?	III negative
Viprinex (ancrod)	Fibrinogen-lowering	3–6 hours/iv	III terminated
GV150526 (gavestinel)	Glycine site antagonist	6 hours/iv	III negative

Notes:
iv, intravenous; po, orally; ICAM, intercellular adhesion molecule.

in order to "wall off" and sequester injurious agents and protect and repair the tissue [4]. Over the past one to two decades, stroke researchers have inspected brain tissue at various times after stroke, and inflammatory cells (neutrophils, monocytes) have been indisputably noted at the site of injury. Moreover, with the development of highly specific molecular, biochemical and immunohistochemical techniques, the presence of numerous inflammatory mediators in and around the ischemic brain have been documented. A dual role of inflammatory mediators has been noted in focal stroke and after brain injury, of which the time, location and extent of their expression may be essential for dictating the nature of either neuroprotection or neurotoxicity.

Expression of inflammatory cytokines and chemokines after ischemic brain injury

Several cell types within the brain are able to secrete cytokines and chemokines, including microglia, astrocytes, endothelial cells and neurons. In addition, there is also evidence to support the involvement of peripherally derived cytokines in brain inflammation. Peripherally derived mononuclear phagocytes, T lymphocytes, natural killer cells and polymorphonuclear neutrophils (PMNs), which produce and secrete cytokines, can all contribute to central nervous system (CNS) inflammation and gliosis. Brain injury is associated with the expression of inflammatory mediators, e.g., inflammatory cytokines (interleukin-1 (IL-1) and tumor necrosis factor-α (TNF-α)), chemokines (interleukin-8 (IL-8), monocyte chemoattractant protein-1 (MCP-1) and interferon-inducible protein-10) and intercellular adhesion molecules (ICAM-1 and selectins).

TNF-α is a proinflammatory cytokine with a diverse array of biological activities. Elevated TNF-α has been repeatedly demonstrated in various experimental models of brain injury. Systemic kainic acid administration induces TNF-α mRNA within 2 to 4 hours in the cerebral cortex, hippocampus and hypothalamus. Systemic or intracerebroventricular administration of the lipopolysaccharide (LPS) endotoxin has also been shown to increase brain TNF-α levels as determined by bioassay [5]. In a model of non-penetrating head injury, Shohami et al. reported an early increase in TNF-α peptide at the site of the focal insult [6]. Also, in rat traumatic head injury, TNF-α mRNA and protein levels are rapidly elevated [1]. Furthermore, in mice challenged with particles of charcoal injected into the hippocampus, an increase in striatal levels of TNF-α mRNA was observed [6].

Elevated expression of TNF-α mRNA and protein occurred shortly after (1 to 3 hours) middle cerebral artery occlusion (MCAO) in rats [7,8]. In the ischemic cortex, TNF-α mRNA levels were elevated as early as 1 hour postocclusion (i.e., prior to significant influx of PMNs), peaked at 12 hours and persisted for about 5 days. The early expression of TNF-α mRNA preceding leukocyte infiltration suggests that TNF-α may be involved in this response. Double-labeling immunofluorescence studies localized the de novo synthesized TNF-α to neurons but not to astroglia. Five days after the ischemic insult, neuronally associated TNF-α was diminished, and TNF-α immunoreactivity was localized in the inflammatory cells. The significance of TNF-α expression in the brain was studied by microinjection of TNF-α into the rat cortex. TNF-α induced leukocyte adhesion to the capillary endothelium, but no evidence for neurotoxicity at the site of injection was found. Buttini et al. [9] identified a rapid upregulation of TNF-α mRNA and protein in activated microglia and macrophages after focal stroke, again suggesting that TNF-α is part of an intrinsic inflammatory reaction of the brain after ischemia. TNF-α may exert a primary effect on microvascular inflammatory response, as reflected by TNF-α-induced neutrophil adhesion to the brain capillary endothelium [7]. Furthermore, intracerebroventricular injection of TNF-α 24 hours prior to MCAO exacerbates ischemia-induced tissue injury [10]. This effect was reversed by ventricular administration of anti-TNF-α monoclonal antibody. Further evidence for the involvement of TNF-α in stroke-induced injury is supported by findings in spontaneously hypertensive rats that are stroke prone and have higher levels of TNF-α production in the brain compared with normotensive rats [5]. These data suggest that TNF-α may prime the brain for subsequent damage by activating the capillary endothelium to a pro-adhesive state.

Similar to TNF-α, IL-1β has many pro-inflammatory properties. IL-1β is produced in the CNS by various cellular elements including microglia, astrocytes, neurons and endothelia [11]. An increase in IL-1β mRNA expression has been shown to occur after several types of injury to the brain, including excitotoxicity and LPS [12,13]. Furthermore, mechanical damage after implantation of a microdialysis probe has been shown to induce expression of IL-1β. A rapid increase in IL-1β mRNA expression has been reported after fluid percussion brain trauma in the rat. Microglial IL-1α expression has also been observed in human head injury. IL-1β mRNA expression has been shown to increase after transient brain ischemia in the rat [14]. The exacerbation of ischemic brain injury due to exogenous IL-1β administered into the brain has been observed [15]. A rapid increase (3 to 6 hours postischemia) in IL-1β mRNA after MCAO peaked at 12 hours but returned to basal values at 5 days [8,16]. Early IL-1β expression after focal stroke has also been demonstrated using in situ hybridization. The recent development of tools such as specific antibodies to rat IL-1β has permitted the identification (by immunohistochemistry) of IL-1β peptide in cerebral vessels, microglia and macrophages after focal stroke.

Interleukin-1 receptor antagonist (IL-1ra) is a naturally occurring inhibitor of IL-1 activity by competing with IL-1 for occupancy of the IL-1RI without inducing a signal of its own. IL-1ra is produced by many different cellular sources including monocytes/macrophages, endothelial cells, fibroblasts, neurons and glial cells. The expression of IL-1ra and IL-1R mRNA after focal stroke has also been reported [17]. The level of IL-1α mRNA was markedly increased in the ischemic cortex at 6 hours, then reached a significantly elevated level from 12 hours to 5 days following MCAO. The presence of IL-1ra in the normal brain and the upregulation of IL-1ra mRNA after ischemic injury suggest that IL-1ra may serve as a defense system to attenuate IL-1-mediated brain injury. It is interesting to observe that the temporal induction profile of IL-1ra after MCAO virtually parallels that of IL-1β [17], except that IL-1ra mRNA exhibited prolonged elevation beyond that of IL-1β. Thus, the balance between the levels of IL-1β and its antagonist, IL-1ra, expressed postischemia may be more critical to the degree of tissue injury than IL-1 levels per se.

In addition to their direct actions, the cytokines TNF-α and IL-1β may be able to stimulate the expression and release of a number of chemokines. In vitro studies have shown that IL-1β may produce similar increases in IL-8 and MCP-1 mRNA expression and release from human cerebrovascular endothelial cells to those of ischemia [18]. Direct studies have demonstrated that ischemia induces production of a number of chemokines including IL-8 [19], MCP-1 [20], cytokine-induced neutrophil chemoattractant (CINC) [21], macrophage inflammatory protein-1 (MIP-1) [22], interferon-inducible protein-10 [23] and MCP-3 [24].

After an ischemic insult, increased expression of MCP-1 mRNA has been reported by 6 hours [20,25]. Peak expression appears to occur from 12 to 48 hours with levels still elevated at 5 days. In comparison, CINC expression declined by day 5 [21], whereas levels of MIP-1 mRNA increased as early as 1 hour postischemia, with a peak between 8 and 16 hours. This differential expression may be reflected in the different time courses of the postischemic, infiltration of neutrophils and monocytes, a process in which chemokines play an important role.

Expression of inflammatory cytokines in brain ischemic tolerance

A short duration of ischemia (i.e., ischemic preconditioning) was shown to result in significant tolerance to subsequent ischemic injury. The expression of TNF-α and IL-1β mRNA was significantly induced after ischemic preconditioning in the brain by means of a quantitative real-time TaqMan polymerase chain reaction [26,27]. However, the peak expression of IL-1β mRNA was significantly less after preconditioning than after permanent occlusion of the MCA, i.e., 87 and 546 copies of RNA per microgram tissue at peak levels for preconditioning (6 hours) and focal stroke (12 hours), respectively [26]. The maximal expression of IL-1β was observed during the first week after preconditioning, showing a marked parallelism with the duration of ischemic tolerance [26]. This observation is in agreement with reports that show that pretreatment of rats with low doses of bacterial LPS induces cytokines and inhibits subsequent ischemic damage [28]. A more direct role for IL-1β in the induction of neuroprotection was revealed by direct administration of IL-1β prior to brain ischemia. This IL-1β-stimulated neuroprotection could be reversed by treatment with the endogenous IL-1 antagonist, IL-1ra [29].

Role of inflammatory cytokines and chemokines in ischemic brain injury

Inhibitors of IL-1 or TNF-α have now been shown repeatedly to result in reduced deficits in focal stroke and head trauma models. The detrimental effects of TNF-α and its role as a mediator of focal ischemia may involve several mechanisms. For example, TNF-α increases blood–brain barrier permeability and produces pial artery constriction that can contribute to focal ischemic brain injury. TNF-α was shown also to augment pulmonary arterial transendothelial albumin flux in vitro [30]. Furthermore, by stimulating the production of matrix-degrading metalloproteinase (gelatinase B) [31,32], TNF-α may further exacerbate capillary integrity. TNF-α also causes damage to myelin and oligodendrocytes [33] and increases astrocytic proliferation, thus potentially contributing to demyelination and reactive gliosis. In addition, TNF-α activates the endothelium for leukocyte adherence and procoagulation activity (i.e., increased tissue factor, von Willebrand factor and platelet-activating factor) that can exacerbate ischemic damage. Indeed, increased

TNF-α in the brain and blood in response to LPS appears to contribute to increased stroke sensitivity/risk in hypertensive rats [5]. TNF-α activates neutrophils and increases leukocyte–endothelial cell adhesion molecule expression, leukocyte adherence to blood vessels and subsequent infiltration into the brain [2].

Several studies have shown that blocking TNF-α results in improved outcome in brain trauma and stroke. Pentoxifyline (a methylxanthine that reduces TNF-α production at the transcriptional level) or soluble TNF receptor I (which acts by competing with TNF-α at the receptor) improves neurological outcome, reduces the disruption of the blood–brain barrier and protects hippocampal cells from delayed cell death after closed head injury in the rat [34]. In rat focal ischemia, an anti-TNF-α monoclonal antibody and the soluble TNF-α receptor I were neuroprotective [10]. In the latter studies, TNF-α was blocked by repeated intracerebroventricular administration before and during focal stroke, which significantly reduced infarct size. In murine focal stroke, topical application of soluble TNF-α receptor I on the brain surface significantly reduced ischemic brain injury [35,36]. In addition, in another study evaluating TNF-α blockade on focal stroke in hypertensive rats, soluble TNF receptor I administered intravenously pre- or post-MCAO significantly reduced impairment in ischemic cortex microvascular perfusion and the degree of cortical infarction, strongly suggesting an inflammatory/vascular mechanism for TNF-α in focal stroke [37].

Many studies have demonstrated the protective effects of IL-1ra in brain injury. Administration of recombinant IL-1ra produced a marked reduction in brain damage induced by focal stroke [38,39] or brain hypoxia [40]. This neuronal protective effect of IL-1ra in focal stroke was further supported using an adenoviral vector that overexpressed IL-1ra in the brain [41]. The excess of IL-1ra significantly reduced infarct size after focal stroke. In addition, IL-1ra expression increases after ischemic preconditioning in a manner that parallels the development of brain ischemic tolerance [42]. Of interest are data showing that peripheral administration of IL-1ra reduces brain injury [38], suggesting a potential use of IL-1ra as a neuroprotective agent in human stroke and/or neurotrauma.

In contrast to the cytokines, there is little evidence to directly connect chemokines with brain pathology. One study with an anti-IL-8 antibody reported reductions in both cerebral edema and ischemic damage [43] but the exact mechanisms involved were not determined. The upregulation of chemokines by ischemia precedes the documented leukocyte responses, and IL-8 and MCP-1 are known to upregulate integrin affinity, thus promoting leukocyte infiltration and accumulation. Whilst this seems a plausible explanation, the absence of specific chemokine inhibitors limits the conclusions which may be drawn.

Role of adhesion molecules in ischemic brain injury

Leukocyte adhesion receptors, P-selectin, ICAM-1 and E-selectin are expressed in sequence by microvascular endothelium within the ischemic territory [44–47]. P-selectin is seen within 60 to 90 minutes following MCAO [44], indicating the rapid reactivity of microvascular endothelium to the ischemic insult. P-selectin and E-selectin receptors are continually expressed within the ischemic territory [47].

The significance of these adhesion molecules in stroke is demonstrated by studies with selective inhibitors to these molecules. For example, rats treated with an antibody against MAC-1 (the leukocyte counterpart to ICAM-1) had smaller lesions (reduction in infarct size by 45% to 50%) after transient MCAO [48]. Similarly, administration of an anti-ICAM-1 antibody demonstrated a 40% reduction of infarct size in a focal stroke model [49]. Blocking adhesion molecules can also reduce apoptosis induced by focal ischemia [50]. Other studies verified these effects but also illustrated that these antibodies could not reduce infarct size when the ischemia was permanent [51,52]. However, this strategy may work only when both leukocyte and endothelial cell adhesion proteins are blocked. The combination of tissue plasminogen activator and anti-CD18 provides significantly improved outcome, and may increase the therapeutic time window in stroke [53]. In a rabbit embolic model of stroke, anti-ICAM-1 antibody was shown to increase the amount of clot necessary to produce permanent damage [54]. In addition, in a baboon model of transient focal ischemia, anti-CD18 monoclonal antibody administered 25 minutes prior to reperfusion led to an increase in reflow in microvessels of various sizes [55]. However, in contrast to the demonstrated anti-ischemic effect of anti-adhesion molecules in animal models, the recent failure of the murine anti-ICAM monoclonal antibody (Enlimomab) in human stroke [3] and its ability to activate human neutrophils [56] demonstrate the difficulties in extrapolating encouraging data obtained in some animal models to clinical reality.

Anti-inflammatory strategies in stroke

Because of the dual nature of some mediators in reformatting brain cells for resistance or sensitivity to injury, it may be critical to carefully balance pharmacological interventions based on anti-inflammatory strategies. The literature is replete with reports of "wrong doing" of such mediators and "beneficial" effect of leukocyte depletion, adhesion molecule antagonists (ICAM-1, E- or P-selectins), anticytokines and interleukin antagonists. The minority of dissenting reports has been ignored. However, careful inspection of the evolution of the sentiments regarding the detrimental role of inflammation in stroke reveals the following potential pitfalls:

1 Pharmacological studies where mediators are injected acutely into the brain (normal or ischemic) are highly artificial; the doses are unrealistic (industrial if not military), with no correlation between the spatial, temporal and contextual and the disease condition.

2 Transgenic animal models that were subjected to discrete deletion of certain cytokine or cytokine receptor genes and were subjected to brain ischemia showed more extensive injury and poorer long-term recovery than wild-type mice – a result opposite to the expected "protection." Most notable are the TNF-$\alpha^{-/-}$ mice where deletion of the cytokine or the cytokine receptors resulted in a significantly worse outcome, as with the IL-6$^{-/-}$ mice [57–59].

3 Cytokines have a "reputation" (i.e., pro-inflammatory), yet the cytokine IL-10 has been shown to possess neuroprotective efficacy in various models of brain injury, including stroke [60,61]. TNF-α and IL-1β, two cytokines most often cited as "bad guys" in stroke, have been shown to provide neuroprotection and, in fact, reformat brain tissue into a state of "tolerance" to ischemic insults when administered in sufficient time before the ischemic insult [28,29].

4 While activated macrophages are viewed as villains when spotted in the brain, the growth-promoting and neuroprotective potential of factors released from activated macrophages has been grossly overlooked. This is evidenced by the remarkable recovery induced by the application of homologous activated macrophages to spinal cord injury in rats [62]. Furthermore, the salutary effect of immune/inflammatory cells in CNS injury has also been shown in studies where neuroprotection (retinal neurons) has been conveyed by myelin basic protein-activated T cells [63].

5 From the clinical perspective, it is well established that glucocorticoids, the most potent and fast-acting anti-inflammatory drugs known to medicine, are of no therapeutic benefit in stroke patients [64]. Likewise, none of the common non-steroidal anti-inflammatory agents (e.g., aspirin, indomethacin, ibuprofen, etc.) have proven to be beneficial in the acute treatment of stroke.

6 Most recently, anti-ICAM-1 antibody clinical trials in acute stroke patients have been terminated after analysis showed the futility of using this antibody [3]. In fact, a trend toward an adverse outcome was noted. While the cause of this situation is still being analyzed, the failure of the ICAM-1 trials in stroke is consistent with a lack of efficacy in the broad spectrum anti-inflammatory agents in stroke treatment.

Conclusion

It is important to point out the need to more carefully analyze the role of inflammation in ischemic brain injury. It is indeed crucial that the salutary role of inflammatory cells and mediators in tissue repair, an evolutionary mechanism of fundamental survival, be acknowledged. It is highly likely that some inflammatory cell-derived mediators may be critical in proper repair and recovery of neuronal networks, enhancement of plasticity and reformatting of circuitries necessary for taking over tasks for which the lost brain tissue was responsible.

REFERENCES

1 Fan L, Young PR, Barone FC, Feuerstein GZ, Smith DH & McIntosh TK (1996) Experimental brain injury induces differential expression of tumor necrosis factor-α mRNA in the CNS. *Molecular Brain Research*, **36**, 287–91.

2 Feuerstein GZ, Wang X & Barone FC (1998) Inflammatory mediators of ischemic injury: cytokine gene regulation in stroke. In *Cerebrovascular Disease: Pathophysiology, Diagnosis and Management*, eds. MD Ginsberg & J Bogousslavsky, pp. 507–31. Malden, MA: Blackwell Science.

3 DeGraba TJ (1998) The role of inflammation after acute stroke: utility of pursuing anti-adhesion molecule therapy. *Neurology*, **51** (Suppl 3), S62–S68.

4 Gallin JI, Goldstein IM & Snyderman R (1988) *Inflammation: Basic Principles and Clinical Correlates*. New York: Raven Press.

5 Siren AL, Heldman E, Doron D, Lysko PG, Yue TL, Liu Y, Feuerstein G & Hallenbeck JM (1992) Release of proinflammatory and prothrombotic mediators in the brain and peripheral circulation in spontaneously hypertensive and normotensive Wistar–Kyoto rats. *Stroke*, **23**, 1643–51.

6 Shohami E, Novikov M, Bass R, Yamin A & Gallily R (1994) Closed head injury triggers early production of TNF-α and IL-6 by brain tissue. *Journal of Cerebral Blood Flow & Metabolism*, **14**, 615–19.

7 Liu T, Clark RK, McDonnell PC, Young PR, White RF, Barone FC & Feuerstein GZ (1994) Tumor necrosis factor-α expression in ischemic neurons. *Stroke*, **25**, 1481–8.

8 Wang X, Yue TL, Barone FC, White RF, Gagnon RC & Feuerstein GZ (1994) Concomitant cortical expression of TNF-α and IL-1β mRNAs follows early response gene expression in transient focal ischemia. *Molecular and Chemical Neuropathology*, **23**, 103–14.

9 Buttini M, Appel K, Sauter A, Gebicke-Haerter PJ & Boddeke HW (1996) Expression of tumor necrosis factor alpha after focal cerebral ischaemia in the rat. *Neuroscience*, **71**, 1–16.

10 Barone FC, Arvin B, White RF, Miller A, Webb CL, Willette RN, Lysko PG & Feuerstein GZ (1997) Tumor necrosis factor-α: a mediator of focal ischemic brain injury. *Stroke*, **28**, 1233–44.

11 Rothwell NJ (1991) Functions and mechanisms of interleukin 1 in the brain. *Trends in Pharmacological Sciences*, **12**, 430–6.

12 Minami M, Kuraishi Y & Satoh M (1991) Effects of kainic acid on messenger RNA levels of IL-1β, IL-6, TNF-α and LIF in the rat brain. *Biochemical and Biophysical Research Communications*, **176**, 593–8.

13 Buttini M & Boddeke H (1995) Peripheral lipopolysaccharide stimulation induces interleukin-1β messenger RNA in rat brain microglial cells. *Neuroscience*, **65**, 523–30.

14 Minami M, Kuraishi Y, Yabuuchi K, Yamazaki A & Satoh M (1992) Induction of interleukin-1 beta mRNA in rat brain after transient forebrain ischemia. *Journal of Neurochemistry*, **58**, 390–2.

15 Yamasaki Y, Matsuura N, Shozuhara H, Onodera H, Itoyama Y & Kogure K (1995) Interleukin-1 as a pathogenetic mediator of ischemic brain damage in rats. *Stroke*, **26**, 676–81.

16 Liu T, McDonnell PC, Young PR, White RF, Siren AL, Hallenbeck JM, Barone FC & Feuerstein GZ (1993) Interleukin-1β mRNA expression in ischemic rat cortex. *Stroke*, **24**, 1746–50.

17 Wang X, Barone FC, Aiyar NV, Feuerstein GZ & del Zoppo GJ (1997) Interleukin-1 receptor and receptor antagonist gene expression after focal stroke in rats. *Stroke*, **28**, 155–62.

18 Zhang W, Smith C, Shapiro A, Monette R, Hutchison J & Stanimirovic D (1999) Increased expression of bioactive chemokines in human cerebromicrovascular endothelial cells and astrocytes subjected to simulated ischemia in vitro. *Journal of Neuroimmunology*, **101**, 148–60.

19 Kostulas N, Kivisäkk P, Huang Y, Matusevicius D, Kostulas V & Link H (1998) Ischemic stroke is associated with a systemic increase of blood mononuclear cells expressing interleukin-8 mRNA. *Stroke*, **29**, 462–66.

20 Wang X, Yue T-L, Barone FC & Feuerstein GZ (1995) Monocyte chemoattractant protein-1 messenger RNA expression in rat ischemic cortex. *Stroke*, **26**, 661–6.

21 Liu T, Young PR, McDonnell PC, White RF, Barone FC & Feuerstein GZ (1993) Cytokine-induced neutrophil chemoattractant mRNA expressed in cerebral ischemia. *Neuroscience Letters*, **164**, 125–8.

22 Kim JS, Gautam SC, Chopp M, Zaloga C, Jones ML, Ward PA & Welch KM (1995) Expression of monocyte chemoattractant protein-1 and macrophage inflammatory protein-1 after focal cerebral ischemia in the rat. *Journal of Neuroimmunology*, **56**, 127–34.

23 Wang X, Ellison JA, Siren AL, Lysko PG, Yue TL, Barone FC, Shatzman A & Feuerstein GZ (1998) Prolonged expression of interferon-inducible protein-10 in ischemic cortex after permanent occlusion of the middle cerebral artery in rat. *Journal of Neurochemistry*, **71**, 1194–1204.

24 Wang X, Li X, Yaish-Ohad S, Sarau HM, Barone FC & Feuerstein GZ (1999) Molecular cloning and expression of the rat monocyte chemotactic protein-3 gene: a possible role in stroke. *Molecular Brain Research*, **71**, 304–12.

25 Yamagami S, Tamura M, Hayashi M, Endo N, Tanabe H, Katsuura Y & Komoriya K (1999) Differential production of MCP-1 and cytokine-induced neutrophil chemoattractant in the ischemic brain after transient focal ischemia in rats. *Journal of Leukocyte Biology*, **65**, 744–9.

26 Wang X, Li X, Currie RW, Willette RN, Barone FC & Feuerstein GZ (2000) Application of real-time polymerase chain reaction to quantitate induced expression of interleukin-1β mRNA in ischemic brain tolerance. *Journal of Neuroscience Research*, **59**, 238–46.

27 Wang X, Li X, Erhardt JA, Barone FC & Feuerstein GZ (2000) Detection of tumor necrosis factor-α mRNA induction in ischemic brain tolerance by means of real-time polymerase chain reaction. *Journal of Cerebral Blood Flow & Metabolism*, **20**, 15–20.

28 Tasaki K, Ruetzler CA, Ohtsuki T, Martin D, Nawashiro H & Hallenbeck JM (1997) Lipopolysaccharide pre-treatment induces resistance against subsequent focal cerebral ischemic damage in spontaneously hypertensive rats. *Brain Research*, **748**, 267–70.

29 Ohtsuki T, Ruetzler CA, Tasaki K & Hallenbeck JM (1996) Interleukin-1 mediates induction of tolerance to global ischemia in gerbil hippocampal CA1 neurons. *Journal of Cerebral Blood Flow & Metabolism*, **16**, 1137–42.

30 Goldblum SE & Sun WL (1990) Tumor necrosis factor-alpha augments pulmonary arterial transendothelial albumin flux in vitro. *American Journal of Physiology*, **258**, L57–L67.

31 Romanic AM, White RF, Arleth AJ, Ohlstein EH & Barone FC (1998) Matrix metalloproteinase expression increases after cerebral focal ischemia in rats: inhibition of matrix metalloproteinase-9 reduces infarct size. *Stroke*, **29**, 1020–30.

32 Rosenberg GA, Estrada EY, Dencoff JE, & Stetler-Stevenson WG (1995) Tumor necrosis factor-α-induced gelatinase B causes delayed opening of the blood–brain barrier: an expanded therapeutic window. *Brain Research*, **703**, 151–5.

33 Robbins DS, Shirazi Y, Drysdale BE, Lieberman A, Shin HS & Shin ML (1987) Production of cytotoxic factor for oligodendrocytes by stimulated astrocytes. *Journal of Immunology*, **139**, 2593–7.

34 Shohami E, Bass R, Wallach D, Yamin A & Gallily R (1996) Inhibition of tumor necrosis factor alpha (TNF-α) activity in rat brain is associated with cerebroprotection after closed head injury. *Journal of Cerebral Blood Flow & Metabolism*, **16**, 378–84.

35 Nawashiro H, Martin D & Hallenbeck JM (1997) Inhibition of tumor necrosis factor and amelioration of brain infarction in mice. *Journal of Cerebral Blood Flow & Metabolism*, **17**, 229–32.

36 Nawashiro H, Tasaki K, Ruetzler CA & Hallenbeck JM (1997) TNF-alpha pretreatment induces protective effects against focal cerebral ischemia in mice. *Journal of Cerebral Blood Flow & Metabolism*, **17**, 483–90.

37 Dawson DA, Martin D & Hallenbeck JM (1996) Inhibition of tumor necrosis factor-alpha reduces focal cerebral ischemic injury in the spontaneously hypertensive rat. *Neuroscience Letters*, **218**, 41–4.

38 Relton JK, Martin D, Thompson RC & Russell DA (1996) Peripheral administration of interleukin-1 receptor antagonist inhibits brain damage after focal cerebral ischemia in the rat. *Experimental Neurology*, **138**, 206–13.

39 Loddick SA & Rothwell NJ (1996) Neuroprotective effects of human recombinant interleukin-1 receptor antagonist in focal cerebral ischaemia in the rat. *Journal of Cerebral Blood Flow & Metabolism*, **16**, 932–40.

40 Martin D, Chinookoswong N & Miller G (1995) The interleukin-1 receptor antagonist (rhIL-1ra) protects against cerebral infarction in a rat model of hypoxia-ischemia. *Experimental Neurology*, **130**, 362–7.

41 Betz AL, Yang GY & Davidson BL (1995) Attenuation of stroke size in rats using an adenoviral vector to induce overexpression of interleukin-1 receptor antagonist in brain. *Journal of Cerebral Blood Flow & Metabolism*, **15**, 547–51.

42 Barone FC, White RF, Spera PA, Ellison J, Currie RW, Wang X & Feuerstein GZ (1998) Ischemic preconditioning and brain tolerance: temporal histological and functional outcomes, protein synthesis requirement, and interleukin-1 receptor antagonist and early gene expression. *Stroke*, **29**, 1937–50.

43 Matsumoto T, Ikeda K, Mukaida N, Harada A, Matsumoto Y, Yamashita J & Matsushima K (1997) Prevention of cerebral edema and infarct in cerebral reperfusion injury by an antibody to interleukin-8. *Laboratory Investigation*, **77**, 119–25.

44 Okada Y, Copeland BR, Mori E, Tung MM, Thomas WS & del Zoppo GJ (1994) P-selectin and intercellular adhesion molecule-1 expression after focal brain ischemia and reperfusion. *Stroke*, **25**, 202–11.

45 Wang X, Siren A-L, Yue T-L, Barone FC & Feuerstein GZ (1994) Upregulation of intercellular adhesion molecule 1 (ICAM-1) on brain microvascular endothelial cells in rat ischemic cortex. *Molecular Brain Research*, **26**, 61–8.

46 Wang X, Yue T-L, Barone FC & Feuerstein GZ (1995) Demonstration of increased endothelial-leukocyte adhesion molecule-1 mRNA expression in rat ischemic cortex. *Stroke*, **26**, 1665–9.

47 Haring H-P, Akamine BS, Habermann R, Koziol JA & Del Zoppo GJ (1996) Distribution of integrin-like immunoreactivity on primate brain microvasculature. *Journal of Neuropathology & Experimental Neurology*, **55**, 236–45.

48 Chen H, Chopp M, Zhang RL, Bodzin G, Chen Q, Rusche JR & Todd RF III (1994) Anti-CD11b monoclonal antibody reduces ischemic cell damage after transient focal cerebral ischemia in rat. *Annals of Neurology*, **35**, 458–63.

49 Zhang RL, Chopp M, Li Y, Zaloga C, Jiang N, Jones ML, Miyasaka M & Ward PA (1994) Anti-ICAM-1 antibody reduces ischemic cell damage after transient middle cerebral artery occlusion in the rat. *Neurology*, **44**, 1747–51.

50 Chopp M, Li Y, Jiang N, Zhang RL & Prostak J (1996) Antibodies against adhesion molecules reduce apoptosis after transient middle cerebral artery occlusion in rat brain. *Journal of Cerebral Blood Flow & Metabolism*, **16**, 578–84.

51 Chopp M, Zhang RL, Chen H, Li Y, Jiang N & Rusche JR (1994) Postischemic administration of an anti-Mac-1 antibody reduces ischemic cell damage after transient middle cerebral artery occlusion in rats. *Stroke*, **25**, 869–76.

52 Zhang RL, Chopp M, Jiang N, Tang WX, Prostak J, Manning AM & Anderson DC (1995) Anti-intercellular adhesion molecule-1 antibody reduces ischemic cell damage after transient but not permanent middle cerebral artery occlusion in the Wistar rat. *Stroke*, **26**, 1438–43.

53 Zhang RL, Zhang ZG & Chopp M (1999) Increased therapeutic efficacy with rtPA and anti-CD18 antibody treatment of stroke in the rat. *Neurology*, **52**, 273–9.

54 Bowes MP, Zivin JA & Rothlein R (1993) Monoclonal antibody to the ICAM-1 adhesion site reduces neurological damage in a rabbit cerebral embolism stroke model. *Experimental Neurology*, **119**, 215–19.

55 Mori E, del Zoppo GJ, Chambers JD, Copeland BR & Arfors KE (1992) Inhibition of polymorphonuclear leukocyte adherence suppresses no-reflow after focal cerebral ischemia in baboons. *Stroke*, **23**, 712–18.

56 Vuorte J, Lindsberg PJ, Kaste M, Meri S, Jansson S-E, Rothlein R & Repo H (1999) Anti-ICAM-1 monoclonal antibody R6.5 (Enlimomab) promotes activation of neutrophils in whole blood. *Journal of Immunology*, **162**, 2353–7.

57 Scherbel U, Raghupathi R, Nakamura M, Saatman KE, Trojanowski JQ, Neugebauer E, Marino MW & McIntosh TK (1999) Differential acute and chronic responses of tumor necrosis factor-deficient mice to experimental brain injury. *Proceedings of the National Academy of Sciences, USA*, **96**, 8721–6.

58 Bruce AJ, Boling W, Kindy MS, Peschon J, Kraemer PJ, Carpenter MK, Holtsberg FW & Mattson MP (1996) Altered neuronal and microglial responses to excitotoxic and ischemic brain injury in mice lacking TNF receptors. *Nature Medicine,* 2, 788–94.

59 Stahel PF, Shohami E, Younis FM, Kariya K, Otto VI, Lenzlinger PM, Grosjean MB, Eugster HP, Trentz O, Kossmann T & Morganti-Kossmann MC (2000) Experimental closed head injury: analysis of neurological outcome, blood–brain barrier dysfunction, intracranial neutrophil infiltration, and neuronal cell death in mice deficient in genes for pro-inflammatory cytokines. *Journal of Cerebral Blood Flow & Metabolism,* 20, 369–80.

60 Spera PA, Ellison JA, Feuerstein GZ & Barone FC (1998) IL-10 reduces rat brain injury following focal stroke. *Neuroscience Letters,* 251, 189–92.

61 Dietrich WD, Busto R & Bethea JR (1999) Postischemic hypothermia and IL-10 treatment provide long-lasting neuroprotection of CA1 hippocampus following transient global ischemia in rats. *Experimental Neurology,* 158, 444–50.

62 Rapalino O, Lazarov-Spiegler O, Agranov E, Velan GJ, Yoles E, Fraidakis M, Solomon A, Gepstein R, Katz A, Belkin M, Hadani M & Schwartz M (1998) Implantation of stimulated homologous macrophages results in partial recovery of paraplegic rats. *Nature Medicine,* 4, 814–21.

63 Moalem G, Leibowitz-Amit R, Yoles E, Mor F, Cohen IR & Schwartz M (1999) Autoimmune T cells protect neurons from secondary degeneration after central nervous system axotomy. *Nature Medicine,* 5, 49–55.

64 Millikan CH, McDowell F & Easton JD (1987) Chapter 8. In *Stroke,* pp. 117–30. Philadelphia: Lea & Febiger.

19

TNF-α and ceramide are involved in the mediation of neuronal tolerance to brain ischemia

Irene Ginis[1]*, Jie Liu[2]*, Maria Spatz[3] & John M. Hallenbeck[4]

[1–4] Stroke Branch, National Institute of Neurological Disorders and Stroke, National Institutes of Health, Bethesda, MD

Introduction

We have been interested in models of tolerance to hypoxia and ischemia as potential guides to appropriate therapeutic targets because of the complexity and multifactorality of the process that causes progressive brain damage during the early hours of a stroke. After having been exposed to single or repetitive episodes of sublethal ischemic stress, brain cells acquire resistance to subsequent, otherwise lethal, ischemic insults [1]. A number of biochemical changes, such as cytokine release, that trigger activation of multiple signaling pathways are caused by ischemic stress and other forms of stress.

Tumor necrosis factor-alpha (TNF-α), a cytokine with pleiotropic activity, affects many different types of cell. Whole brain, neurons [2,3], microglia, astrocytes [4,5] and brain endothelium [6] are not only capable of TNF-α synthesis in response to stress, but also express TNF-α receptors and amplify the TNF-α response through paracrine and autocrine mechanisms [7]. In addition, this cytokine has been implicated in both detrimental [8] and neuroprotective [9] actions in brain cells, depending on the experimental conditions. This dual function of TNF-α has also been observed in vivo. The TNF-α-binding protein that neutralizes TNF-α had a protective effect against focal ischemia [10,11]. However, in a model of permanent middle cerebral artery occlusion, transgenic mice lacking TNF-α receptors developed significantly larger infarcts than did littermate controls [12]. An inference from these data is that TNF-α has the potential to function either as a stressor or as a molecule with a homeostatic function. It can also act as a preconditioning stimulus for induction of tolerance. Intravenous pretreatment of SHR

---

* These two investigators made equal contributions to this work.

rats with the TNF-α-inducing agent, lipopolysaccharide [13], or intracisternal pre-treatment of mice with TNF-α [14] have been shown in recent studies to substitute for ischemic preconditioning and to protect animals from ischemic injury in the middle cerebral artery occlusion model.

In cultured cortical neurons from 2-day-old Sprague–Dawley rats, we have recently developed an in vitro model of ischemic preconditioning. When these cells are preconditioned with mild hypoxia (8% oxygen in the medium for 20 minutes) they become more resistant to severe hypoxia (2% to 5% oxygen for 2.5 hours) or to in vitro ischemia (similar to hypoxia plus no glucose in the medium) applied 24 hours later. TNF-α pretreatment of cultured cells (25 ng/ml for 24 hours) protected neurons to the same degree as hypoxic preconditioning (about 50% protection) and thus resembled the animal studies. This in vitro paradigm of adaptation to hypoxic–ischemic stress permitted the direct demonstration that TNF-α is a key mediator of tolerance. No tolerance developed when preconditioning was performed in the presence of an antibody known to neutralize the biological activity of TNF-α.

Ceramide, a sphingolipid, has been implicated as a second messenger in many of the multiple signaling pathways initiated upon binding of TNF-α to its p55 receptor [15,16]. In addition to studies that have implicated ceramide in induction of apoptosis and cell cycle control [17,18], there is also evidence that ceramide can cause cytoprotection [15]. We hypothesized that ceramide could play a role in the induction of ischemic tolerance. We tested this hypothesis in our in vitro model of tolerance. This chapter presents evidence that preconditioning of cortical neurons with mild hypoxia results in upregulation of intracellular ceramide that is mediated by TNF-α, and that these intracellular signaling molecules are necessary and sufficient for induction of tolerance in this model.

Methods

Cortical neuronal cultures

Cortical neuronal cultures were established from 2-day-old Sprague–Dawley rats. Cerebral cortices without meninges were placed into a dissection medium (0.3% (w/v) glucose, 0.75% (w/v) sucrose, 28 mM Hepes in Hanks' balanced salt solution, pH 7.3, osmolarity 320 mM/kg), cut into small pieces, treated with 0.25% (w/v) trypsin for 20 minutes at 37 °C and then resuspended in Dulbecco's modified Eagle's medium (DMEM)/high glucose (4500 mg/l), 2 mM glutamine, 1% antibiotic/antimycotic (all from Gibco Life Technology), 10% (v/v) fetal bovine serum (Summit Biotechnology) and 40 μg DNase/ml (Boehringer Mannheim), and triturated 20 times in culture medium. The cell suspension was centrifuged at low speed (1000 rpm) to get rid of cell debris, resuspended in culture medium (Neurobasal-A with 2% B27 supplement, 1 mM L-glutamine (all from Gibco Life Technology),

0.2% (v/v) horse serum (Sigma)) at $5.5 \sim 5.8 \times 10^5$/ml (one brain yielded a 24 ml cell suspension) and plated 500 μl/well in 24-well plates (Costar) precoated with 2.5 μg/cm^2 of poly-L-lysine. The glucose concentration in Neurobasal-A was 4500 mg/l. Non-neuronal cells were eliminated by changing the medium 20 minutes after plating and by addition of 15 μg 5'-fluoro-2'-deoxyuridine/ml (Sigma) in the culture medium. Immunostaining of neurons with an antibody against neuron-specific enolase (Chemicon International, Inc., Temecula, CA) and astrocytes with glial fibrillary acidic protein-specific antibody (Boehringer Mannheim) demonstrated that astrocyte contamination was less than 5%.

Hypoxic pretreatment

Hypoxic pretreatment was performed on day 4 in vitro after withdrawal of 200 μl (out of 400 μl/well) of culture medium. Neuronal cultures were placed in modular incubator chambers (Billups Rothenberg, Del Mar, CA) and flushed with a gas mixture of 5% CO_2/95% N_2 for 20 minutes at room temperature (when the cells were grown in 60 mm dishes, the flushing time was 15 minutes). The chambers were sealed and incubated at 37 °C for 20 minutes. Oxygen concentration in the culture medium was monitored with an oxygen meter (Microelectrodes, Inc., Bedford, NH) and reached 8% at the end of pretreatment. After pretreatment, 200 μl/well of normoxic medium was added back to the cultures and they were incubated under normoxic conditions (5% CO_2, 100% humidity at 37 °C) for 24 hours and then subjected to severe hypoxia.

Severe hypoxic treatment

Severe hypoxic treatment was performed on day 5 in vitro. Culture medium was completely removed from naïve and preconditioned cells and substituted with 200 μl Neurobasal-A medium/well plus 1 mM L-glutamine (no B27 supplement and horse serum). The plates were flushed with a 5% CO_2/95% N_2 gas mixture in hypoxic chambers until oxygen concentrations dropped to 2% (about 40 minutes). Chambers were agitated every 5 minutes to ensure maximal gas exchange in the culture medium. The chambers were sealed and incubated for 2.5 hours at 37 °C (oxygen concentration in the medium was 5% at the end of incubation). For reoxygenation 200 μl of normoxic culture medium containing double concentrations of B27 supplement and horse serum was added per well to the cells, which were placed in a regular tissue culture incubator; cell viability was measured at indicated times. Control cells were subjected to the same washing and feeding procedures with normoxic medium. For glucose deprivation studies, cells were incubated in 200 μl DMEM/well containing no glucose, and 200 μl/well DMEM containing double concentrations of glucose were added to the cultures upon reoxygenation.

Pretreatment of neuronal cultures with TNF-α and C-2 ceramide and blocking reagents

TNF-α (25 ng/ml) was added to neuronal cultures on day 4 in Neurobasal-A plus 1 mM L-glutamine and 2% B27 supplement and 0.2% horse serum for 24 hours (it was washed out just before the severe hypoxic treatment). *N*-acetylceramide (C-2 ceramide) (10 μM) was added to the cultures at the beginning of severe hypoxia (day 5 in vitro) and remained in the medium during the entire reoxygenation period. Anti-TNF-α neutralizing antibody (8 μg/ml at $ND_{50} = 3$ to 6 μg/ml; R & D Systems) or fumonisin B_1 (50 μM; Alexis Biochemicals, San Diego, CA) was added to neuronal cultures at the time of preconditioning. Both reagents were washed out just before incubation of the cells in severe hypoxia.

Quantitation of neuronal injury

Quantification of neuronal injury was performed by means of an ethidium homodimer fluorescence exclusion test [18]. In order to quantify fluorescence changes, neurons were plated in 24-well plates and, at the end of each experiment, culture medium was withdrawn and cells were incubated with 6 μM ethidium homodimer (Molecular Probes, Eugene, OR) in Hanks' buffer at 300 μl/well for 30 minutes at 37° C. Cell fluorescence was measured with a CytoFluor 4000 fluorescent plate reader (PerSeptive Biosystems, Framingham, MA) at excitation/emission wavelengths of 530/620 nm. Background fluorescence was measured on each plate and subtracted. The percentage of dead cells was calculated by means of the following formula:

$$\% \text{ dead cells} = \frac{F - F_{min}}{F_{max} - F_{min}} \times 100\%$$

where F was fluorescence of unknown sample, F_{min} was fluorescence of untreated healthy control cultures and F_{max} was fluorescence of the same cultures treated with 0.03% (w/v) saponin for 1 hour at 37 °C. In order to estimate the percentage of cells that had already detached from the dish, saponin was added to all the wells at the end of incubation with an ethidium homodimer, and fluorescence of each sample ($F_{saponin}$) was related to that of the control, untreated samples (F_{max}) using the following formula:

$$\% \text{ lost cells} = \frac{F_{max} - F_{saponin}}{F_{max}} \times 100$$

To take into account uneven distribution of cells on the surface of any well, the fluorescent plate reader was programmed to read five different areas of each well, and the mean signal was calculated. In order to overcome variability in cell plating density each experimental value was obtained as an average of measurements performed in eight wells.

Intracellular ceramide levels

Intracellular ceramide levels were measured in neurons, which were grown in 60 mm culture dishes and subjected to preconditioning hypoxia or to TNF-α pretreatment. Zero, 16, 20, 24, 28 and 32 hours after reoxygenation cells were washed twice with cold phosphate-buffered saline, scraped off and pelleted. Cell pellets were subjected to lipid extraction and intracellular ceramide was quantified by means of reversed phase high performance liquid chromatography, according to Santana et al. [19], as has been described in detail elsewhere [15]. Ceramide values were normalized per lipid phosphate as described [15].

Measurements of TNF-α concentrations

Neuronal cultures in 24-well plates were covered with 0.4 ml of culture medium and subjected to hypoxic pretreatment. Aliquots of culture medium were withdrawn 4, 8 and 24 hours after preconditioning and TNF-α levels were measured in these samples using an enzyme-linked immunosorbent assay (ELISA) kit for rat TNF-α (Endogen, Woburn, MA) according to the manufacturer's instructions.

Statistical analysis

Statistical analysis was carried out by two-factor analysis of variance for repeated measurements, and by the paired t test using Excel software.

Results

Description of the in vitro model of hypoxia tolerance

Hypoxia-induced injury of neuronal cells had already begun during the severe hypoxic exposure, as demonstrated by measurements of number of dead cells, and it then progressed after reoxygenation. About 13% of the cells were dead ($P=0.004$, $n=4$) at the end of the 2.5-hour hypoxic incubation period. The number of dead cells doubled during 8 hours of reoxygenation ($P=0.0001$, $n=6$). Progression of hypoxia-initiated cell death continued up to 24 hours of observation. In the control cultures maintained in normoxia and in the sham-washed cultures, no significant cell death was apparent during the entire period of observation. Hypoxic preconditioning of neuronal cultures 24 hours prior to the hypoxic insult inhibited cell death. Neuronal death was reduced by 50% during the period of incubation in the hypoxic environment ($P=0.044$, $n=4$) and during progression of neuronal injury after reoxygenation by 52% at 8 hours ($P=0.0003$, $n=7$) and 39% 24 hours ($P=0.0013$, $n=7$) after reoxygenation.

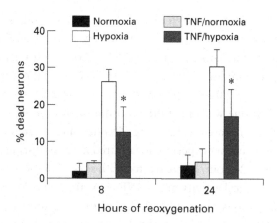

Figure 19.1   This displays the percentage of dead neurons 8 and 24 hours after severe (2.5 hours) hypoxia exposure in TNF-α preconditioned (TNF/hypoxia) neuronal cultures compared with naïve (hypoxia) neuronal cultures. Also shown is percentage of dead neurons from cultures maintained in a normoxic atmosphere with (TNF/normoxia) and without (normoxia) TNF-α preconditioning.

Glucose deprivation (GD) without hypoxia did not affect cell viability, but when superimposed on hypoxic (O) treatment (O/GD), it resulted in a higher death toll (33.4% vs. 23.6% dead cells; $P=0.03$, $n=4$). Hypoxic preconditioning, however, was as effective in protection against O/GD as it was against hypoxia alone (52% 8 hours after reoxygenation and addition of glucose; $P=0.045$, n = 4). On the basis of these observations we have chosen to study molecular mechanisms of hypoxic preconditioning in the model of hypoxic injury of neurons, rather than in the more complicated model of O/GD.

TNF-α as a mediator of hypoxic preconditioning of neurons

TNF-α (25 ng/ml) was added to neuronal cultures at 24 hours prior to hypoxic treatment. Immediately before placement of the cells into hypoxic chambers, the culture medium with TNF-α was completely exchanged for the culture medium containing no TNF-α, and cells were subjected to 2.5 hours of hypoxia treatment. Measurements of the number of dead cells 0, 8 and 24 hours after cell reoxygenation demonstrated that pretreatment with TNF-α protected neurons from a hypoxic insult to the same degree as did hypoxic preconditioning by: 40% ($P=0.004$, $n=3$), 53% ($P=0.002$, $n=5$) and 44% ($P=0.002$, $n=5$), respectively (Figure 19.1).

We hypothesized that hypoxic preconditioning is at least partially mediated by TNF-α because the time course for the TNF-α pretreatment and the magnitude of its protective effect were shown to be very similar to that for hypoxic preconditioning. This hypothesis has been tested in two ways: first, we investigated whether preconditioned neurons released TNF-α in culture medium, and, second, we examined whether inhibition of TNF-α activity during preconditioning would compromise the tolerant state. An increase in TNF-α concentrations could be detected 4 hours after preconditioning by means of the TNF-α ELISA. Eight hours after preconditioning, 6.15 ± 2.0 pg TNF-α was released by 2.5×10^5 preconditioned neurons (plated in one well) in contrast to the same number of control, untreated neurons, which released 1.0 ± 1.2 pg TNF-α (mean ± standard error (SEM); $P < 0.05$, $n = 3$). In another experiment, cultured neurons during the entire period of preconditioning (24 hours) were treated with sheep polyclonal antibody, which neutralizes the biological activity of rat TNF-α. As the severe hypoxic treatment began, the antibody was washed out with the culture medium. Hypoxic preconditioning decreased the percentage of dead cells in severe hypoxia-treated cultures from 20.2% to 7.4% ($P = 0.01$, $n = 4$) and from 27.2% to 14.7% ($P = 0.002$, $n = 4$) when measured 8 and 24 hours after reoxygenation, respectively. When preconditioning was performed in the presence of anti-TNF-α antibody, however, it had no protective effect, resulting in 17.7% (P vs. tolerant cells 0.026, $n = 4$) and 23.8% ($P = 0.017$, $n = 4$) dead cells, respectively. Sheep immunoglobulin G with no specificity against TNF-α contrasted with the above results in that it did not block the effect of preconditioning on neuronal survival.

Ceramide is a downstream mediator of hypoxic tolerance

Just before the hypoxic insult, cell permeable C-2 ceramide (10 μM) was added to neuronal cultures. Cells were subjected to 2.5 hours of hypoxia and the number of dead cells was measured by an ethidium homodimer exclusion test 8 and 24 hours after reoxygenation. The presence of C-2 ceramide in the culture medium decreased the cell death rate from 30.1% to 13.5% ($P = 0.001$, $n = 4$) and from 34.1% to 16.1% ($P = 0.009$, $n = 4$) 8 and 24 hours after reoxygenation, respectively (Figure 19.2). The efficacy of ceramide-induced protection (55% and 54%, respectively) was similar to that of hypoxic preconditioning (52% and 39%, respectively) and that of TNF-α (53% and 44%, respectively).

At time intervals to 32 hours after hypoxic preconditioning and after TNF-α pretreatment, ceramide concentrations in neuronal cells were measured. Increased intracellular ceramide levels 120% to 140% over baseline (0.7 ± 0.1 pmol lipid phosphate/nmol) were observed by 16 hours ($P = 0.018$, $n = 3$) and reached 180% to 200% 24 hours after preconditioning ($P = 0.035$, $n = 3$). Ceramide accumulation peaked at 20 hours in two out of five experiments. A similar ceramide time course was observed in TNF-α-pretreated neurons. Neither of the preconditioning exposures, hypoxia or TNF-α, induced ceramide accumulation in the presence of fumonisin B$_1$, a mycotoxin produced by *Fusarium monileforme*, which inhibits ceramide synthetase (sphingosine-N-acyl transferase) in many cell types including neurons [4].

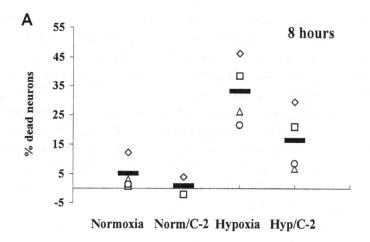

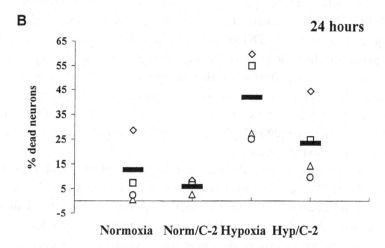

Figure 19.2 This shows the percentage of dead neurons 8 and 24 hours after severe (2.5 hours) hypoxia exposure in C-2 ceramide-treated (Hyp/C-2) neuronal cultures compared with naïve (Hypoxia) neuronal cultures. Also shown is percentage of dead neurons from cultures maintained in a normoxic atmosphere with (Norm/C-2) and without (Normoxia) C-2 ceramide treatment. Differences between Hyp/C-2 and Hypoxia cultures were highly significant at both time points.

The ability of fumonisin B_1 to attenuate tolerance paralleled its inhibitory effect on ceramide levels in preconditioned cells. Hypoxic preconditioning without fumonisin B_1 rescued 45.8% ($P=0.0013$, $n=4$) and 51.8% ($P=0.023$; $n=4$) of cells subjected to 2.5 hours of hypoxic insult, which would otherwise have died 8 and 24 hours, respectively, after reoxygenation. The percentage of dead cells in the cultures preconditioned in the presence of fumonisin B_1 was not significantly different from that of the naïve cultures: 17.9% vs. 17.4% at 8 hours and 20.8% vs. 25.4% 24 hours after reoxygenation (P values vs. tolerant cells were 0.01 and 0.026 for 8 and 24 hours, respectively, $n=4$). These studies indicate that ceramide de novo synthesis is required for induction of tolerance to severe hypoxia by hypoxic or TNF-α preconditioning.

Discussion

The data indicate that exogenous TNF-α and exogenous C-2 ceramide were able to substitute for hypoxic pretreatment in making cortical neurons resistant to a subsequent hypoxic insult. TNF-α and C-2 ceramide protected neurons to the same degree as did hypoxic preconditioning. Hypoxic preconditioning resulted in no tolerance if it was performed in the presence of a TNF-α-neutralizing antibody (but not in the presence of a non-specific antibody) or in the presence of the inhibitor of ceramide de novo synthesis, fumonisin B_1. The ability of fumonisin B_1 to block hypoxic preconditioning suggests that de novo synthesis of ceramide contributes to induction of tolerance.

Measurements of ceramide levels in cells preconditioned with hypoxia or pretreated with TNF-α provide further evidence that ceramide is a TNF-α messenger during induction of ischemic tolerance. Both treatments resulted in a delayed increase of intracellular ceramide levels that coincided with development of resistance to the severe hypoxic insult. These data are consistent with our previous observation that astrocytes and brain endothelial cells preconditioned with TNF-α also exhibit delayed ceramide responses, which coincide with a tolerant state [20]. The ability of fumonisin B_1 to abolish ceramide synthesis parallels its effect on ischemic tolerance and strongly argues for a role of ceramide as a mediator of tolerance.

Mechanisms controlling apoptosis/survival in neuronal cells through stabilization of $[Ca^{2+}]_i$, increase of the density of the outward potassium currents and induction of antioxidants [21–23] involve activation of nuclear factor-kappa B (NF-κB). Which of these mechanisms is involved in ceramide-mediated hypoxic preconditioning in neuronal cells is not clear. Participation of NF-κB in adaptation to ischemia is suggested by recent studies of myocardial preconditioning [24,25]. In support of this hypothesis, loss of NF-κB activity was observed during brain ischemia and inhibition of NF-κB sensitized brain cells to cytotoxic effects of TNF-α in vitro [26].

REFERENCES

1 Chen J & Simon R (1997) Ischemic tolerance in the brain. *Neurology*, **48**, 306–11.

2 Hallenbeck JM, Dutka AJ, Vogel SN, Heldman E, Doron DA & Feuerstein G (1991) Lipopolysaccharide-induced production of tumor necrosis factor activity in rats with and without risk factors for stroke. *Brain Research*, **541**, 115–20.

3 Liu T, Clark RK, McDonnell PC, Young PR, White RF, Barone FC & Feuerstein GZ (1994) Tumor necrosis factor-alpha expression in ischemic neurons. *Stroke*, **25**, 1481–8.

4 Yamasaki Y, Itoyama Y & Kogure K (1996) Involvement of cytokine production in pathogenesis of transient cerebral ischemic damage. *Keio Journal of Medicine*, **45**, 225–9.

5 Uno H, Matsuyama T, Akita H, Nishimura H & Sugita M (1997) Induction of tumor necrosis factor-alpha in the mouse hippocampus following transient forebrain ischemia. *Journal of Cerebral Blood Flow & Metabolism*, **17**, 491–9.

6 Botchkina GI, Meistrell ME III, Botchkina IL & Tracey KJ (1997) Expression of TNF and TNF receptors (p55 and p75) in the rat brain after focal cerebral ischemia. *Molecular Medicine*, **3**, 765–81.

7 Smith RA & Baglioni C (1992) Characterization of TNF receptors. *Immunology Series*, **56**, 131–47.

8 Arvin B, Neville LF, Barone FC & Feuerstein GZ (1996) The role of inflammation and cytokines in brain injury. *Neuroscience & Biobehavioral Reviews*, **20**, 445–52.

9 Mattson MP (1997) Neuroprotective signal transduction: relevance to stroke. *Neuroscience & Biobehavioral Reviews*, **21**, 193–206.

10 Dawson DA, Martin D & Hallenbeck JM (1996) Inhibition of tumor necrosis factor-alpha reduces focal cerebral ischemic injury in the spontaneously hypertensive rat. *Neuroscience Letters*, **218**, 41–4.

11 Nawashiro H, Tasaki K, Ruetzler CA & Hallenbeck JM (1997) TNF-alpha pretreatment induces protective effects against focal cerebral ischemia in mice. *Journal of Cerebral Blood Flow & Metabolism*, **17**, 483–90.

12 Bruce AJ, Boling W, Kindy MS, Peschon J, Kraemer PJ, Carpenter MK, Holtsberg FW & Mattson MP (1996) Altered neuronal and microglial responses to excitotoxic and ischemic brain injury in mice lacking TNF receptors. *Nature Medicine*, **2**, 788–94.

13 Tasaki K, Ruetzler CA, Ohtsuki T, Martin D, Nawashiro H & Hallenbeck JM (1997) Lipopolysaccharide pre-treatment induces resistance against subsequent focal cerebral ischemic damage in spontaneously hypertensive rats. *Brain Research*, **748**, 267–70.

14 Nawashiro H, Martin D & Hallenbeck JM (1997) Inhibition of tumor necrosis factor and amelioration of brain infarction in mice. *Journal of Cerebral Blood Flow & Metabolism*, **17**, 229–32.

15 Ghosh S, Strum JC & Bell RM (1997) Lipid biochemistry: functions of glycerolipids and sphingolipids in cellular signaling. *FASEB Journal*, **11**, 45–50.

16 Kolesnick R & Golde DW (1994) The sphingomyelin pathway in tumor necrosis factor and interleukin-1 signaling. *Cell*, **77**, 325–8.

17 Pena LA, Fuks Z & Kolesnick R (1997) Stress-induced apoptosis and the sphingomyelin pathway. *Biochemical Pharmacology*, **53**, 615–21.

18 Smyth MJ, Obeid LM & Hannun YA (1997) Ceramide: a novel lipid mediator of apoptosis. *Advances in Pharmacology*, **41**, 133–54.

19 Santana P, Pena LA, Haimovitz-Friedman A, Martin S, Green D, McLoughlin M, Cordon-Cardo C, Schuchman EH, Fuks Z & Kolesnick R (1996) Acid sphingomyelinase-deficient human lymphoblasts and mice are defective in radiation-induced apoptosis. *Cell*, **86**, 189–99.

20 Ginis I, Schweizer U, Brenner M, Liu J, Azzam N, Spatz M & Hallenbeck JM (1999) TNF-a pretreatment prevents subsequent activation of cultured brain cells with TNF-a and hypoxia via ceramide. *American Journal of Physiology*, **276**, C1171–C1183.

21 Barger SW, Hörster D, Furukawa K, Goodman Y, Krieglstein J & Mattson MP (1995) Tumor necrosis factors a and b protect neurons against amyloid b-peptide toxicity: evidence for involvement of a kB-binding factor and attenuation of peroxide and Ca^{2+} accumulation. *Proceedings of the National Academy of Sciences, USA*, **92**, 9328–32.

22 Furukawa K & Mattson MP (1998) The transcription factor NF-kappaB mediates increases in calcium currents and decreases in NMDA- and AMPA/kainate-induced currents induced by tumor necrosis factor-alpha in hippocampal neurons. *Journal of Neurochemistry*, **70**, 1876–86.

23 Mattson MP, Goodman Y, Luo H, Fu W & Furukawa K (1997) Activation of NF-kB protects hippocampal neurons against oxidative stress-induced apoptosis: evidence for induction of manganese superoxide dismutase and suppression of peroxynitrite production and protein tyrosine nitration. *Journal of Neuroscience Research*, **49**, 681–97.

24 Maulik N, Sasaki H & Galang N (1999) Differential regulation of apoptosis by ischemia-reperfusion and ischemic adaptation. *Annals of the New York Academy of Sciences*, **874**, 401–11.

25 Xuan Y-T, Tang X-L, Banerjee S, Takano H, Li RCX, Han H, Qiu Y, Li J-J & Bolli R (1999) Nuclear factor-kB plays an essential role in the late phase of ischemic preconditioning in conscious rabbits. *Circulation Research*, **84**, 1095–109.

26 Botchkina GI, Geimonen E, Bilof ML, Villarreal O & Tracey KJ (1999) Loss of NF-kappaB activity during cerebral ischemia and TNF cytotoxicity. *Molecular Medicine*, **5**, 372–81.

20

Sites and mechanisms of IL-1 action in ischemic and excitotoxic brain damage

Stuart M. Allan[1], Robert I. Grundy[2], Lisa C. Parker[3] &
Nancy J. Rothwell[4]

[1-4] School of Biological Sciences, University of Manchester, Manchester, England

Cytokines and ischemic brain damage

Cytokines are polypeptides that include the families of interleukins (IL-1), tumor necrosis factors (TNF), interferons and growth factors with diverse actions on development, inflammation, tissue injury and repair in almost all cells in the body. The past decade has witnessed increasing interest in the functions and importance of cytokines in central nervous system biology and pathology.

Most cytokines are produced at low levels in healthy adult brains, but many are upregulated rapidly in response to injury, infection or inflammation in the brain including cerebral ischemia [1,2]. The influence of cytokines on ischemic brain damage appears to be diverse and complex. While several cytokines have clearly identified neurotrophic or neuroprotective effects (e.g., IL-6, insulin-like growth factor (IGF), nerve growth factor (NGF), fibroblast growth factor (FGF), transforming growth factor-β (TGF-β)), others have been implicated as mediators of cell damage (most notably IL-1), while for some (such as TNF-α) both neuroprotective and neurotoxic effects have been identified. This review will focus on the actions of IL-1 on ischemic brain damage and recent findings about its mechanisms of action.

IL-1 expression in stroke

IL-1, IL-1α and IL-1β, and IL-1 receptor antagonist (IL-1ra) are all rapidly produced in response to experimental stroke and excitotoxic and traumatic brain injury in rodents [3–5]. Temporal studies on expression indicate that IL-1β is produced most extensively and rapidly, initially by microglia and meningeal macrophages and later by astrocytes and invading immune cells [6–9]. IL-1α appears to be induced slightly later than IL-1β, but by the same cells, while IL-1ra expression occurs later, predominantly in neurons [10,11].

IL-1β, the major ligand, is produced as an inactive precursor (pro-IL-1β) which must be cleaved by the enzyme caspase-1 to yield the mature, active form of IL-1β. Thus, bioactive IL-1β will be produced only where and when caspase-1 is expressed and activated – reportedly predominantly in microglia [12]. All other components of the IL-1 family have also been identified in the central nervous system, including the signaling receptor (IL-1RI) and its accessory protein, which is required for signal transduction, as well as the RII receptor, which is non-signaling, but can act as a shield "decoy" receptor [13]. However, there is considerable debate about the cells and regions that express IL-1RI; astrocytes certainly express this receptor, but its location on microglia, neurons and cerebrovascular cells is less well defined, though all of these can respond to IL-1.

Evidence for IL-1 involvement in stroke

The evidence that IL-1 participates directly in ischemic, excitotoxic and traumatic brain damage derives from three sets of observations. First, as described above, IL-1 (immunoreactive and bioactive) is produced rapidly after induction of cerebral ischemia in rodents in a temporal and spatial pattern that is consistent with the emergence of cell injury and death [6–9].

IL-1 itself is not directly neurotoxic to healthy neurons in vivo or in vitro. Indeed, IL-1 can, at low concentrations, *protect* primary cultured neurons from excitotoxic injury [14]. However, injection (intracerebroventricular (icv)) of low doses (< 10 ng) of recombinant IL-1β, or injection into specific brain regions of the rat dramatically enhances ischemic and excitotoxic brain damage [15–18].

Most importantly, blocking the release or actions of endogenous IL-1 markedly attenuates ischemic brain damage in rodents [11,17,19–22]. The majority of studies have used recombinant IL-1ra injected icv into rodents, though IL-1ra is also effective, at much higher doses, when administered intravenously or intraperitoneally [20,23]. IL-1ra has been shown to reduce infarct volume by over 50% in rats or mice exposed to permanent or reversible middle cerebral artery occlusion (MCAO), and also reduces neuronal loss caused by global ischemia in gerbils [24] or hypoxia–ischemia in neonatal rats [25]. This neuroprotection by IL-1ra is associated with reduced edema and neutrophil invasion, increased numbers of surviving neurons and improved neurological function [20,23]. The therapeutic window for protection by IL-1ra varies according to the type of injury, ranging from 1 hour in permanent MCAO, to at least 4 hours after lateral fluid percussion injury (brain trauma) [26]. Additional studies have demonstrated that injection of caspase inhibitors or genetic deletion of caspase-1 (which limit IL-1β release) or administration of antibodies to IL-1β, also reduce ischemic brain damage, supporting the studies with IL-1ra and suggesting that IL-1β is the predominant ligand [19,27,28].

Mechanisms of IL-1 action

At the time of writing, the mechanism(s) by which IL-1 contributes to ischemic brain damage is largely unknown, but may involve multiple actions of the cytokine on neurons, glia and the vasculature. It has been established that IL-1 is induced by N-methyl-D-aspartate (NMDA), α-amino-3-hydroxy-5-methyl-4-isoxazole propionic acid (AMPA) or kainate receptor activation, and contributes to neuronal death induced by these excitotoxins [7–9,16]. Several actions of IL-1 have been reported that may contribute to ischemic damage.

IL-1 is a potent pyrogen, and an increase in body temperature could exacerbate neuronal loss after ischemia [29,30]. However, several studies suggest that this is unlikely to be a primary mediator of IL-1 effects [18,31]. Similarly, reported effects of IL-1 on release of prostanoids, kinins, free radicals and nitric oxide, induction of adhesion molecules, acute phase proteins and complement and induction of vascular injury are all likely to influence the outcome after stroke, but the specific contributions of these pathways have not been clearly demonstrated.

Specific sites of IL-1 action

Our recent data suggest that IL-1 may act at specific sites within the brain to influence damage at distant regions. In rats subjected to permanent MCAO, injection of IL-1β into the striatum markedly exacerbates cortical injury, while injection of IL-1ra at this site inhibits both striatal and cortical damage. In contrast, IL-1β or IL-1ra infused directly into the cortex fail to influence infarct volume at either site [18,22]. Similar site-specific actions have been identified in excitotoxic damage. Striatal infusion of the excitotoxin S-AMPA induces local injury that is attenuated by IL-1ra [16]. While IL-1β alone fails to induce neuronal damage, co-infusion with S-AMPA into the striatum leads to massive cortical damage and edema (Figure 20.1). These drastic effects are not obvious when IL-1β is co-infused with an excitotoxin directly into the cortex, and are not mimicked by striatal infusion of the excitotoxin with TNF-α or IL-6 ([16] and S.M. Allan & N.J. Rothwell, unpublished observations).

Although IL-1β does cause an increase in body temperature, this is unlikely to be the cause of the distant cortical damage for several reasons. Icv injection of IL-1β with striatal S-AMPA causes similar fever, but no cortical damage. IL-6, a similar pyrogen, has no such effect [31]. There are no direct striatocortical pathways and we now believe that IL-1 activates complex polysynaptic pathways to cause distant cortical injury.

More detailed localization studies have identified specific responses within the striatum at which co-injection of IL-1β and S-AMPA are most effective in causing

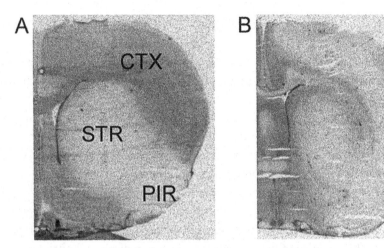

Figure 20.1   Representative coronal brain sections to demonstrate the effect of intrastriatal co-injection of vehicle (A) or hrIL-1β (10 ng) (B) with S-AMPA (7.5 nmol) on neuronal damage. The pale (white) region is non-viable neuronal tissue and the dark region represents viable tissue. Note the extensive region of the cortex damaged after treatment with hrIL-1β. CTX, parietal cortex; STR, striatum; PIR, piriform cortex.

cortical injury (predominantly in the parietal region) – notably the lateral shell of the nucleus accumbens and the ventrolateral striatum (Figure 20.2). These regions have connections with the limbic system [32] and the hypothalamus [33]. The hypothalamus is a known site of IL-1 action [13,34,35] and it is possible that connections to this brain area from the ventral striatum and nucleus accumbens may contribute to effects of IL-1β on AMPA receptor-mediated cell death. Importantly, there are direct and indirect (via the basal ganglia and related structures such as the thalamus and amygdala) afferent projections from the hypothalamus to the entire cortical mantle [33,36], and these could influence cortical cell excitability and survival.

Involvement of the hypothalamus in IL-1 actions

In view of the striatal outputs described above, which may contribute to IL-1β effects on cortical injury, we investigated the possible role of the hypothalamus in these distant actions of IL-1β. A marked increase in IL-1β mRNA was observed in the hypothalamus 3 hours after striatal injection of hrIL-1β or S-AMPA plus hrIL-1β, compared to naïve, sham, vehicle- or S-AMPA-treated animals (data not shown). This increase was maintained at 8 hours. In addition, a marked increase in IL-1β mRNA in the ipsilateral cortex of S-AMPA- plus hrIL-1β-treated animals was seen (Figure 20.3). Similar changes in immunoreactive IL-1β levels were detected with enzyme-linked immunosorbent assay.

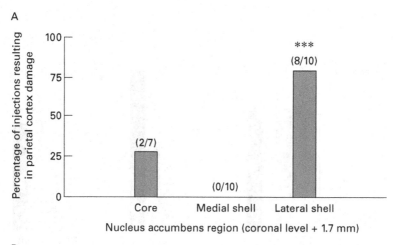

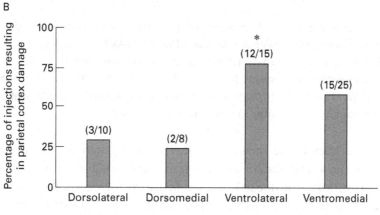

Figure 20.2 Bar graphs showing effect of injection site on the cortical cell death produced by intrastriatal injection of hrIL-1β and S-AMPA. (A) Percentage of animals displaying marked cell death in the parietal cortex after injection of S-AMPA (6 nmol) and hrIL-1β (10 ng) into the core, medial shell, and lateral shell of the nucleus accumbens at +1.7 mm anterior to bregma. ***$P<0.001$ vs. medial shell (Fisher's exact test). (B) Percentage of animals displaying marked cell death in the parietal cortex after injection of S-AMPA (6 nmol) and hrIL-1β (10 ng) into the dorsolateral, dorsomedial, ventrolateral and ventromedial quadrants of the striatum at +0.7 mm anterior to bregma. Data represented as the percentage of animals displaying distinct cell death in the parietal cortical region compared to the number injected (actual numbers indicated in parentheses). *$P<0.05$ vs. dorsolateral and dorsomedial (Fisher's exact test).

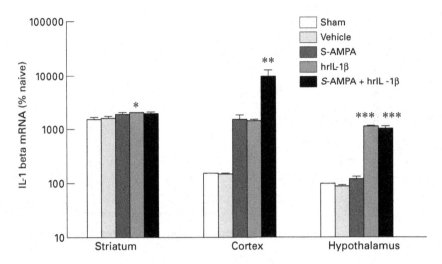

Figure 20.3 Expression of IL-1β mRNA (as a percentage of naïve values) in different regions of the rat brain 8 hours after intrastriatal injection of vehicle, S-AMPA (7.5 nmol), hrIL-1β (10 ng) or S-AMPA (7.5 nmol) + hrIL-1β (10 ng). Values are from three or four rats at each time point and are expressed as mean ± SEM. *$P < 0.05$ vs. sham; **$P < 0.01$ vs. sham, vehicle, S-AMPA + hrIL-1β; ***$P < 0.001$ vs. sham, vehicle and S-AMPA (one-way analysis of variance followed by Tukey's multiple comparison test).

Subsequently, we showed that IL-1β injected into the hypothalamus alone caused no local or distant cell damage, but when combined with excitotoxin injection (S-AMPA) into the striatum, resulted in extensive cortical injury similar to that observed in response to co-infusion of IL-1β and S-AMPA into the striatum (Figure 20.4A). In order to determine whether endogenous IL-1 in the hypothalamus contributes to distant cortical injury, the effects of IL-1ra were studied. Intrastriatal co-infusion of IL-1β and S-AMPA again led to massive cortical injury that was markedly attenuated by hypothalamic injection of IL-1ra (Figure 20.4B). Thus we propose that IL-1 synergizes with other insults in the striatum to cause expression of IL-1 in the hypothalamus, and that this in turn leads to distant cortical injury. The resulting cortical death occurs slightly after the striatal injury and is dependent on local activation of NMDA receptors, since cortical infusion of a selective NMDA receptor antagonist inhibits the cortical infarct (S.M. Allan & N.J. Rothwell, unpublished data).

These site-specific effects of IL-1, which cause distant cortical injury, remain to be fully explained. At present, the exact nature of the striatohypothalamic pathways or hypothalamic-cortical pathways are not identified, and the involvement of additional pathways with the thalamus and amygdala require investigation. Similarly, it is not known why IL-1 synergizes with S-AMPA at these striatal sites that do not correlate with the reported distribution of IL-1RI receptors.

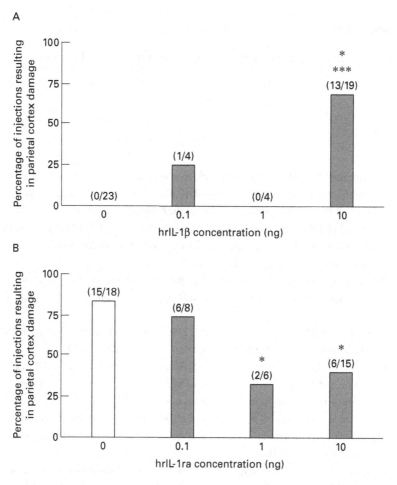

Figure 20.4 (A) Effect of hypothalamic IL-1β treatment on cortical cell death produced by intrastriatal injection of S-AMPA in the rat brain. Groups of animals were injected in the striatum with S-AMPA (7.5 nmol), immediately followed by injection of hrIL-1β (0.1, 1 or 10 ng) or vehicle (0 ng) in the lateral hypothalamus. *P<0.05 vs. 0.1 ng; ***P<0.001 vs. vehicle (0 ng; Fisher's exact test). (B) Effect of hypothalamic IL-1ra treatment on cortical cell death produced by intrastriatal injection of IL-1β plus S-AMPA in the rat brain. Groups of animals were injected in the striatum with S-AMPA (7.5 nmol) + hrIL-1β (10 ng), followed immediately by injection of hrIL-1ra (0.1, 1 or 10 μg) or vehicle (0 μg) in the lateral hypothalamus. Data represented as the percentage of animals displaying distinct cell death in the parietal cortical region as compared with the number injected (actual numbers indicated in parentheses). *P<0.05 vs. vehicle (0 ng; Fisher's exact test).

Acknowledgments

We are grateful to MRC and EU Biomed for supporting this work.

REFERENCES

1 Benveniste EN (1997) Cytokines: influence on glial cell gene expression and function. In *Neuroimmunoendocrinology*, vol. 69, ed. JE Blalock, pp. 31–75. Basel: Karger.

2 Rothwell NJ (1999) Cytokines – killers in the brain? *Journal of Physiology*, **514**, 3–17.

3 Yabuuchi K, Minami M, Katsumata S, Yamazaki A & Satoh M (1994) An in situ hybridization study on interleukin-1 beta mRNA induced by transient forebrain ischemia in the rat brain. *Molecular Brain Research*, **26**, 135–42.

4 Yabuuchi K, Minami M, Katsumata S & Satoh M (1993) In situ hybridization study of interleukin-1β mRNA induced by kainic acid in the rat brain. *Molecular Brain Research*, **20**, 153–61.

5 Buttini M, Sauter A & Boddeke HWGM (1994) Induction of interleukin-1β mRNA after focal cerebral ischaemia in the rat. *Molecular Brain Research*, **23**, 126–34.

6 Davies CA, Loddick SA, Toulmond S, Stroemer RP, Hunt J & Rothwell NJ (1999) The progression and topographic distribution of interleukin-1β expression after permanent middle cerebral artery occlusion in the rat. *Journal of Cerebral Blood Flow & Metabolism*, **19**, 87–98.

7 Pearson VL, Rothwell NJ & Toulmond S (1999) Excitotoxic brain damage in the rat induces interleukin-1β protein in microglia and astrocytes: correlation with the progression of cell death. *Glia*, **25**, 311–23.

8 Vezzani A, Conti M, De Luigi A, Ravizza T, Moneta D, Marchesi F & De Simoni MG (1999) Interleukin-1β immunoreactivity and microglia are enhanced in the rat hippocampus by focal kainate application: functional evidence for enhancement of electrographic seizures. *Journal of Neuroscience*, **19**, 5054–65.

9 Eriksson C, Van Dam AM, Lucassen PJ, Bol JGJM, Winblad B & Schultzberg M (1999) Immunohistochemical localization of interleukin-1β, interleukin-1 receptor antagonist and interleukin-1β converting enzyme/caspase-1 in the rat brain after peripheral administration of kainic acid. *Neuroscience*, **93**, 915–30.

10 Toulmond S & Rothwell NJ (1995) Time-course of IL-1 receptor antagonist (IL-1ra) expression after brain trauma in the rat. *Society for Neuroscience Abstracts*, **21**, 200.2.

11 Loddick SA, Wong M-L, Bongiorno PB, Gold PW, Licinio J & Rothwell NJ (1997) Endogenous interleukin-1 receptor antagonist is neuroprotective. *Biochemical and Biophysical Research Communications*, **234**, 211–15.

12 Bhat RV, DiRocco R, Marcy VR, Flood DG, Zhu Y, Dobrzanski P, Siman R, Scott R, Contreras PC & Miller M (1996) Increased expression of IL-1β converting enzyme in hippocampus after ischemia: selective localization in microglia. *Journal of Neuroscience*, **16**, 4146–54.

13 Dinarello CA (1996) Biologic basis for interleukin-1 in disease. *Blood*, **87**, 2095–147.

14 Strijbos PJLM & Rothwell NJ (1995) Interleukin-1β attenuates excitatory amino acid-induced neurodegeneration in vitro: involvement of nerve growth factor. *Journal of Neuroscience,* 15, 3468–74.

15 Yamasaki Y, Matsuura N, Shozuhara H, Onodera H, Itoyama Y & Kogure K (1995) Interleukin-1 as a pathogenetic mediator of ischemic brain damage in rats. *Stroke,* 26, 676–81.

16 Lawrence CB, Allan SM & Rothwell NJ (1998) Interleukin-1β and the interleukin-1 receptor antagonist act in the striatum to modify excitotoxic brain damage in the rat. *European Journal of Neuroscience,* 10, 1188–95.

17 Loddick SA & Rothwell NJ (1996) Neuroprotective effects of human recombinant interleukin-1 receptor antagonist in focal cerebral ischaemia in the rat. *Journal of Cerebral Blood Flow & Metabolism,* 16, 932–40.

18 Stroemer RP & Rothwell NJ (1998) Exacerbation of ischemic brain damage by localized striatal injection of interleukin-1β in the rat. *Journal of Cerebral Blood Flow & Metabolism,* 18, 833–9.

19 Betz AL, Yang G-Y & Davidson BL (1995) Attenuation of stroke size in rats using an adenoviral vector to induce overexpression of interleukin-1 receptor antagonist in brain. *Journal of Cerebral Blood Flow & Metabolism,* 15, 547–51.

20 Garcia JH, Liu KF & Relton JK (1995) Interleukin-1 receptor antagonist decreases the number of necrotic neurons in rats with middle cerebral artery occlusion. *American Journal of Pathology,* 147, 1477–86.

21 Relton JK & Rothwell NJ (1992) Interleukin-1 receptor antagonist inhibits ischaemic and excitotoxic brain damage in the rat. *Journal of Physiology,* 452, 122P.

22 Stroemer RP & Rothwell NJ (1997) Cortical protection by localized striatal injection of IL-1ra following cerebral ischemia in the rat. *Journal of Cerebral Blood Flow & Metabolism,* 17, 597–604.

23 Relton JK, Martin D, Thompson RC & Russell DA (1996) Peripheral administration of interleukin-1 receptor antagonist inhibits brain damage after focal cerebral ischemia in the rat. *Experimental Neurology,* 138, 206–13.

24 Martin D, Relton JK, Muller G, Bendele A, Fischer N & Russell D (1996) Cytokines as therapeutic agents in neurological disorders. In *Cytokines in the Nervous System,* ed. NJ Rothwell, pp. 162–78. Boston, MA: Chapman & Hall.

25 Martin D, Chinookoswong N & Miller G (1994) The interleukin-1 receptor antagonist (rhIL-1ra) protects against cerebral infarction in a rat model of hypoxia–ischemia. *Experimental Neurology,* 130, 362–7.

26 Toulmond S & Rothwell NJ (1995) Interleukin-1 receptor antagonist inhibits neuronal damage caused by fluid percussion injury in the rat. *Brain Research,* 671, 261–6.

27 Loddick SA, MacKenzie A & Rothwell NJ (1996) An ICE inhibitor, z-VAD-DCB, attenuates ischaemic brain damage in the rat. *Neuroreport,* 7, 1465–8.

28 Hara H, Fink K, Endres M, Friedlander RM, Gagliardini V, Yuan J & Moskowitz MA (1997) Attenuation of transient focal cerebral ischemic injury in transgenic mice expressing a mutant ICE inhibitory protein. *Journal of Cerebral Blood Flow & Metabolism,* 17, 370–5.

29 Busto R, Dietrich WD, Globus MYT, Valdés I, Scheinberg P & Ginsberg MD (1987) Small differences in intraischemic brain temperature critically determine the extent of ischemic neuronal injury. *Journal of Cerebral Blood Flow & Metabolism,* 7, 729–38.

30 Malberg JE & Seiden LS (1998) Small changes in ambient temperature cause large changes in 3,4-methylenedioxymethamphetamine (MDMA)-induced serotonin neurotoxicity and core body temperature in the rat. *Journal of Neuroscience,* 18, 5086–94.

31 Grundy RI, Rothwell NJ & Allan SM (1999) Dissociation between the effects of interleukin-1 on excitotoxic brain damage and body temperature in the rat. *Brain Research,* 830, 32–7.

32 Heimer L, Alheid GF, de Olmos JS, Groenewegen HJ, Haber SN, Harlan RE & Zahm DS (1997) The accumbens: beyond the core-shell dichotomy. *Journal of Neuropsychiatry and Clinical Neurosciences,* 9, 354–81.

33 Risold PY, Thompson RH & Swanson LW (1997) The structural organization of connections between hypothalamus and cerebral cortex. *Brain Research Reviews,* 24, 197–254.

34 Rothwell NJ & Hopkins SJ (1995) Cytokines and the nervous system. II: Actions and mechanisms of action. *Trends in Neurosciences,* 18, 130–6.

35 Rothwell NJ & Luheshi G (1994) Pharmacology of interleukin-1 actions in the brain. *Advances in Pharmacology,* 25, 1–20.

36 Saper CB (1985) Organization of cerebral cortical afferent systems in the rat. II. Hypothalamocortical projections. *Journal of Comparative Neurology,* 237, 21–46.

21

Protease generation, inflammation and cerebral microvascular activation

Gregory J. del Zoppo

Department of Molecular and Experimental Medicine, The Scripps Research Institute, La Jolla, CA

Introduction

Middle cerebral artery occlusion (MCAO) promotes occlusion of downstream microvessels, which leads to microvascular perfusion defects [1–6], and initiates cellular inflammation, which requires the sequential expression of leukocyte adhesion receptors on microvascular endothelial cells [7,8]. Changes in microvascular integrity and permeability [9,10], loss of basal lamina integrity [11,12], simultaneous decreases in specific endothelial cell and astrocyte integrins [13,14] and changes in astrocyte ultrastructure [2,15] also occur during early ischemia. Endothelial cell leukocyte adhesion receptors respond to ischemia in a rapid and orderly way, to initiate the cellular inflammatory response. P-selectin appears on the endothelium by 2 hours of MCAO, followed by intercellular adhesion molecule-1 by 4 hours and E-selectin between 7 and 24 hours after MCAO (during reperfusion) [7,8]. Also, integrin $\alpha_V\beta_3$ is rapidly expressed by microvascular myointimal smooth muscle cells within 2 hours of MCAO [16,17]. Those findings are consistent with the view that both microvascular and neuron injury may occur much more rapidly than the time frame for the appearance of cellular inflammatory cells in the primate basal ganglia.

Cerebral capillaries consist of endothelial cells, basal lamina (a portion of the extracellular matrix (ECM)) and astrocyte end-feet. Anatomical and functional relationships support their consideration as unique ternary complexes [1,18]. In the adult brain, the ECM is found as the basal lamina in microvessels and within the meninges, in addition to other sites [19]. In non-capillary microvessels, individual smooth muscle cells are encased in the ECM, which is continuous with the basal lamina [18]. The basal lamina is also one important barrier to the transmigration of circulating blood cells [11,12].

The microvascular basal lamina and ECM

The ECM is a fabric of laminins, type IV collagen, fibronectin and heparan sulfates studded with entactin, thrombospondin and nidogen [20]. Although less well appreciated, selected proteoglycans have been identified between neurons and neighboring cells [19]. Generated by endothelial cells and astrocytes in concert during development, the basal lamina forms a biologically active connection between these two cell compartments. Organotypic tissue cultures have shown that the intact basal lamina requires the juxtaposition of microvascular endothelium and astrocytes [21,22]. Microvascular endothelial cells and astrocytes play reciprocal roles in the generation of matrix proteins. In culture, astrocytes secrete laminin, fibronectin and chondroitin sulfate proteoglycan, while collagens stimulate astrocyte-induced endothelial cell maturation [23–25]. Conversely, endothelial cell-derived ECM components stimulate astrocyte growth and function (e.g., glutamine synthetase activity) [26,27]. The blood–brain barrier also relies upon the interdependence of endothelial cells and astrocytes. This has been elegantly shown in chick–quail adrenal vascular tissue/brain tissue xenografts [28] and fetal–adult hippocampal/neocortex allograft preparations [29]. Soluble factor(s) generated by astrocytes are necessary to maintain endothelial blood–brain barrier characteristics, including the induction of tight junctions, transendothelial resistance and glucose/amino acid transport polarity [29–31]. The basal lamina and blood–brain barriers, then, depend exquisitely upon cooperation between these two unrelated cell types. Disruption of both barriers, as during focal cerebral ischemia, contributes to edema formation and hemorrhagic transformation.

Endothelial cell–astrocyte–neuron interrelationships

The proximity of the endothelium to neighboring astrocytes in cerebral capillaries and postcapillary venules suggests a close functional relationship for communication and nutrient supply. Adhesion receptors on endothelial cells and on astrocyte end-feet are presumed to maintain close cell–cell apposition [10,13,14]. The association of astrocytes with neurons suggests the presence of direct interactions between cerebral microvessels and the neurons they serve.

The endothelium and astrocyte end-feet attach to matrix laminins and collagen IV by integrin receptors. Integrins are $\alpha\beta$ heterodimeric transmembrane glycoproteins that participate in vascular development, structural integrity and intercellular communication [32–34]. The matrix attachments of individual cells occur at focal contact points [35]. In one formulation, when cells attach to the matrix via integrin receptors, the respective matrix metalloproteinase (MMP) is not secreted; but, with detachment, the MMP is secreted and the receptor is not expressed at the contact point [36,37]. It might be predicted that, in cerebral microvessels where the endothelium and astrocyte end-feet detach from the matrix, connections with neurons may be lost.

Focal cerebral ischemia and microvascular responses

During early focal ischemia, subtle changes in endothelial cell ultrastructure and increases in endothelial permeability coincide with swelling of astrocyte end-foot processes and astrocyte cytoplasmic reorganization. The rapidity of these changes, together with the onset of neurological symptoms, the loss of integrin receptors on endothelial cells and astrocytes, the appearance of MMPs and neuron injury suggest that both microvascular and neuron injury are related.

Markers of neuron injury

Incorporation of labeled deoxyuridine 5'-triphosphate (dUTP) into sites of nuclear DNA scission, which reflect DNA damage and repair events, provides a reliable index of neuron and non-vascular cell injury in the primate ischemic basal ganglia [38–41]. By 2 hours of MCAO the extent of the regions of most severe ischemic injury (dUTP$^+$, Ic) can be easily distinguished from regions peripheral to the ischemic center (dUTP$^-$, Ip). The number and density of dUTP$^+$ cells within the ischemic region increase with time after MCAO significantly faster in the non-human primate than in the Wistar rat [41]. In the primate basal ganglia, by 2 hours of MCAO, $80.0 \pm 6.6\%$ of dUTP$^+$ cells are microtubule-associated protein-2$^+$ neurons. By 24 hours of reperfusion, $<2\%$ of endothelial and vascular myointimal cells are dUTP$^+$ [41]. These findings imply that dUTP incorporation can define the region of ischemic injury in the primate basal ganglia by 2 hours of MCAO, when neuron injury is detectable. This allows coordination of microvascular events with early evidence of neuron injury.

The microvascular basal lamina and integrin receptors

During focal cerebral ischemia, microvascular basal lamina antigens are lost. The ECM components of the basal lamina (laminin-1, laminin-5, collagen IV and fibronectin) disappear together during MCAO [11,12]. The intermediate filaments, laminin-1 and laminin-5, codistribute in the basal lamina and show identical responses to MCAO [12,14]. These changes are most prominent in the region of most severe ischemic neuron injury, and may be detectable as early as 2 hours after MCAO (e.g., laminin-5).

Endothelial cell and astrocyte responses to ischemia also have a highly significant temporal and topographical relationship to neuron injury. This is most evident in how microvessel integrin receptors respond to ischemia [13,14]. Integrin $\alpha_1\beta_1$ colocalizes with endothelium (CD31, platelet/endothelial cell adhesion molecule-1

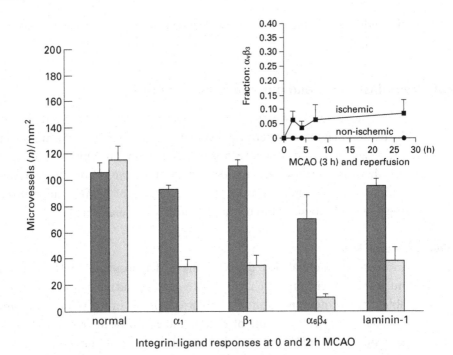

Figure 21.1   Responses of integrin subunits α_1 and β_1, integrin $\alpha_6\beta_4$ and laminin 2 hours after MCAO in the ischemic zone (light gray) compared with the contralateral non-ischemic basal ganglia (dark gray). Normal data represent integrin β_1 expression in unoperated animals. The time course and relative expression (fraction of microvessels) of integrin $\alpha_v\beta_3$ are represented (inset). All data points are $n \geq 3$ and error bars depict standard deviations.

(PECAM-1)), lying luminal to the basal lamina and vascular medial smooth muscle cells (SMC) (demonstrated by SMC α-actin antigen), while integrin $\alpha_6\beta_4$ colocalizes with astrocyte end-feet [10,13,14]. Integrins $\alpha_1\beta_1$ and $\alpha_6\beta_4$ appear to link endothelial cells and astrocytes to their ligands in the basal lamina [13,14]. There is a rapid and significant loss of integrin $\alpha_1\beta_1$ from microvascular endothelium as early as 2 hours of MCAO in the ischemic region (2 $P<0.007$) (Figure 21.1) [13]. This is accompanied by a comparable and highly significant abrupt loss of subunit β_1 from astrocyte fibers in the same time frame [13]. The decreased expression of integrin subunit β_1 parallels blockade of β_1 transcription, which also is evident by 2 hours of MCAO [13]. Ischemia also alters the close relationship between the astrocyte end-feet and the basal lamina endothelium [14]. In the ischemic region, the number of microvessels expressing integrin $\alpha_6\beta_4$ falls rapidly by 2 hours of MCAO (2 $P<0.01$), exceeding the fall in expression of the ligand laminin-5 (Figure 21.1). Integrins $\alpha_1\beta_1$ and $\alpha_6\beta_4$ are, then, equally sensitive to ischemia. The changes in integrin expression are graded with respect to the degree of neuron injury, being most pronounced in the regions of most severe ischemic neuron damage, and less severe at a distance (Ic > Ip > N, where N is the non-ischemic region) [42].

The appearance of these integrin antigens in the face of increased endothelial cell polymorphonuclear (PMN) leukocyte adhesion receptor expression indicates (i) the viability of selected microvascular endothelial cells during ischemia, (ii) the rapid responsiveness to injury of endothelial cells in proximity to injured neurons and (iii) their active participation in the transition from ischemia to the cellular inflammatory phase of brain infarction. The coincidence in time and distribution of the rapid downregulation of both microvascular astrocyte integrins and neuron injury after MCAO suggests, but does not prove, a potential interaction of the two cell types in the setting of ischemia.

Causes of matrix degradation during MCAO

The progressive loss of microvascular basal lamina during ischemia is greatest in the region where neuron injury is maximal [12,14]. The disappearance of matrix proteins may be due to proteolysis, blockade of transcription, inhibition of translation, or a combination of these. Remodeling of the microvascular basal lamina occurs when secreted proteases such as the matrix metalloproteinases (MMPs) and plasminogen activators, which are associated with the cerebral microvasculature, degrade laminin, collagen or fibronectin [43,44]. Activated serine proteases generated during ischemia may augment these processes. Among serine proteases, thrombin is interesting because it has multiple actions and targets. For instance, thrombin stimulates MMP-2 and MMP-9 secretion by vascular smooth muscle cells [45,46]. Also, PMN leukocyte granule enzymes, including collagenase (MMP-8), gelatinase (MMP-9), elastase and cathepsin G are released during the inflammatory phase after ischemia and degrade laminins and collagens [43,47–50].

Anthony et al. [51] reported the marked expression of latent MMP-9 by PMN leukocytes in human brain within 1 week of stroke, and MMP-2 from macrophages thereafter. In anesthetized Wistar–Kyoto and spontaneously hypertensive rats, Rosenberg et al. [52] showed that pro-MMP-9 increases by 12 to 24 hours and MMP-2 by 5 days after MCAO. Those findings have been variably corroborated by others [53–55]. Those studies suggest that in rodents subjected to MCAO increased pro-MMP-2 and MMP-9 expression precedes that of pro-MMP-2. By contrast, a significant rapid increase in the expression of the latent form of MMP-2 occurs 1 to 2 hours after MCAO in the ischemic basal ganglia of the non-human primate, which correlates significantly with the size of the ischemic region [56] (Figure 21.2). Those findings suggest that MMP-2 secretion may be directly related to early neuron injury. Moreover, in situ hybridization experiments have demonstrated the appearance of MMP-2 mRNA transcripts in both microvessels and non-vascular

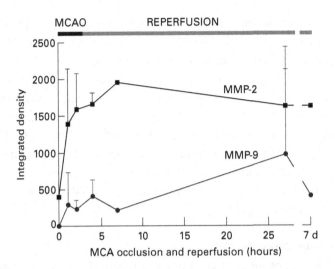

Figure 21.2   Expression of latent MMP-2 and latent MMP-9 activities during MCAO and reperfusion. The data are represented as the integrated density of respective lysis bands from successive gel zymographic studies. The expression of latent MMP-2 activity increased significantly from baseline constitutive levels (2 $P = 0.001$), while no difference in MMP-9 expression was detected. Error bars depict standard deviations. See text and ref. 16 for further explanation.

non-neuronal cell nuclei in the ischemic region by 2 hours of MCAO (G.J. del Zoppo, unpublished data). Furthermore, evidence of coexpression of the activators of latent MMP-2 has been obtained. Hence, MMP-2 may be synthesized de novo by microvascular cells in direct association with neuron injury, in the same time and location as microvascular matrix and integrin loss.

In contrast, pro-MMP-9 activity was not increased except in the ischemic regions of those subjects displaying hemorrhagic transformation compared with those without hemorrhage (2 $P = 0.018$). A clear dichotomy between the expression of pro-MMP-2 and pro-MMP-9 has been seen in the following MCAO in the primate, which is differentially related to neuron injury.

Microvascular activation after MCAO

Within 2 hours after MCAO, cerebral microvessels within the ischemic region express integrin $\alpha_V\beta_3$ [16]. Integrin $\alpha_V\beta_3$ is a receptor for multiple ligands including (fibrin)ogen, fibronectin, vitronection, osteopontin and von Willebrand factor. Given the known relationships between integrin $\alpha_V\beta_3$ and the vascular remodeling that can occur in preparation for new vessel formation, factors known to promote integrin $\alpha_V\beta_3$ expression were studied [16]. Predominantly in the ischemic region, vascular endothelial growth factor (VEGF) and integrin $\alpha_V\beta_3$ were coexpressed in microvessels displaying activation antigens (proliferating cell nuclear antigen) in a highly significant association beginning 1 hour after MCAO [16]. The co-appearance of these antigens was predominantly seen on non-capillary microvessels resembling precapillary arterioles (7.5 to 30.0 μm diameter), where the primary immunoreactivity was associated with the smooth muscle. These events coincided with evidence of neuron injury and, while spatially codistributed, were independent of time. These findings further support the idea of very rapid activation of microvessels following MCAO.

Rapid microvascular activation and cellular inflammation

VEGF transcripts also appeared on cells with the morphology of PMN leukocytes that had penetrated the vascular wall or histiocyte-appearing cells localized within the vascular wall of select microvessels [16]. These cells were identified in the ischemic region within 2 hours after MCAO on select microvessels [16], indicating that transmigration could occur substantially earlier than previously recorded in this model [2,8]. Of relevance, VEGF can be expressed by activated leukocytes, presumably as participants in the inflammatory process [57–59]. To what degree they contribute to the VEGF antigen observed in the microvascular wall during ischemia is unknown. Furthermore, the exact purposes of the activities of VEGF generated by either smooth muscle cells or inflammatory cells early during cerebral ischemia remain unclear. It is certain that these events coincide with early evidence of neuron injury.

Conclusion

Rapidly following MCAO in the non-human primate, microvascular cells within the ischemic zone express activation antigens, VEGF and specific leukocyte adhesion receptors. Alterations in the expression of integrin–matrix constituents, including integrin receptors on endothelial cells and astrocyte end-feet are observed within 1 to 2 hours of MCAO. These coincide exactly with clear evidence of neuron injury. In addition, select MMPs are acutely generated in the ischemic zone from microvascular and parenchymal cells. In this preparation it is unlikely that latent MMP-2 and its activators are generated by leukocytes at those early moments. However, the demonstration that leukocytes are associated with select microvessels and appear to generate VEGF transcripts as early as 1 to 2 hours after MCAO indicates that microvascular reactivity and leukocyte activation may be overlapping events even as neuron injury is occurring. Whether and how microvascular activation, integrin–matrix alterations and leukocyte activation contribute to neuron injury during ischemia is a question of significance.

Acknowledgments

The work described in this chapter is supported in part by grants RO1 NS 26945 and NS 38710 from the National Institute of Neurological Disorders and Stroke. This is manuscript 13428–MEM of The Scripps Research Institute.

REFERENCES

1 del Zoppo GJ (1994) Microvascular changes during cerebral ischemia and reperfusion. *Cerebrovascular & Brain Metabolism Reviews*, 6, 47–96.

2 del Zoppo GJ, Schmid-Schönbein GW, Mori E, Copeland BR & Chang C-M (1991) Polymorphonuclear leukocytes occlude capillaries following middle cerebral artery occlusion and reperfusion in baboons. *Stroke*, 22, 1276–83.

3 Little JR, Kerr FWL & Sundt TM Jr (1975) Microcirculatory obstruction in focal cerebral ischemia. Relationship to neuronal alterations. *Mayo Clinic Proceedings*, 50, 264–70.

4 Little JR, Kerr FWL & Sundt TM Jr (1976) Microcirculatory obstruction in focal cerebral ischemia: an electron microscopic investigation in monkeys. *Stroke*, 7, 25–30.

5 Mori E, del Zoppo GJ, Chambers JD, Copeland BR & Arfors K-E (1992) Inhibition of polymorphonuclear leukocyte adherence suppresses no-reflow after focal cerebral ischemia in baboons. *Stroke*, 23, 712–18.

6 Thomas WS, Mori E, Copeland BR, Yu J-Q, Morrissey JH & del Zoppo GJ (1993) Tissue factor contributes to microvascular defects following cerebral ischemia. *Stroke*, 24, 847–53.

7 Haring H-P, Berg EL, Tsurushita N, Tagaya M & del Zoppo GJ (1996) E-selectin appears in non-ischemic tissue during experimental focal cerebral ischemia. *Stroke*, 27, 1386–91.

8 Okada Y, Copeland BR, Mori E, Tung M-M, Thomas WS & del Zoppo GJ (1994) P-selectin and intercellular adhesion molecule-1 expression after focal brain ischemia and reperfusion. *Stroke*, 25, 202–11.

9 del Zoppo GJ, Copeland BR, Harker LA, Waltz TA, Zyroff J, Hanson SR & Battenberg E (1986) Experimental acute thrombotic stroke in baboons. *Stroke*, 17, 1254–65.

10 Haring H-P, Akamine BS, Habermann R, Koziol JA & del Zoppo GJ (1996) Distribution of integrin-like immunoreactivity on primate brain microvasculature. *Journal of Neuropathology & Experimental Neurology*, 55, 236–45.

11 Hamann GF, Okada Y & del Zoppo GJ (1996) Hemorrhagic transformation and microvascular integrity during focal cerebral ischemia/reperfusion. *Journal of Cerebral Blood Flow & Metabolism*, 16, 1373–8.

12 Hamann GF, Okada Y, Fitridge R & del Zoppo GJ (1995) Microvascular basal lamina antigens disappear during cerebral ischemia and reperfusion. *Stroke*, 26, 2120–6.

13 del Zoppo GJ, Haring H-P, Tagaya M, Wagner S, Akamine P & Hamann GF (1996) Loss of $\alpha_1\beta_1$ integrin immunoreactivity on cerebral microvessels and astrocytes following focal cerebral ischemia/reperfusion. *Cerebrovascular Diseases*, 6, 9.

14 Wagner S, Tagaya M, Koziol JA, Quaranta V & del Zoppo GJ (1997) Rapid disruption of an astrocyte interaction with the extracellular matrix mediated by integrin $\alpha_6\beta_4$ during focal cerebral ischemia/reperfusion. *Stroke*, **28**, 858–65.

15 Garcia JH, Mitchem HL, Briggs L, Morawetz R, Hudetz AG, Hazelrig JB, Halsey JH Jr & Conger KA (1983) Transient focal ischemia in subhuman primates. Neuronal injury as a function of local cerebral blood flow. *Journal of Neuropathology & Experimental Neurology*, **42**, 44–60.

16 Abumiya T, Lucero J, Heo JH, Tagaya M, Koziol JA, Copeland BR & del Zoppo GJ (1999) Activated microvessels express vascular endothelial growth factor and integrin $\alpha_V\beta_3$ during focal cerebral ischemia. *Journal of Cerebral Blood Flow & Metabolism*, **19**, 1038–50.

17 Okada Y, Copeland BR, Hamann GF, Koziol JA, Cheresh DA & del Zoppo GJ (1996) Integrin $\alpha_V\beta_3$ is expressed in selected microvessels after focal cerebral ischemia. *American Journal of Pathology*, **149**, 37–44.

18 Peters A, Palay BL & Webster H (1991) *The Fine Structure of the Nervous System. Neurons and Their Supporting Cells*, 3rd edn. New York: Oxford University Press.

19 Carlson SS & Hockfield S (1996) Central nervous system. In *Extracellular Matrix*, vol. 1, ed. WD Comper, pp. 1–23. Amsterdam: Harwood Academic Publishers.

20 Yurchenko PD & Schittny JC (1986) Molecular architecture of basement membranes. *Journal of Biological Chemistry*, **261**, 1577–90.

21 Bernstein JJ, Getz R, Jefferson M & Kelemen M (1985) Astrocytes secrete basal lamina after hemisection of rat spinal cord. *Brain Research*, **327**, 135–41.

22 Kusaka H, Hirano A, Bornstein MB & Raine CS (1985) Basal lamina formation by astrocytes in organotypic cultures of mouse spinal cord tissue. *Journal of Neuropathology & Experimental Neurology*, **44**, 295–303.

23 Ard MD & Faissner A (1991) Components of astrocytic extracellular matrix are regulated by contact with axons. *Annals of the New York Academy of Sciences*, **633**, 566–9.

24 Tagami M, Yamagata K, Fujino H, Kubota A, Nara Y & Yamori Y (1992) Morphological differentiation of endothelial cells co-cultured with astrocytes on type-I or type-IV collagen. *Cell and Tissue Research*, **268**, 225–32.

25 Webersinke G, Bauer H, Amberger A, Zach O & Bauer HC (1992) Comparison of gene expression of extracellular matrix molecules in brain microvascular endothelial cells and astrocytes. *Biochemical and Biophysical Research Communications*, **189**, 877–84.

26 Kozlova M, Kentroti S & Vernadakis A (1993) Influence of culture substrata on the differentiation of advanced passage glial cells in cultures from aged mouse cerebral hemispheres. *International Journal of Developmental Neuroscience*, **11**, 513–19.

27 Nagano N, Aoyagi M & Hirakawa K (1993) Extracellular matrix modulates the proliferation of rat astrocytes in serum-free culture. *Glia*, **8**, 71–6.

28 Janzer RC & Raff MC (1987) Astrocytes induce blood–brain barrier properties in endothelial cells. *Nature*, **325**, 253–7 (Letter).

29 Hurwitz AA, Berman JW, Rashbaum WK & Lyman WD (1993) Human fetal astrocytes induce the expression of blood–brain barrier specific proteins by autologous endothelial cells. *Brain Research*, **625**, 238–43.

30 Estrada C, Bready JV, Berliner JA, Pardridge WM & Cancilla PA (1990) Astrocyte growth stimulation by a soluble factor produced by cerebral endothelial cells in vitro. *Journal of Neuropathology & Experimental Neurology*, **49**, 539–49.

31 Minakawa T, Bready J, Berliner J, Fisher M & Cancilla PA (1991) in vitro interaction of astrocytes and pericytes with capillary-like structures of brain microvessel endothelium. *Laboratory Investigation*, **65**, 32–40.

32 Albelda SM & Buck CA (1990) Integrins and other cell adhesion molecules. *FASEB Journal*, **4**, 2868–80.

33 Luscinskas FW & Lawler J (1994) Integrins as dynamic regulators of vascular function. *FASEB Journal*, **8**, 929–38.

34 Ruoslahti E (1991) Integrins. *Journal of Clinical Investigation*, **87**, 1–5.

35 Pasqualini R & Hemler ME (1994) Contrasting roles for integrin β_1 and β_5 cytoplasmic domains in subcellular localization, cell proliferation, and cell migration. *Journal of Cell Biology*, **125**, 447–60.

36 Chintala SK, Sawaya R, Gokaslan ZL & Rao JS (1996) Modulation of matrix metalloprotease-2 and invasion in human glioma cells by $\alpha_3\beta_1$ integrin. *Cancer Letters*, **103**, 201–8.

37 Partridge CA, Phillips PG, Niedbala MJ & Jeffrey JJ (1997) Localization and activation of type IV collagenase/gelatinase at endothelial focal contacts. *American Journal of Physiology*, **272**, L813–L822.

38 Gottlieb RA, Burleson KO, Kloner RA, Babior BM & Engler RL (1994) Reperfusion injury induces apoptosis in rabbit cardiomyocytes. *Journal of Clinical Investigation*, **94**, 1621–8.

39 MacManus JP, Hill IE, Huang ZG, Rasquinha I, Xue D & Buchan AM (1994) DNA damage consistent with apoptosis in transient focal ischaemic neocortex. *Neuroreport*, **5**, 493–6.

40 Seekamp A, Till GO, Mulligan MS, Paulson JC, Anderson DC, Miyasaka M & Ward PA (1994) Role of selectins in local and remote tissue injury following ischemia and reperfusion. *American Journal of Pathology*, **144**, 592–8.

41 Tagaya M, Liu K-F, Copeland B, Seiffert D, Engler R, Garcia JH & del Zoppo GJ (1997) DNA scission after focal brain ischemia. Temporal differences in two species. *Stroke*, **28**, 1245–54.

42 Tagaya M, Haring H-P, Stuiver I, Wagner S, Abumiya T, Lucero J, Lee P, Copeland BR, Seiffert D and del Zoppo GJ (2001) Rapid loss of microvascular integrin expression during focal brain ischemia reflects neuron injury. *Journal of Cerebral Blood Flow & Metabolism*, **21**, 835–46.

43 Krane SM (1994) Clinical importance of metalloproteinases and their inhibitors. *Annals of the New York Academy of Sciences*, **732**, 1–10.

44 Levin EG & del Zoppo GJ (1994) Localization of tissue plasminogen activator in the endothelium of a limited number of vessels. *American Journal of Pathology*, **144**, 855–61.

45 Fabunmi RP, Baker AH, Murray EJ, Booth RFG & Newby AC (1996) Divergent regulation by growth factors and cytokines of 95 kDa and 72 kDa gelatinases and tissue inhibitors or metalloproteinases-1, -2, and -3 in rabbit aortic smooth muscle cells. *Biochemical Journal*, **315**, 335–42.

46 Galis ZS, Kranzhöfer R, Fenton JW II & Libby P (1997) Thrombin promotes activation of matrix metalloproteinase-2 produced by cultured vascular smooth muscle cells. *Arteriosclerosis, Thrombosis, and Vascular Biology*, **17**, 483–9.

47 Heck LW, Blackburn WD, Irwin MH & Abrahamson DR (1990) Degradation of basement membrane laminin by human neutrophil elastase and cathepsin G. *American Journal of Pathology*, **136**, 1267–74.

48 Murphy G, Reynolds JJ, Bretz U & Baggiolini M (1987) Collagenase is a component of the specific granules of human neutrophil leukocytes. *Biochemical Journal*, **162**, 195–7.

49 Pike MC, Wicha MS, Yoon P, Mayo L & Boxer LA (1989) Laminin promotes the oxidative burst in human neutrophils via increased chemoattractant receptor expression. *Journal of Immunology*, **142**, 2004–11.

50 Watanabe H, Hattori S, Katsuda S, Nakanishi I & Nagai Y (1990) Human neutrophil elastase: degradation of basement membrane components and immunolocalization in the tissue. *Journal of Biochemistry*, **108**, 753–9.

51 Anthony DC, Ferguson B, Matyzak MK, Miller KM, Esiri MM & Perry VH (1997) Differential matrix metalloproteinase expression in cases of multiple sclerosis and stroke. *Neuropathology and Applied Neurobiology*, **23**, 406–15.

52 Rosenberg GA, Navratil M, Barone F & Feuerstein G (1996) Proteolytic cascade enzymes increase in focal cerebral ischemia in rat. *Journal of Cerebral Blood Flow & Metabolism*, **16**, 360–6.

53 Clark AW, Krekoski CA, Bou S-S, Chapman KR & Edwards DR (1997) Increased gelatinase A (MMP-2) and gelatinase B (MMP-9) activities in human brain after focal ischemia. *Neuroscience Letters*, **238**, 53–6.

54 Fujimura M, Gasche Y, Morita-Fujimura Y, Massengale J, Kawase M & Chan PH (1999) Early appearance of activated matrix metalloproteinase-9 and blood–brain barrier disruption in mice after focal cerebral ischemia and reperfusion. *Brain Research*, **842**, 92–100.

55 Gasche Y, Fujimura M, Morita-Fujimura Y, Copin J-C, Kawase M, Massengale J & Chan PH (1999) Early appearance of activated matrix metalloproteinase-9 after focal cerebral ischemia in mice: a possible role in blood–brain barrier dysfunction. *Journal of Cerebral Blood Flow & Metabolism*, **19**, 1020–8.

56 Heo JH, Lucero J, Abumiya T, Koziol JA, Copeland BR & del Zoppo GJ (1999) Matrix metalloproteinases increase very early during experimental focal cerebral ischemia. *Journal of Cerebral Blood Flow & Metabolism*, **19**, 624–33.

57 Salven P, Orpana A & Joensuu H (1999) Leukocytes and platelets of patients with cancer contain high levels of vascular endothelial growth factor. *Clinical Cancer Research*, **5**, 487–91.

58 Scalia R, Booth G & Lefer DJ (1999) Vascular endothelial growth factor attenuates leukocyte–endothelium interaction during acute endothelial dysfunction: essential role of endothelium-derived nitric oxide. *FASEB Journal*, **13**, 1039–46.

59 Webb NJ, Myers CR, Watson CJ, Bottomley MJ & Brenchley PE (1998) Activated human neutrophils express vascular endothelial growth factor (VEGF). *Cytokine*, **10**, 254–7.

Part VII

Gene transfer and therapy

Co-Chairs: Gary K. Steinberg & Nicolas G. Bazan

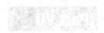

22

Adenoviral vectors for gene therapy in stroke

A. Lorris Betz[1] & Guo-Yuan Yang[2]

[1] Departments of Pediatrics and Neurobiology and Anatomy, University of Utah, Salt Lake City, UT
[2] Department of Surgery, Section of Neurosurgery, University of Michigan, Ann Arbor, MI

Introduction

Over the past decade, knowledge in two areas has been converging toward a new era in the treatment of acute cerebral injuries such as stroke. From one direction, there have been remarkable new insights into the basic mechanisms at the molecular, cellular and tissue levels that cause ischemic brain injury and the repair processes that follow the acute injury. From another area of science, there have been major advances in our ability to introduce foreign genes into cells and cause the expression of specific proteins that affect tissue function. Knowledge in these two areas will inevitably result in the use of gene therapy to treat strokes.

While clinical trials of gene therapy in stroke are not imminent at the time of writing, the ground work is being established through studies using experimental animals and through efforts to perfect gene delivery vehicles known collectively as vectors. The purpose of this report is to review the development of a particularly promising vector, the adenovirus, and to outline some of the logistical issues that must be addressed before adenoviral vectors can be used in humans to treat stroke.

The adenovirus

The use of viruses to deliver genes to cells in vivo has progressed to the point where numerous clinical trials have been approved and many are ongoing. The most commonly used viruses for gene therapy are retroviruses, herpes simplex viruses and adenoviruses [1]. While each type has properties that make it useful for a given application, the adenoviruses are particularly attractive as vectors for gene therapy in the brain.

Adenoviruses are double-stranded DNA viruses that infect a wide variety of cells with high efficiency. Entry of adenoviruses into cells is dependent upon interaction with specific receptors and integrins on the cell surface [2]. Following cellular entry, the adenovirus enters the cell nucleus, but, in contrast to other viral vectors, its DNA does not become incorporated into the host chromosomes, a process that could introduce mutations into the host cell genome. For gene therapy, portions of the adenoviral genome are deleted to make the viruses incapable of replicating and to create space for insertion of a gene of interest. The first generation of adenoviral vectors have the E1 region deleted, which allows the introduction of about 8 kb of foreign DNA, including regulatory elements [1,3,4]. Because the E1-deleted adenovirus does stimulate a mild inflammatory reaction and there is a finite risk of the E1 gene being reinserted during the course of virus production thus making the virus capable of replicating, a number of investigators are testing adenoviral vectors that have had other viral genes deleted, up to and including essentially the entire viral genome [1,3,4]. These newer generations of vectors will accommodate more foreign DNA and they also should lead to more prolonged expression of their gene products in transfected cells.

Adenoviruses are useful for gene therapy in the brain because they infect virtually all cell types present in the central nervous system (CNS) [5]. The consequences of an adenoviral infection of the brain are minimal as is the reaction to the first-generation adenoviral vectors used for gene therapy. Nevertheless, the expression of the foreign gene is generally limited to several months or less, probably owing to a low-grade inflammatory process directed at viral epitopes or the product of the foreign gene [1,5]. While transient expression may be a limitation in the use of adenoviral vectors to treat hereditary or degenerative diseases of the brain, it could be an advantage in treating acute injuries such as stroke.

Delivery of adenoviral vectors to the brain

Because the course of a natural infection is too unpredictable, an invasive approach for virus administration is necessary to achieve the desired effect. Possible routes include intravascular, intraventricular or intraparenchymal injections or administration of virus to a peripheral site where the virus may enter the CNS by retrograde axonal transport. Each of these routes has advantages and limitations that must be considered in relation to the location of injury and the nature of the injury mechanism that is to be modified by gene therapy.

Intravascular

Since blood vessels are distributed throughout the brain, they seem like a useful pathway for global delivery of adenoviral vectors. In the normal brain, the rapid passage of blood through intracerebral vessels limits the ability of an adenovirus to consistently infect even the endothelial cells of the brain after either intravascular injection or intracarotid infusion [6]. The reduced blood flow rate that exists during cerebral ischemia may improve the opportunity for virus delivery and may even favor delivery to the ischemic zone; however, this has not been investigated.

The blood–brain barrier (BBB) formed by the endothelium normally restricts direct penetration of a virus into the brain substance. Osmotic disruption of the BBB permits the penetration of virus-sized particles [7] and intracarotid infusion of adenovirus after osmotic BBB disruption results in foreign gene expression in cells beyond the vasculature. But consistent with the fact that astrocytic foot processes surround brain microvessels in nearly all parts of the brain [8] and are the first extravascular cellular elements to be contacted by a virus that has penetrated the disrupted BBB, the transfected cells appear to be primarily astrocytes [6]. Since BBB integrity is also compromised during the evolution of a stroke [9], this may provide a disease-related opportunity for adenoviral uptake. Nevertheless, the intravascular route, either with or without BBB disruption, is likely to result in delivery of genes only to the endothelium and/or astrocytes.

Intraventricular

The brain is bathed in cerebral spinal fluid (CSF) located both within the cerebral ventricles and in the subarachnoid space, and this fluid could provide ready access to the brain. However, the injection of adenovirus into the cerebral ventricles results in the expression of viral gene products primarily in the ependymal cells, which line the ventricles, and in the choroid plexus [10–13]. Only a few scattered cells within about 1mm of the ventricular surface express the gene product. Injection of adenovirus into the cisterna magna results in gene expression in the leptomeningeal cells and a few scattered adventitial and smooth muscle cells of blood vessels [13]. Thus the intraventricular route is not a good approach to deliver adenovirus to injured brain cells. However, despite the limited distribution of transfected cells after intraventricular injection of a virus, transduced proteins are secreted into the CSF and penetrate into the brain [12]. This offers an effective delivery system for expression of proteins that function at extracellular sites and at a distance from the cells that are transduced.

Intraparenchymal

Injection of adenovirus into the brain's parenchyma offers the most direct access to brain cells. The virus infects virtually all cell types immediately adjacent to the injection site [5,10] and, therefore, it is an effective means for delivery of genes to specific localized areas of the brain. While injection of adenovirus into ischemic or reperfused brain also results in production of the transgene product, it may be at a lower level or delayed by comparison with expression in the normal brain [14].

The spread of a virus away from the injection site is limited both by the size of the viral particles by comparison with the size of the extracellular spaces of the

brain and by the tortuosity of the extracellular spaces [15], which results in fre-
quent contact between virus and cell. Since the extracellular space of the brain represents about 15% to 20% of the entire brain volume and because the virus enters
cells while the injection fluid does not, the volume of transfected cells is considerably smaller than the vehicle fluid volume. The volume of brain that is infected
with the virus is dependent upon the dose and concentration of the virus in the
injection fluid and the presence of non-infective viral particles, but rate, time or
volume of the infusion has little effect [15]. The entry of adenoviruses into cells
involves specific receptors and integrins on the cell surface [2], and this may
provide an opportunity for manipulating the virus–cell interaction to produce
selectivity.

Delivery through peripheral nerves

Highly targeted expression of foreign genes in neurons can be accomplished by
taking advantage of retrograde axonal transport. After adenovirus injection into
peripheral tissues such as muscle, foreign gene products are expressed centrally in
the motor and sensory neurons that innervate the muscle [16]. Similarly, after
intranasal administration, viral genes are expressed in the olfactory bulb as well as
in the locus ceruleus and area postrema [17]. This process is likely to be too slow
and the area of brain that is transfected too small to be a practical approach for gene
therapy in stroke.

Measurement and timing of therapeutic gene expression

There is inevitably some time delay between the injection of the viral vector and the
expression of the foreign gene product (Figure 22.1A). Therefore, to determine
when and where a gene is expressed, it is necessary to assay for the gene product. In
animal studies, the *Escherichia coli* β-galactosidase gene (*lacZ*) is commonly used
to identify transfected cells because the activity of β-galactosidase can be readily
localized with a simple staining procedure. In other studies, the gene product itself
was directly assayed using samples of brain tissue or CSF [12]. Immunostaining
may also be used to verify gene expression [18–20].

These techniques, however, require samples of brain tissue and, therefore, are
not feasible for monitoring gene expression in humans. For this purpose, safe, non-
invasive techniques must be developed. Tjuvajev et al. [21] demonstrated the feasibility of using positron emission tomography to non-invasively monitor the
enzymatic activity of thymidine kinase that was overexpressed by gene transfer into
glioma cells. This approach, with appropriate marker genes and marker substrates,
could permit non-invasive monitoring of gene expression in humans.

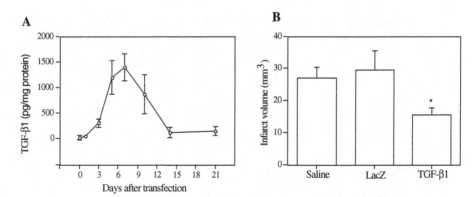

Figure 22.1   (A) Concentration of active TGF-β1 in brain tissue. Following AdRSVTGF-β1 transfer, mice were anesthetized and sacrificed from day 1 to day 21 (*n* = 5 to 7 in each group). The brains were rapidly removed and immediately homogenized. The homogenates were assayed using a human TGF-β1 enzyme-linked immunosorbent assay kit that cross-reacts with human and mouse TGF-β1. The optical density was determined and the results were expressed as picograms of TGF-β1 per mg of tissue protein. (B) Infarct volume in saline-treated, AdRSVlacZ and AdRSVTGF-β1 transduced mice following 30 minutes of transient middle cerebral artery occlusion with 24 hours of reperfusion. The animals were killed and the brains were immediately frozen on dry ice. Twenty coronal sections 20 μm thick were cut from the frontal pole and mounted on slides. Cresyl violet staining was used to identify the infarct area. Infarct volume is calculated by summing the infarct areas multiplied by the distance between the sections. Saline, saline-treated; LacZ, AdRSVlacZ transduced; TGF-β1, AdRSVTGF-β1 transduced mice. Data are shown as mean ± SD (*n* = 5 to 7 in each group). * $P < 0.05$, AdRSVTGF-β1 mice vs. saline-treated and AdRSVlacZ transduced mice.

Therapeutic genes in stroke

Due to the involvement of multiple biochemical processes in stroke, there are many potential genes to explore as therapies for stroke. Although protein synthesis in general is suppressed by ischemia [22], a reporter gene (*lacZ*) transferred into the ischemic or reperfused brain using adenoviral vectors is expressed as early as 8 hours after introduction [14].

If gene therapy is used after a stroke has already occurred, the goal may necessarily be focused on enhancing the repair process rather than blocking injury mechanisms because there may be a delay of many hours to a day before the protein product of the foreign gene is produced. To date, all studies of the efficacy of adenoviral-mediated transfer of therapeutic genes have involved delivery of the gene 1 to 7 days prior to ischemia. Whether adenoviral-mediated gene therapy would be

Table 22.1. Therapeutic genes that reduce ischemic brain injury

Target	Mediator	Vector	Reference
Anti-inflammatory	IL-1ra	Ad	12,25,26
	TGF-β	Ad	24
Anti-apoptotic	Bcl-2	HSV	18
		HSV	19,23
	NAIP	Ad	27
Metabolism	GLUT1	HSV	20
Stress proteins	HSP72	HSV	28
Neurotrophins	GDNF	Ad	29

Notes:
IL, interleukin; TGF, transforming growth factor; NAIP, neural apoptosis inhibiting protein; GLUT, glucose transporter; HSP, heat shock protein; GDNF, glial cell-derived neurotrophic factor; Ad, adenovirus; HSV, herpes simplex virus.

effective when administered after a stroke is yet to be determined; however, herpes simplex-mediated gene transfer has been shown to improve neuronal survival even when the virus is injected 30 minutes into the reperfusion period [23].

Table 22.1 summarizes the genes that have been shown to have a beneficial effect on ischemic brain injury. Adenovirus has served as the vector in many of these studies, while herpes simplex was used in the others. Since all but one of these studies used pretreatment to maximize gene expression at the time of ischemia, it remains to be determined whether any of these genes will be effective when used in the clinical setting. Nevertheless, these studies have provided useful models for exploring the role of various biochemical pathways in ischemic brain injury. For example, adenoviral-mediated delivery of the human transforming growth factor-β1 (TGF-β1) gene significantly reduces the volume of injured brain in a mouse model of temporary ischemia [24] (Figure 22.1B). By studying how the inflammatory cascade has been altered as a result of overexpression of TGF-β1, it should be possible to gain insights into the mechanism by which TGF-β1 reduces stroke, as well as the role of the inflammatory cascade in ischemic brain injury.

REFERENCES

1 Hermens WTJMC & Verhaagen J (1998) Viral vectors, tools for gene transfer in the nervous system. *Progress in Neurobiology,* 55, 399–432.

2 Nemerow GR & Stewart PL (1999) Role of α_v integrins in adenovirus cell entry and gene delivery. *Microbiology and Molecular Biology Reviews,* **63**, 725–34.

3 Kovesdi I, Brough DE, Bruder JT & Wickham TJ (1997) Adenoviral vectors for gene transfer. *Current Opinion in Biotechnology,* **8**, 583–9.

4 Benihoud K, Yeh P & Perricaudet M (1999) Adenovirus vectors for gene delivery. *Current Opinion in Biotechnology,* **10**, 440–7.

5 Davidson BL, Allen ED, Kozarsky KF, Wilson JM & Roessler BJ (1993) A model system for in vivo gene transfer into the central nervous system using an adenoviral vector. *Nature Genetics,* **3**, 219–23.

6 Doran SE, Ren XD, Betz AL, Pagel MA, Neuwelt EA, Roessler BJ & Davidson BL (1995) Gene expression from recombinant viral vectors in the central nervous system after blood-brain barrier disruption. *Neurosurgery,* **36**, 965–70.

7 Neuwelt EA, Weissleder R, Nilaver G, Kroll RA, Roman-Goldstein S, Szumowski J, et al. (1994) Delivery of virus-sized iron oxide particles to rodent CNS neurons. *Neurosurgery,* **34**, 777–84.

8 Betz AL, Goldstein GW & Katzman R (1994) Blood-brain-cerebrospinal fluid barriers. In *Basic Neurochemistry,* 5th edn, eds. GJ Siegel, B Agranoff, RW Albers & P Molinoff, pp. 681–99. New York: Raven Press.

9 Betz AL & Dietrich WD (1998) Blood-brain barrier dysfunction in cerebral ischemia. In *Cerebrovascular Disease: Pathophysiology, Diagnosis, and Management,* eds. MD Ginsberg & J Bogousslavsky, pp. 358–70. Malden, MA: Blackwell Science.

10 Akli S, Caillaud C, Vigne E, Stratford-Perricaudet LD, Poenaru L, Perricaudet M, Kahn A & Peschanski MR (1993) Transfer of a foreign gene into the brain using adenovirus vectors. *Nature Genetics,* **3**, 224–8.

11 Bajocchi G, Feldman SH, Crystal RG & Mastrangeli A (1993) Direct in vivo gene transfer to ependymal cells in the central nervous system using recombinant adenovirus vectors. *Nature Genetics,* **3**, 229–34.

12 Betz AL, Yang G-Y & Davidson BL (1995) Attenuation of stroke size in rats using an adenoviral vector to induce overexpression of interleukin-1 receptor antagonist in brain. *Journal of Cerebral Blood Flow & Metabolism,* **15**, 547–51.

13 Ooboshi H, Welsh MJ, Rios CD, Davidson BL & Heistad DD (1995) Adenovirus-mediated gene transfer in vivo to cerebral blood vessels and perivascular tissue. *Circulation Research,* **77**, 7–13.

14 Abe K, Setoguchi Y, Hayashi T & Itoyama Y (1997) In vivo adenovirus-mediated gene transfer and the expression in ischemic and reperfused rat brain. *Brain Research,* **763**, 191–201.

15 Betz AL, Shakui P & Davidson BL (1998) Gene transfer to rodent brain with recombinant adenoviral vectors: effects of infusion parameters, infectious titer, and virus concentration on transduction volume. *Experimental Neurology,* **150**, 136–42.

16 Ghadge GD, Roos RP, Kang UJ, Wollmann R, Fishman PS, Kalynych AM, Barr E & Leiden JM (1995) CNS gene delivery by retrograde transport of recombinant replication-defective adenoviruses. *Gene Therapy,* **2**, 132–7.

17 Draghia R, Caillaud C, Manicom R, Pavirani A, Kahn A & Poenaru L (1995) Gene delivery into the central nervous system by nasal instillation in rats. *Gene Therapy,* **2**, 418–23.

18 Linnik MD, Zahos P, Geschwind MD & Federoff H J (1995) Expression of bcl-2 from a defective herpes simplex virus-1 vector limits neuronal death in focal cerebral ischemia. *Stroke*, **26**, 1670–4.

19 Lawrence MS, Ho DY, Sun GH, Steinberg GK & Sapolsky RM (1996) Overexpression of Bcl-2 with herpes simplex virus vectors protects CNS neurons against neurological insults in vitro and in vivo. *Journal of Neuroscience*, **16**, 486–96.

20 Lawrence MS, Sun GH, Kunis DM, Saydam TC, Dash R, Ho DY, Sapolsky RM & Steinberg GK (1996) Overexpression of the glucose transporter gene with a herpes simplex viral vector protects striatal neurons against stroke. *Journal of Cerebral Blood Flow & Metabolism*, **16**, 181–5.

21 Tjuvajev JG, Stockhammer G, Desai R, Uehara H, Watanabe K, Gansbacher B & Blasberg RG (1995) Imaging the expression of transfected genes in vivo. *Cancer Research*, **55**, 6126–32.

22 Xie Y, Mies G & Hossmann K-A (1989) Ischemic threshold of brain protein synthesis after unilateral carotid artery occlusion in gerbils. *Stroke*, **20**, 620–6.

23 Lawrence MS, McLaughlin JR, Sun G-H, Ho DY, McIntosh L, Kunis DM, Sapolsky RM & Steinberg GK (1997) Herpes simplex viral vectors expressing Bcl-2 are neuroprotective when delivered after a stroke. *Journal of Cerebral Blood Flow & Metabolism*, **17**, 740–4.

24 Pang L, Yang G-Y, Roessler BJ, Ye W & Betz AL (1999) The protective effects of adenovirus-mediated transforming growth factor-beta 1 expression in ischemic mouse brain. *Journal of Cerebral Blood Flow & Metabolism*, **19**, S137.

25 Yang G-Y, Liu X-H, Kadoya C, Zhao YJ, Mao Y, Davidson BL & Betz AL (1998) Attenuation of ischemic inflammatory response in mouse brain using an adenoviral vector to induce overexpression of interleukin-1 receptor. *Journal of Cerebral Blood Flow & Metabolism*, **18**, 840–7.

26 Yang GY, Mao Y, Zhou LF, Ye W, Liu XH, Gong C & Betz AL (1999) Attenuation of temporary focal cerebral ischemic injury in the mouse following transfection with interleukin-1 receptor antagonist. *Brain Research Molecular Brain Research*, **72**, 129–37.

27 Xu DG, Crocker SJ, Doucet J-P, St. Jean M, Tamai K, Hakim AM, Ikeda J-E, Liston P, Thompson CS, Korneluk RG, MacKenzie A & Robertson GS (1997) Elevation of neuronal expression of NAIP reduces ischemic damage in the rat hippocampus. *Nature Medicine*, **3**, 997–1004.

28 Yenari MA, Fink SL, Sun GH, Chang LK, Patel MK, Kunis DM, Onley D, Ho DY, Sapolsky RM & Steinberg GK (1998) Gene therapy with HSP72 is neuroprotective in rat models of stroke and epilepsy. *Annals of Neurology*, **44**, 584–91.

29 Kitagawa H, Sasaki C, Sakai K, Mori A, Mitsumoto Y, Mori T, Fukuchi Y, Setoguchi Y & Abe K (1999) Adenovirus-mediated gene transfer of glial cell line-derived neurotrophic factor prevents ischemic brain injury after transient middle cerebral artery occlusion in rats. *Journal of Cerebral Blood Flow & Metabolism*, **19**, 1336–44.

Gene transfer of glial cell line-derived neurotrophic factor prevents ischemic brain injury

Hisashi Kitagawa[1], Takeshi Hayashi[2] & Koji Abe[3]

[1] Department of Neurology, Okayama University Medical School, Okayama, and Second Institute of New Drug Research, Otsuka Pharmaceutical Co. Ltd., Tokushima, Japan
[2,3] Department of Neurology, Okayama University Medical School, Okayama, Japan

Topical application of glial cell line-derived neurotrophic factor reduces ischemic brain injury after permanent middle cerebral artery occlusion in rats

Glial cell line-derived neurotrophic factor (GDNF), a member of the transforming growth factor-β (TGF-β) superfamily [1], plays important roles not only in the differentiation of neurons during normal development, but also in the survival and recovery of many populations of mature neurons. It has been reported that GDNF has protective effects on various injuries of the central and peripheral nervous systems in vitro and in vivo [2–4]. However, a possible protective effect of GDNF in focal cerebral ischemia, and the exact mechanism of the ameliorative effect of GDNF in brain ischemic injury are not fully understood.

Caspase-1 (interleukin-1β converting enzyme (ICE)), caspase-2 and caspase-3 have been thought to play important roles in ischemic neuronal injury. Expression or upregulation of caspase mRNAs have been reported in some ischemic injury models [5,6]. Inhibition of caspase family proteases reduced ischemic and excito-toxic neuronal damage [7], and expression of a dominant negative mutant of ICE or a mutant ICE inhibitory protein in transgenic mice prevented or attenuated ischemic brain injury [8,9]. Therefore, the progression of ischemic neuronal injuries may be greatly associated with activation of these caspases through an apoptotic process. However, it has been uncertain whether caspases are also induced during, or involved in, neuronal death after permanent middle cerebral artery occlusion (MCAO). In this section, we show the possible protective effect of GDNF on the infarct area and brain edema in association with modification of DNA fragmentation and immunoreactivity for caspases after permanent MCAO in rats.

Adult male Wistar rats (250 to 280 g) were anesthetized with an intraperitoneal injection of pentobarbital (10 mg/250 g), and a burr hole with a diameter of 2 mm was carefully made in the skull with an electric dental drill, avoiding traumatic brain injury. The location of the burr hole was 3 mm dorsal and 4 mm lateral to the right from the bregma, which is located in the upper part of the MCA territory. The dura mater was preserved at this time. The animals recovered in an ambient atmosphere.

Approximately 24 hours after the drilling, the rats were anesthetized by inhalation of a nitrous oxide/oxygen/halothane (69%/30%/1%) mixture during surgical preparation. The origin of the right MCA was occluded by inserting a nylon thread through the common carotid artery according to a previous report [10]. Body temperature was maintained at $37 \pm 0.3\,°C$ during the surgical procedure for MCAO. Immediately after MCAO, the vehicle or GDNF was topically applied on the surface of the cerebral cortex with a small piece (8 mm^3) of Spongel (Yamanouchi Pharma. Co. Ltd., Japan) presoaked in 9 µl of Ringer's solution (Otsuka Pharma. Co. Ltd., Tokushima, Japan) as the vehicle, or GDNF (2.5 µg in 9 µl of vehicle; RBI, Natick, MA). Sham control animals were treated in the same way without MCAO. The animals recovered in an ambient temperature (21 °C to 24 °C) until sampling.

For estimation of ischemic brain injury, the infarct size 24 hours after permanent MCAO with the vehicle ($n=7$) or GDNF ($n=9$) treatment was measured by 2,3,5-triphenyltetrazolium chloride (TTC) staining according to a previous report [11]. In this experiment, regional cerebral blood flow (CBF) of the right frontoparietal cortex region was also measured through the burr hole with a laser blood flowmeter (Flo-C1; Omegawave, Tokyo, Japan) before or 0, 8 and 24 hours after MCAO. Brain edema in the sham-operated ($n=6$), vehicle-treated ($n=5$) or GDNF-treated ($n=7$) groups was measured by the dry-weight method according to our previous report [10]. Statistical analyses were performed using Student's t test.

For histochemical staining for DNA fragmentation and caspases, the rat forebrains were removed and quickly frozen after 12 hours of occlusion with the vehicle ($n=4$) or GDNF ($n=4$). Coronal sections at the caudate putamen and dorsal hippocampal levels were cut into a thickness of 10 µm on a cryostat at $-18\,°C$ and collected on slide glass coated with poly-L-lysine. Sham control sections were also obtained. Histochemical staining for terminal deoxynucleotidyl transferase-mediated dUTP-biotin nick end labeling (TUNEL) was performed with a TACS TdT in situ apoptosis detection kit (no. 80–4625–00; Genzyme, Cambridge, MA) according to our previous report [10]. After detection of double-stranded breaks in genomic DNA with 2,3'-diaminobenzidine (DAB) tetrahydrochloride (0.5 mg/ml in 50 mmol/l Tris-HCl buffer, pH 7.4), the sections were counterstained with methyl green according to the protocol in the kit. Immunostainings for caspases were performed using the avidin-biotin–peroxidase method (ABC kit, PK-6102;

Vector Laboratories, Burlingame, CA, USA) according to our previous report [10]. The sections were examined by light microscope, and the stained cells in $0.25\,mm^2$ of three random MCA areas were counted, summed and categorized into four grades in the following manner: no staining, or a small (2 to 50), moderate (50 to 200) or large (200 to 500 or more) number of stained cells.

While an infarct volume in the brain sections of the sham control group was not detected, the infarct volumes of the vehicle- and GDNF-treated groups 24 hours after permanent MCAO were $343.3 \pm 112.4\,mm^2$ (mean $\pm$ standard deviation (SD), $n = 7$) and $176.5 \pm 119.8\,mm^2$ ($n = 9$), respectively ($P = 0.01$ vs. the vehicle-treated group) (Figure 23.1A). The infarct area of four coronal sections (4, 6, 8 and 10 mm caudal from the frontal pole) in the GDNF-treated group was significantly smaller than in the vehicle-treated group (Figure 23.1B). Sham control cortices showed $80.6 \pm 0.4\%$ (mean $\pm$ SD, $n = 6$) water content, while those with vehicle or GDNF treatment 24 hours after permanent MCAO showed 86.5 ± 0.6 ($n = 5$; $P < 0.001$ vs. sham control group) and 84.7 ± 1.4 ($n = 7$; $P = 0.01$ vs. the vehicle-treated group, and $P < 0.001$ vs. sham control group), respectively (Figure 23.1C). Regional CBF in both the vehicle- and GDNF-treated groups was reduced to less than 50% of the control immediately after MCAO, and persisted to 24 hours (Figure 23.1D). There was no significant difference between the two groups (Figure 23.1D).

TUNEL staining was negative in the sham control brain sections, but was strongly present in the vehicle-treated sections 12 hours after permanent MCAO (Figure 23.2a, arrowheads). TUNEL-positive cells were distributed mainly in the ischemic core of the cerebral cortex and dorsal caudate putamen of the occluded MCA area. Approximately 50% to 70% of cells were positive for TUNEL in this area, and the staining was essentially found in the nucleus of neuronal cells. Treatment with GDNF greatly reduced the number of TUNEL-positive cells 12 hours after permanent MCAO (Figure 23.2e, arrowhead).

Immunoreactivity for caspases was not detectable in the sham control brain sections (data not shown). However, caspases -1 and -3 became markedly present 12 hours after permanent MCAO in the neuronal cytoplasm of the cerebral cortex (Figure 23.2b and c, arrowheads), especially in the inner boundary zone of the infarct and caudate putamen in the MCA territory. The staining cells for both caspases -1 and -3 were apparently reduced by GDNF treatment (Figure 23.2f and g, arrowheads). Immunoreactivity for caspase-2 was also induced after MCAO, but was more widely distributed in the cerebral cortex and caudate putamen in the MCA territory than for caspase-1 and -3 immunoreactivity. The staining was only slightly more reduced with the GDNF treatment (Figure 23.2h, arrowheads) than with the vehicle treatment (Figure 23.2d, arrowheads).

Neurotrophic factors have recently been classified into several groups, such as neurotrophins, cytokines, the fibroblast growth factor family and the TGF-β

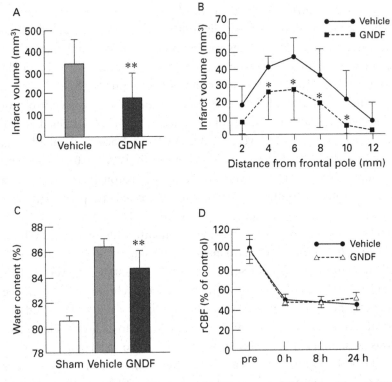

Figure 23.1   Effects of GDNF on (A) infarct volume, (B) infarct area, (C) brain edema and (D) regional CBF, 24 hours after permanent MCAO. (A) Infarct volume in the brain sections was significantly reduced by GDNF treatment (** $P=0.01$). (B) Infarct volume of four coronal sections from the GDNF-treated group were also significantly smaller than in the vehicle group (* $P<0.05$). (C) Increase in water content was significantly reduced by GDNF treatment as compared with vehicle treatment (** $P=0.01$). (D) There was no significant difference in CBF between vehicle and GDNF treatments. Data are mean ± SD (A, B and D = vehicle, $n=7$ and GDNF, $n=9$; C = sham, $n=6$, vehicle, $n=5$ and GDNF, $n=7$). (From Kitagawa H, Hayashi T, Mitsumoto Y, Koga N, Itoyama Y & Abe K (1998) Reduction of ischemic brain injury by topical application of glial cell line-derived neurotrophic factor after permanent middle cerebral artery occlusion in rats. *Stroke*, **29**, 1417–22, with permission.)

superfamily [12]. GDNF, a member of the TGF-β superfamily, is thought to be the most potent among the neurotrophic factors for the survival of cultured neurons [12]. It has also been reported that GDNF has a protective effect on various injuries of the central and peripheral nervous systems in vitro and in vivo [2–4]. In this study, we showed that topical application of GDNF significantly ameliorated both infarction and brain edema formation in the MCA region (48% and 30% decreases, respectively) after permanent MCAO. There was no difference in regional CBF

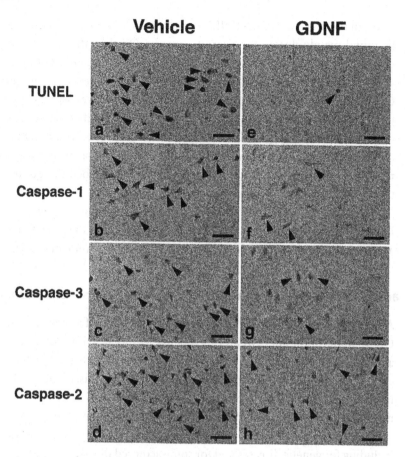

Figure 23.2 Representative stainings of TUNEL (a and e), caspase-1 (b and f), caspase-3 (c and g) and caspase-2 (d and h) treated with the vehicle (a–d) or GDNF (e–h). Magnification × 100. Bars = 0.04 mm. (From Kitagawa H, Hayashi T, Mitsumoto Y, Koga N, Itoyama Y & Abe K (1998) Reduction of ischemic brain injury by topical application of glial cell line-derived neurotrophic factor after permanent middle cerebral artery occlusion in rats. *Stroke*, **29**, 1417–22, with permission.)

between the vehicle- and GDNF-treated groups (Figure 23.1D), suggesting that the ameliorative effect of GDNF was less involved in the improvement of CBF.

Interestingly, the effect was greatly associated with the marked reduction of TUNEL staining (Figure 23.2e), which was predominantly located in the ischemic core region rather than in the ischemic penumbra. Apoptotic neurons were localized primarily in the inner boundary zone of the infarct, whereas necrotic cells were distributed mainly in the ischemic core after transient focal ischemia in rats [13,14]. Furthermore, DNA fragmentation in both apoptotic and necrotic neurons in the brain sections after transient MCAO was detected by the TUNEL method [13].

Thus, in the present study, TUNEL-positive cells located in the ischemic core may be found mainly during the necrotic process. On the other hand, the moderate decrease in immunoreactivity for caspases -1 and -3 (Figure 23.2f and g) and the slight decrease in caspase-2 staining (Figure 23.2h) were also observed in the GDNF-treated group. The distribution of immunoreactive caspases were mainly in the ischemic penumbra and not colocalized with TUNEL-positive cells (data not shown). These data suggest that the mechanism of the ameliorative effect of GDNF on brain ischemic injury after permanent MCAO may be related not only to the reduction of necrotic cells, but also to the reduction of the apoptotic process through the inhibition of the caspase-1 and -3 pathways.

In conclusion, this study demonstrated the ameliorative effect of GDNF on ischemic brain injury, which was strongly associated with the reduction of both the apoptotic and necrotic processes but not with the improvement of regional CBF.

Effect of adenovirus-mediated gene transfer of GDNF on ischemic brain injury

Although several reports demonstrate the amelioration of ischemic brain injury by GDNF application after MCAO in rodents [3,10,15], with regard to the clinical application of this protein, administration remains difficult. GDNF cannot be effectively delivered to a brain parenchymal lesion after vascular injection owing to the blood–brain barrier. Furthermore, intracerebroventricular or intraparenchymal injections are frequently not applicable in the clinical setting.

Gene delivery systems using virus vectors have been reported in many fields, including for genetic diseases and for some acquired diseases such as cancer or cardiovascular disease [16,17]. Recently, our group demonstrated a successful adenovirus-mediated lacZ gene transfer into the normal or ischemic rodent brain [18–20]. Other genes have also been successfully transferred into the brain, and have shown protective effects against ischemic brain injury [21–26]. Therefore, gene therapy for cerebrovascular disease could become one potential therapy in the near future [27]. We therefore prepared an adenovirus vector containing the GDNF gene (Ad-GDNF) and examined the possible protective effect of Ad-GDNF transfer into the rat brain after transient MCAO in association with modifications of apoptotic signals.

Male adult Wistar rats (250–280 g) were anesthetized by inhalation of a nitrous oxide/oxygen/halothane (68%/30%/2%) mixture, and their heads were fixed in a stereotactic frame (SR-5N; Narishige, Tokyo, Japan). Ad-GDNF, Ad-LacZ (10^8 plaque-forming units (pfu) in 10 μl of the vector vehicle consisting of 10 mM Tris-HCl, pH 7.4, 1 mM $MgCl_2$, and 10% (v/v) glycerol) or the vehicle solution was administered to the ipsilateral cortex via a burr hole through the dura mater. Twenty-four hours after the virus vector injection, the rats were again anesthetized by inhalation of a nitrous oxide/oxygen/halothane (69%/30%/1%) mixture during the surgical procedure. The right MCA was occluded by the insertion of a nylon thread through the common carotid artery as described in our previous report [10]. The blood flow was restored by removal of the nylon thread after 90 minutes of transient ischemia. The animals were allowed to recover in an ambient temperature (21 °C to 24 °C) until the time of sampling.

To examine the effect of Ad-GDNF on infarct size after transient MCAO, the rat forebrains were removed and divided into six coronal sections (2 mm each) after 24 hours of reperfusion with the vehicle ($n=9$), Ad-LacZ ($n=6$) or Ad-GDNF ($n=9$) treatments. The coronal sections were stained with saline containing 2% (v/v) TTC at 37 °C for 30 minutes, after which the sections were fixed in 10% (v/v) neutralized formalin, according to a previously reported technique [11]. The five infarct areas between each adjoining slice were measured by Scion Image software, version 1.62a (Frederick, MD), and then the infarct areas on each slice were summed and multiplied by slice thickness to find the infarct volume. In this experiment, regional CBF of the right frontoparietal cortex was measured through the burr hole using a laser blood flowmeter (Flo-C1, Omegawave) before or immediately after occlusion (-1.5 hours) or reperfusion (0 hours), respectively, and at 8 or 24 hours after reperfusion.

For the histological staining of DNA fragmentation, caspase-3 and cytochrome c, the rat forebrains of both the vehicle-treated ($n=3$) and Ad-GDNF-treated ($n=3$) groups were removed and quickly frozen in powdered dry ice 24 hours after transient MCAO (2 days after injection). The sham control samples ($n=2$) were also collected in the same way without the drug injection and MCAO. Coronal sections at the caudate putamen and dorsal hippocampal levels were cut on a cryostat at -18 °C to a thickness of 10 μm and collected on glass slides. For detection of DNA fragmentation, TUNEL was performed according to our previous report [10]. Immunostaining for caspase-3 and cytochrome c was performed by the avidin-biotin–peroxidase method (ABC kits PK-6101 for GDNF or cytochrome c, and PK-6105 for caspase-3; Vector Laboratories) according to our previous report [28]. Staining was developed with DAB and lightly counterstained with Mayer hematoxylin. The sections were examined with a light microscope, and the stained cells in 0.25 mm² of a random three MCA areas were counted, summed and categorized into four grades as follows: no staining ($-$), small (1 to 10; $\pm$), moderate (10 to 100; $+$) or large (100 to 500; $2+$) number of stained cells.

Statistical analysis were performed using one-way analysis of variance (ANOVA) for infarct volume, two-way ANOVA followed by Bonferroni post hoc test for infarct area and ANOVA repeated measure for physiological and regional CBF data.

There were no significant differences in blood gases, pH, and rectal temperature between the vehicle-, Ad-LacZ- and Ad-GDNF-treated groups before MCAO, or 0, 8 or 24 hours after reperfusion (data not shown).

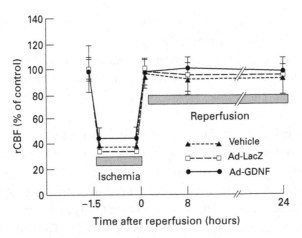

Figure 23.3 Temporal profile of regional CBF (rCBF) after 90 minutes of transient MCAO. Regional CBF was reduced to about 40% of basal line immediately after MCAO (−1.5 hours) and was restored to base line after reperfusion (0 hours) in vehicle- ($n=9$, ---▲---), Ad-LacZ- ($n=6$, − □ −) and Ad-GDNF- ($n=9$, − ● −) treated groups. There was no significant difference in CBF among these three groups. Data are expressed as mean ± SD. (From Kitagawa H, Sasaki C, Sakai K, Mori A, Mitsumoto Y, Mori T, Fukuchi Y, Setoguchi Y & Abe K (1999) Adenovirus-mediated gene transfer of glial cell line-derived neurotrophic factor prevents ischemic brain injury after transient middle cerebral artery occlusion in rats. *Journal of Cerebral Blood Flow & Metabolism*, **19**, 1336–44, with permission.)

Regional CBF for the vehicle-, Ad-LacZ- and Ad-GDNF-treated groups was reduced to about 40% of the control immediately after MCAO and recovered to the base line after reperfusion by withdrawal of the nylon thread (Figure 23.3). There was no significant difference among these three groups (Figure 23.3). While infarction in the brain sections of the sham control group could not be observed, infarct volumes in the vehicle-, Ad-LacZ- and Ad-GDNF-treated groups 24 hours after 90 minutes of transient MCAO were $209.2 \pm 35.8 \, mm^3$ (mean ± SD, $n=9$), $213.3 \pm 59.1 \, mm^3$ ($n=6$) and $97.6 \pm 71.5 \, mm^3$ ($n=9$; $P<0.001$ vs. the vehicle- and Ad-LacZ-treated groups), respectively (Figure 23.4A). Infarct areas in two or three coronal sections (4, 6 and 8 mm caudal from frontal pole) from the Ad-GDNF-treated group were also significantly smaller than those from the vehicle or Ad-LacZ groups (Figure 23.4B), respectively.

There were no TUNEL- or caspase-3-positive cells in the sham control brains, while cytochrome *c*-stained cells were slightly detected in layers IV to V of the ipsilateral or contralateral frontoparietal somatosensory cortex (Table 23.1). TUNEL-, caspase-3- or cytochrome *c*-positive cells were markedly increased in the ipsilateral cortex and caudate putamen in the vehicle-treated group 24 hours after transient MCAO (Table 23.1). In the Ad-GDNF-treated group, the number of positive cells

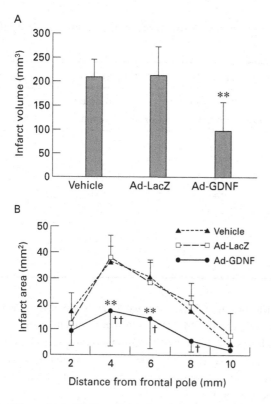

Figure 23.4 Effect of Ad-GDNF on (A) infarct volume and (B) infarct area, 24 hours after 90 minutes of transient MCAO. (A) Infarct volume in the brain sections of the Ad-GDNF-treated group ($n = 9$, ** $P<0.01$) was significantly smaller than in the vehicle- ($n=9$) or Ad-LacZ- ($n=6$) treated groups. (B) Infarct area of three coronal sections (4, 6 and 8 mm caudal from the frontal pole) from the Ad-GDNF- (– ● –) treated group (** $P<0.01$ vs. vehicle group; $^{†}P<0.05$, $^{††}P<0.01$ vs. Ad-LacZ group) was also significantly smaller than in the vehicle- (---▲---) or Ad-LacZ- (– □ –) treated groups. Data are expressed as mean ± SD. (From Kitagawa H, Sasaki C, Sakai K, Mori A, Mitsumoto Y, Mori T, Fukuchi Y, Setoguchi Y & Abe K (1999) Adenovirus-mediated gene transfer of glial cell line-derived neurotrophic factor prevents ischemic brain injury after transient middle cerebral artery occlusion in rats. *Journal of Cerebral Blood Flow & Metabolism*, **19**, 1336–44, with permission.)

was obviously smaller, especially in the cortex (Table 23.1), than in the vehicle group. There was no leukocyte infiltration except for around the needle track in one vehicle-treated rat, and traumatic injury was observed only around the needle track (data not shown).

Adenovirus or adeno-associated virus-mediated GDNF gene transfer prevents dopaminergic neuron degeneration [29–32] and improves behavioral impairment in the rat model of Parkinson's disease [33,34]. Neuroprotective activity of the adenovirus-mediated GDNF gene transfer against axotomy-induced motoneuron

Table 23.1. Changes in TUNEL, caspase-3 and cytochrome c immunoreactivity after transient MCAO in rats

		TUNEL		Caspase-3		Cytochrome c	
Treatment		Cortex	Caudate putamen	Cortex	Caudate putamen	Cortex	Caudate putamen
Sham control	1	−	−	−	−	+	−
	2	−	−	−	−	+	−
Vehicle	1	2+	2+	+	+	+	+
	2	+	2+	2+	2+	2+	2+
	3	2+	2+	2+	+	2+	+
Ad-GDNF	1	+	2+	+	+	+	+
	2	−	±	−	−	±	−
	3	±	+	+	+	+	+

Notes:
TUNEL, terminal deoxynucleotidyl transferase-mediated dUTP-biotin nick end-labeling; MCAO, middle cerebral artery occlusion; Ad-GDNF, adenovirus containing the GDNF gene. Staining was performed 24 hours after transient MCAO and was categorized into the following four grades: no staining (−), or a small (2 to 10; ±), moderate (10 to 100; +) or large (100 to 500; 2+) number of stained cells. Sham control, $n=2$; vehicle- and Ad-GDNF-treated groups, $n=3$. (From ref. 28, with permission.)

death has also been reported [35]. However, there is no report of adenovirus-mediated GDNF gene transfer protecting against more severe types of neuronal death such as in ischemia or stroke. We first demonstrated that the adenovirus-mediated exogenous GDNF gene was successfully transferred into cortical neurons and attenuated ischemic brain injury after transient MCAO [28].

The protective mechanism of GDNF is not fully understood, although previous work has demonstrated that GDNF diminished ischemia-induced nitric oxide release [3] or reduced caspase-immunoreactive neurons [10]. In this study, there was no significant difference in regional CBF among the vehicle-, Ad-LacZ- and Ad-GDNF-treated groups (Figure 23.3), suggesting that the effect of Ad-GDNF is not associated with improvement in regional CBF. GDNF signaling is mediated by the receptor tyrosine kinase encoded by the c-*ret* protooncogene (Ret) [36,37], and GDNF receptor α-1 (GFRα-1), a glycosyl-phosphatidylinositol-linked protein, assists in GDNF binding to Ret [38,39]. Distribution of Ret and GFRα-1 mRNA expression in the rat central nervous system was recently reported. GFRα-1 mRNA was detected in the cerebral cortex, while Ret mRNA was not seen in the normal rat brain [40,41]. However, both GFRα-1 and Ret mRNAs were markedly induced in the pyramidal layer of the cerebral cortex 12 to 24 hours after kainic acid treatment

[40]. Therefore, GDNF/Ret/GFRα-1 interactions may also occur under ischemic conditions. Further study is required to confirm that the interaction between GDNF and its receptors could be essential for the neuroprotective effect in ischemic brain injury.

Our previous study suggests that the protective effect of GDNF on ischemic brain injury is associated with the inhibition of immunoreactive caspases -1 and -3 [10]. Of interest is that one of the most important pathways of neuronal death is related to mitochondrial dysfunction [42]. Recently, it was demonstrated that cytochrome c release from mitochondria to the cytosol activates the caspase cascade in vitro [43,44]. Furthermore, cytosolic redistribution of cytochrome c after transient focal cerebral ischemia in rats has been demonstrated [45], suggesting a vital role in neuronal cell death. In the present study, both immunoreactive caspase-3 and cytochrome c were induced in the cytoplasm of neuronal cells in the penumbral cortex after transient ischemia, and obviously decreased in the Ad-GDNF-treated group, with correspondence in TUNEL staining profiles (Table 23.1). Although the TUNEL method is not specific for apoptotic neurons in the ischemic brain, the TUNEL-positive neurons in the ischemic penumbral region were mainly apoptotic cells, while those in the ischemic core were necrotic [13]. Therefore some of the TUNEL-positive neurons observed in the present study died by the apoptotic process. Thus the apoptotic pathway via cytochrome c and caspase-3 seems to be one of the targets for protection by GDNF. In this study, we have demonstrated the change in the immunoreactive caspase-3 protein after transient MCAO, but the pro- or activated forms of caspase-3 have not been examined. Further study of the change in caspase-3 activity would provide precise information about the protective mechanism of GDNF.

Gene therapeutic studies for stroke have not yet been tried in the clinical situation. Although it has been demonstrated that the adenovirus-mediated neuronal apoptosis inhibitory protein or an interleukin-1 receptor antagonist have a protective effect against ischemic brain injury, adenoviral vectors were injected 5 days before ischemia [21,46]. Herpes simplex virus-mediated *hsp72* gene transfer markedly improved striatal neuron survival in focal ischemia, but the vector was injected 8 hours before occlusion [26]. In this study, the adenoviral vector was also injected 24 hours before MCAO because it takes more than 8 hours to express the gene product using the adenoviral vector in the normal rat brain [18]. However, in the clinical setting, gene therapy should be applied after a stroke. Therefore, therapeutic studies with these vectors, when delivered after ischemia, should be conducted. Furthermore, each vector has some disadvantages, such as toxicity or efficacy of gene expression. Improvement of the vectors or development of a safer vector may be necessary for more practical gene therapy. Finally, the route of administration may be of major concern for gene therapy. In the present study, we administered the vector directly into the cerebral cortex. Of course, direct injection of the vector may not be practical in clinical applications. Although intra-arterial or venous administration could be more suitable for human ischemic diseases, there may be great difficulty in how to deliver the vector specifically to the ischemic area. When these problems are successfully resolved, gene therapy could have great potential for stroke therapy.

Acknowledgments

The authors express their appreciation to Dr. Warita, Dr. Sakai and Dr. Sasaki for their advice and technical support. This work was partly supported by Grants-in-Aid for Scientific Research 09470151 from the Ministry of Education, Japan.

REFERENCES

1 Lin L-FH, Doherty DH, Lile JD, Bektesh S & Collins F (1993) GDNF: a glial cell line-derived neurotrophic factor for midbrain dopaminergic neurons. *Science*, **260**, 1130–2.

2 Beck KD, Valverde J, Alexi T, Poulsen K, Moffat B, Vandlen RA, Rosenthal A & Hefti F (1995) Mesencephalic dopaminergic neurons protected by GDNF from axotomy-induced degeneration in the adult brain. *Nature*, **373**, 339–41.

3 Wang Y, Lin S-Z, Chiou A-L, Williams LR & Hoffer BJ (1997) Glial cell line-derived neurotrophic factor protects against ischemia-induced injury in the cerebral cortex. *Journal of Neuroscience*, **17**, 4341–8.

4 Tomac A, Lindqvist E, Lin L-FH, Ögren SO, Young D, Hoffer BJ & Olson L (1995) Protection and repair of the nigrostriatal dopaminergic system by GDNF in vivo. *Nature*, **373**, 335–9.

5 Kinoshita M, Tomimoto H, Kinoshita A, Kumar S & Noda M (1997) Up-regulation of the *Nedd2* gene encoding an ICE/Ced-3-like cysteine protease in the gerbil brain after transient global ischemia. *Journal of Cerebral Blood Flow & Metabolism*, **17**, 507–14.

6 Asahi M, Hoshimaru M, Uemura Y, Tokime T, Kojima M, Ohtsuka T, Matsuura N, Aoki T, Shibahara K & Kikuchi H (1997) Expression of interleukin-1β converting enzyme gene family and *bcl-2* gene family in the rat brain following permanent occlusion of the middle cerebral artery. *Journal of Cerebral Blood Flow & Metabolism*, **17**, 11–18.

7 Hara H, Friedlander RM, Gagliardini V, Ayata C, Fink K, Huang Z, Shimizu-Sasamata M, Yuan J & Moskowitz MA (1997) Inhibition of interleukin 1β converting enzyme family proteases reduces ischemic and excitotoxic neuronal damage. *Proceedings of the National Academy of Sciences, USA*, **94**, 2007–12.

8 Friedlander RM, Gagliardini V, Hara H, Fink KB, Li W, MacDonald G, Fishman MC, Greenberg AH, Moskowitz MA & Yuan J (1997) Expression of a dominant negative mutant of interleukin-1β converting enzyme in transgenic mice prevents neuronal cell death induced by trophic factor withdrawal and ischemic brain injury. *Journal of Experimental Medicine*, **185**, 933–40.

9 Hara H, Fink K, Endres M, Friedlander RM, Gagliardini V, Yuan J & Moskowitz MA (1997) Attenuation of transient focal cerebral ischemic injury in transgenic mice expressing a mutant ICE inhibitory protein. *Journal of Cerebral Blood Flow & Metabolism*, 17, 370–5.

10 Kitagawa H, Hayashi T, Mitsumoto Y, Koga N, Itoyama Y & Abe K (1998) Reduction of ischemic brain injury by topical application of glial cell line-derived neurotrophic factor after permanent middle cerebral artery occlusion in rats. *Stroke*, 29, 1417–22.

11 Bederson JB, Pitts LH, Germano SM, Nishimura MC, Davis RL & Bartkowski HM (1986) Evaluation of 2,3,5-triphenyltetrazolium chloride as a stain for detection and quantification of experimental cerebral infarction in rats. *Stroke*, 17, 1304–8.

12 Lidsay RM (1995) Neuron saving schemes. *Nature*, 373, 289–90.

13 Charriaut-Marlangue C, Margaill I, Represa A, Popovici T, Plotkine M & Ben-Ari Y (1996) Apoptosis and necrosis after reversible focal ischemia: an in situ DNA fragmentation analysis. *Journal of Cerebral Blood Flow & Metabolism*, 16, 186–94.

14 Li Y, Chopp M, Jiang N, Yao F & Zaloga C (1995) Temporal profile of in situ DNA fragmentation after transient middle cerebral artery occlusion in the rat. *Journal of Cerebral Blood Flow & Metabolism*, 15, 389–97.

15 Abe K, Hayashi T & Itoyama Y (1997) Amelioration of brain edema by topical application of glial cell line-derived neurotrophic factor in reperfused rat brain. *Neuroscience Letters*, 231, 37–40.

16 Nabel EG (1995) Gene therapy for cardiovascular disease. *Circulation*, 91, 541–8.

17 Verma IM & Somia N (1997) Gene therapy – promises, problems and prospects. *Nature*, 389, 239–42.

18 Abe K, Setoguchi Y, Hayashi T & Itoyama Y (1997) In vivo adenovirus-mediated gene transfer and the expression in ischemic and reperfused rat brain. *Brain Research*, 763, 191–201.

19 Kitagawa H, Setoguchi Y, Fukuchi Y, Mitsumoto Y, Koga N, Mori T & Abe K (1998) Induction of DNA fragmentation and HSP72 immunoreactivity by adenovirus-mediated gene transfer in normal gerbil hippocampus and ventricle. *Journal of Neuroscience Research*, 54, 38–45.

20 Kitagawa H, Setoguchi Y, Fukuchi Y, Mitsumoto Y, Koga N, Mori T & Abe K (1998) DNA fragmentation and HSP72 gene expression by adenovirus-mediated gene transfer in postischemic gerbil hippocampus and ventricle. *Metabolic Brain Disease*, 13, 211–23.

21 Betz AL, Yang G-Y & Davidson BL (1995) Attenuation of stroke size in rats using an adenoviral vector to induce overexpression of interleukin-1 receptor antagonist in brain. *Journal of Cerebral Blood Flow & Metabolism*, 15, 547–51.

22 Linnik MD, Zahos P, Geschwind MD & Federoff HJ (1995) Expression of Bcl-2 from a defective herpes simplex virus-1 vector limits neuronal death in focal cerebral ischemia. *Stroke*, 26, 1670–5.

23 Lawrence MS, McLaughlin JR, Sun G-H, Ho DY, McIntosh L, Kunis DM, Sapolsky RM & Steinberg GK (1997) Herpes simplex viral vectors expressing Bcl-2 are neuroprotective when delivered after a stroke. *Journal of Cerebral Blood Flow & Metabolism*, 17, 740–4.

24 Yang G-Y, Zhao Y-J, Davidson BL & Betz AL (1997) Overexpression of interleukin-1 receptor antagonist in the mouse brain reduces ischemic brain injury. *Brain Research*, 751, 181–8.

25 Yang G-Y, Liu X-H, Kadoya C, Zhao Y-J, Mao Y, Davidson BL & Betz AL (1998) Attenuation of ischemic inflammatory response in mouse brain using an adenoviral vector to induce over-expression of interleukin-1 receptor antagonist. *Journal of Cerebral Blood Flow & Metabolism*, 18, 840–7.

26 Yenari MA, Fink SL, Sun GH, Chang LK, Patel MK, Kunis DM, Onley D, Ho DY, Sapolsky RM & Steinberg GK (1998) Gene therapy with HSP72 is neuroprotective in rat models of stroke and epilepsy. *Annals of Neurology*, 44, 584–91.

27 Heistad DD & Faraci FM (1996) Gene therapy for cerebral vascular disease. *Stroke*, 27, 1688–93.

28 Kitagawa H, Sasaki C, Sakai K, Mori A, Mitsumoto Y, Mori T, Fukuchi Y, Setoguchi Y & Abe K (1999) Adenovirus-mediated gene transfer of glial cell line-derived neurotrophic factor prevents ischemic brain injury after transient middle cerebral artery occlusion in rats. *Journal of Cerebral Blood Flow & Metabolism*, 19, 1336–44.

29 Choi-Lundberg DL, Lin Q, Chang Y-N, Chiang YL, Hay CM, Mohajeri H, Davidson BL & Bohn MC (1997) Dopaminergic neurons protected from degeneration by GDNF gene therapy. *Science*, 275, 838–41.

30 Kojima H, Abiru Y, Sakajiri K, Watabe K, Ohishi N, Takamori M, Hatanaka H & Yagi K (1997) Adenovirus-mediated transduction with human glial cell-derived neurotrophic factor gene prevents 1-methyl-4-phenyl-1,2,3,6-tetrahydropyridine-induced dopamine depletion in striatum of mouse brain. *Biochemical and Biophysical Research Communications*, 238, 569–73.

31 Mandel RJ, Spratt SK, Snyder RO & Leff SE (1997) Midbrain injection of recombinant adeno-associated virus encoding rat glial cell line-derived neurotrophic factor protects nigral neurons in a progressive 6-hydroxydopamine-induced degeneration model of Parkinson's disease in rats. *Proceedings of the National Academy of Sciences, USA*, 94, 14083–8.

32 Fan D-s, Ogawa M, Ikeguchi K, Fujimoto K-i, Urabe M, Kume A, Nishizawa M, Matsushita N, Kiuchi K, Ichinose H, Nagatsu T, Kurtzman GJ, Nakano I & Ozawa K (1998) Prevention of dopaminergic neuron death by adeno-associated virus vector-mediated GDNF gene transfer in rat mesencephalic cells in vitro. *Neuroscience Letters*, 248, 61–4.

33 Bilang-Bleuel A, Revah F, Colin P, Locquet I, Robert J-J, Mallet J & Horellou P (1997) Intrastriatal injection of an adenoviral vector expressing glial-cell-line-derived neuro-trophic factor prevents dopaminergic neuron degeneration and behavioral impairment in a rat model of Parkinson disease. *Proceedings of the National Academy of Sciences, USA*, 94, 8818–23.

34 Lapchak PA, Araujo DM, Hilt DC, Sheng J & Jiao S (1997) Adenoviral vector-mediated GDNF gene therapy in a rodent lesion model of late stage Parkinson's disease. *Brain Research*, 777, 153–60.

35 Baumgartner BJ & Shine HD (1997) Targeted transduction of CNS neurons with adenoviral vectors carrying neurotrophic factor genes confers neuroprotection that exceeds the trans-duced population. *Journal of Neuroscience*, 17, 6504–11.

36 Durbec P, Marcos-Gutierrez CV, Kilkenny C, Grigoriou M, Wartiowaara K, Suvanto P, Smith D, Ponder B, Costantini F, Saarma M, Sariola H & Pachnis V (1996) GDNF signalling through the Ret receptor tyrosine kinase. *Nature*, 381, 789–93.

37 Trupp M, Arenas E, Fainzilber M, Nilsson A-S, Sieber B-A, Grigoriou M, Kilkenny C, Salazar-Grueso E, Pachnis V, Arumäe U, Sariola H, Saarma M & Ibáñez CF (1996) Functional receptor for GDNF encoded by the c-ret proto-oncogene. *Nature*, **381**, 785–9.

38 Treanor JJS, Goodman L, Sauvage F, Stone DM, Poulsen KT, Beck CD, Gray C, Armanini MP, Pollock RA, Hefti F, Phillips HS, Goddard A, Moore MW, Buj-Bello A, Davies AM, Asai N, Takahashi M, Vandlen R, Henderson CE & Rosenthal A (1996) Characterization of a multi-component receptor for GDNF. *Nature*, **382**, 80–3.

39 Klein RD, Sherman D, Ho W-H, Stone D, Bennett GL, Moffat B, Vandlen R, Simmons L, Gu Q, Hongo J-A, Devaux B, Poulsen K, Armanini M, Nozaki C, Asai N, Goddard A, Phillips H, Henderson CE, Takahashi M & Rosenthal A (1997) A GPI-linked protein that interacts with Ret to form a candidate neurturin receptor. *Nature*, **387**, 717–21.

40 Trupp M, Belluardo N, Funakoshi H & Ibáñez CF (1997) Complementary and overlapping expression of glial cell line-derived neurotrophic factor (GDNF), c-*ret* proto-oncogene, and GDNF receptor-α indicates multiple mechanisms of trophic actions in the adult rat CNS. *Journal of Neuroscience*, **17**, 3554–67.

41 Glazner GW, Mu X & Springer JE (1998) Localization of glial cell line-derived neurotrophic factor receptor alpha and c-*ret* mRNA in rat central nervous system. *Journal of Comparative Neurology*, **391**, 42–9.

42 Abe K, Aoki M, Kawagoe J, Yoshida T, Hattori A, Kogure K & Itoyama Y (1995) Ischemic delayed neuronal death. A mitochondrial hypothesis. *Stroke*, **26**, 1478–89.

43 Kluck RM, Bossy-Wetzel E, Green DR & Newmeyer DD (1997) The release of cytochrome c from mitochondria: a primary site for Bcl-2 regulation of apoptosis. *Science*, **275**, 1132–6.

44 Yang J, Liu X, Bhalla K, Kim CN, Ibrado AM, Cai J, Peng T-I, Jones DP & Wang X (1997) Prevention of apoptosis by Bcl-2: release of cytochrome c from mitochondria blocked. *Science*, **275**, 1129–32.

45 Fujimura M, Morita-Fujimura Y, Murakami K, Kawase M & Chan PH (1998) Cytosolic redistribution of cytochrome c after transient focal cerebral ischemia in rats. *Journal of Cerebral Blood Flow & Metabolism*, **18**, 1239–47.

46 Xu DG, Crocker SJ, Doucet J-P, St-Jean M, Tamai K, Hakim AM, Ikeda J-E, Liston P, Thompson CS, Korneluk RG, MacKenzie A & Robertson GS (1997) Elevation of neuronal expression of NAIP reduces ischemic damage in the rat hippocampus. *Nature Medicine*, **3**, 997–1004.

24

Vasomotor effects of nitric oxide, superoxide dismutases and calcitonin gene-related peptide

Donald D. Heistad[1] & Frank M. Faraci[2]

[1,2] Departments of Internal Medicine and Pharmacology, University of Iowa and VA Medical Center, Iowa City, IA

Introduction

Several years ago we wrote "after several years of unfettered excitement and hype it is now clear that gene therapy is at a very early stage of development" [1]. That statement, although quite conservative, still seems appropriate.

We remain optimistic, however, about the long-term potential value of gene transfer to cerebral blood vessels. The method has already led to novel insights into vascular biology, and it is likely that gene therapy will ultimately prove to be useful in prevention and treatment of some types of stroke.

In this review, we will first describe several applications of gene transfer to blood vessels that have led to new insights in vascular biology. Second, we will describe a new method to study the cerebral circulation, which involves gene transfer of different isoforms of superoxide dismutase (SOD). Then we will describe studies that suggest that gene therapy may eventually prove to be useful in prevention of cerebral vasospasm after subarachnoid hemorrhage (SAH).

Approaches to gene transfer

We use a replication-deficient recombinant adenovirus to transfer DNA to the nucleus of target cells, which results in transcription of mRNA and translation of the desired protein. We have made most of the recombinant viruses that we use in experiments, by deletion of the portions of the viral genome that are required for replication and then insertion of the gene of interest into the region that has been deleted. We use an adenoviral vector because it is more effective than other vectors in transduction of the slowly dividing cells of blood vessels [2].

Typically, when we have made a new recombinant adenovirus, we test it in tissue culture to determine whether the transgene product is made. Then we generally transfect rings of blood vessels in tissue culture and examine vasomotor responses of the vascular rings [3]. This approach accomplishes gene transfer only to the endothelium and adventitia, and not to smooth muscle of the media, but it has proven effective in altering vasomotor responses [4].

Our next step generally has been to perform gene transfer in vivo. This was a great challenge in intracranial cerebral blood vessels, because the typical approach used previously to accomplish gene transfer in other organs was to inject the vector into blood, and stop blood flow to the organ or vessel for several minutes to accomplish infection by the adenovirus and gene transfer. Clearly, this approach could not be used for intracranial blood vessels.

We therefore developed an alternative method, which did not require intravascular injection of the vector, and did not require interruption of blood flow. We injected the adenoviral vectors into the cisterna magna, which allows the virus to diffuse through the cerebrospinal fluid (CSF), and results in expression of the transgene product in adventitia and perivascular tissues [5]. We also used this extravascular approach to accomplish gene transfer to the femoral and carotid arteries by injecting the vector into the sheath around the vessels [6].

A major concern with gene transfer to the adventitia was whether we would be able to alter vasomotor function. Our concern was that, without transfection of the endothelium or smooth muscle, expression of the transgene product in the adventitia alone would have little effect. We and others have found, however, that transfer of a gene with a diffusible product (such as nitric oxide (NO) or calcitonin gene-related peptide (CGRP)) to adventitia produces marked alteration of vasomotor function, because the gene product diffuses into the smooth muscle [7,8].

To our knowledge, the first study using this approach to study intracranial blood vessels was accomplished with transduction of the adventitia with endothelial nitric oxide synthase (eNOS) in vivo, and demonstration of altered vasomotor tone ex vivo [9]. Our collaborating investigators have used eNOS applied extravascularly to the carotid sinus baroreceptors in vivo to alter function [10].

The approaches described above relied on transduction of adventitia and perivascular tissues to alter vasomotor function. An alternative approach is to use gene transfer to transduce tissues in the subarachnoid space, and then allow the transgene product to bathe the brain. Using this approach, Betz et al. [11] demonstrated that gene transfer of IL-1ra produces a large increase in IL-1ra in brain and CSF and reduces the size of stroke after occlusion of the middle cerebral artery. Recently, we have used this approach with extracellular SOD (ECSOD) and demonstrated that we could produce large increases in SOD activity in the CSF [12].

Gene transfer to study vascular biology

We will describe studies of gene transfer of eNOS, inducible nitric oxide synthase (iNOS) and SODs to blood vessels. An appropriate question is why not simply give NO or an NO donor to study effects on blood vessels, and not go through all the steps that are required for gene transfer of NOS? There are several advantages of gene transfer over simply administering the gene product. First, different isoforms of an enzyme can be given by gene transfer. Thus eNOS, iNOS or neuronal NOS can be given to examine the effects and regulation of the various isoforms of NOS. One can also transduce tissues with the three isoforms of SOD (copper, zinc (CuZnSOD), ECSOD, manganese SOD). This is particularly attractive because the subcellular localization of the three isoforms is different and only ECSOD typically is released into the extravascular space.

Another advantage of gene transfer is that one can transduce only the endothelium or only the adventitia with an enzyme and thus study the role of endothelium and adventitia in vascular biology.

Gene transfer of eNOS to eNOS-deficient mice

Replacement of a disrupted gene is called complementation. Gene complementation by gene transfer has been used previously in ApoE-deficient mice and in low density lipoprotein receptor-deficient mice [13,14]. Gene transfer to blood vessels of gene-targeted mice – or complementation – has not been previously reported. We found that in eNOS-deficient mice, vasomotor function could be restored to essentially normal by gene transfer of eNOS [15]. Relaxation to acetylcholine or A23187, which was absent in eNOS-deficient animals, was restored to normal 24 hours after gene transfer of eNOS (Figure 24.1). This approach allows a unique way to study eNOS in vessels, and it also demonstrates remarkable efficacy of gene transfer to blood vessels.

We have used gene transfer approaches to attempt to improve endothelium-dependent relaxation in several disease states. A large number of studies have shown that responses to acetylcholine and other endothelium-dependent vasodilators are profoundly impaired by atherosclerosis, diabetes and hypertension. It is well known that superoxide anion inactivates NO, and this appears to be the major mechanism for impairment of endothelium-dependent relaxation.

On the basis of this concept, we examined effects of gene transfer of eNOS and SOD to vessels from atherosclerotic, diabetic or hypertensive animals. We expected that gene transfer of SOD, particularly ECSOD, would improve relaxation. To our surprise, gene transfer of SOD failed to improve responses to acetylcholine [16], but gene transfer of eNOS improved relaxation [17] (Figure 24.2).

In atherosclerotic rabbits, we used hydroethidine, a fluorescent dye that turns red

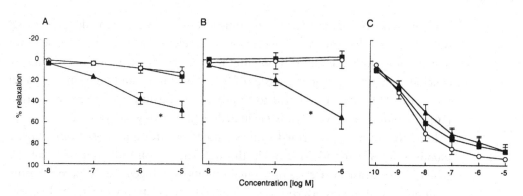

Figure 24.1   Relaxation to (A) acetylcholine, (B) A23187 and (C) nitroprusside, in aorta from eNOS-
deficient mice. Vessels were treated with vehicle (○) or were incubated with Ad-lacZ (■)
or Ad-eNOS (▲). Data are mean ± SE, * $P<0.05$ eNOS-transduced vessels vs. vehicle-
treated and *lacZ*-transduced vessels. (Reproduced from ref. 15.)

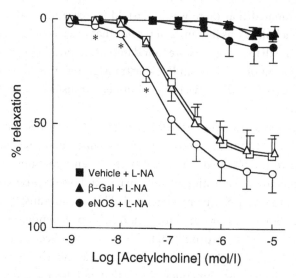

Figure 24.2   Responses of carotid arteries from WHHL rabbits to acetylcholine 1 day after transfection
with Ad-β-gal (β-gal), Ad-eNOS (eNOS) or vehicle alone. Relaxation to acetylcholine was
performed in the presence (●) or absence (□) of N$^\omega$-nitro-L-arginine (L-NA, 100 μmol/l).
Values are mean ± SEM. (Reproduced from ref. 4. Ooboshi H, Toyoda K, Faraci FM, Lang
MG & Heistad DD (1998) Improvement of relaxation in an atherosclerotic artery by gene
transfer of endothelial nitric oxide synthase. *Arteriosclerosis, Thrombosis, and Vascular
Biology*, **18**, 1752–8.)

in the presence of superoxide, to determine localization of superoxide in the vessel wall. We found that superoxide levels were elevated in atherosclerotic vessels, not only in the endothelium, but throughout the vessel wall, including the media. We concluded that because gene transfer of SOD failed to dismute the superoxide in the media, SOD therefore failed to improve endothelium-dependent relaxation [16]. This conclusion was greatly facilitated by the use of gene transfer.

Recently, we have performed similar studies in carotid arteries from diabetic rabbits [18]. We found superoxide throughout the carotid artery in diabetic rabbits, in contrast to arteries of normal rabbits, which generate superoxide only from endothelium and adventitia (Figure 24.3). Relaxation to acetylcholine was impaired in carotid arteries from diabetic rabbits and gene transfer of CuZnSOD failed to improve the relaxation. Gene transfer of eNOS, however, produced a marked improvement in relaxation (Figure 24.4).

We also examined this concept in rabbits that received an infusion of angiotensin II for one week [19]. We found increased levels of superoxide throughout the aortic wall and estimated that there was a 2.5-fold increase in superoxide levels. Relaxation to acetylcholine was impaired in rabbits that received angiotensin II. As in atherosclerotic and diabetic rabbits, we found impaired endothelium-dependent relaxation after infusion of angiotensin II. Gene transfer of CuZn-SOD or ECSOD failed to improve responses to acetylcholine, but gene transfer of eNOS restored responses to normal.

We interpret this series of studies in the following way. Gene transfer of SOD fails to deliver enough SOD to the media to dismute the superoxide, and thus fails to improve responses to the NO that is released from the endothelium. In contrast, NO is extremely effective in activation of superoxide, and overexpression of eNOS results in a large amount of NO being generated. Thus, gene transfer of eNOS is more effective than SOD in improvement of endothelium-dependent relaxation.

The reason that we were surprised that eNOS was so effective was that we thought superoxide anion would inactivate the NO, and thus eNOS would fail to improve responses. In contrast, our conclusion is that NO inactivates the superoxide in the vessel wall, thereby improving responses to acetylcholine. Gene transfer approaches were invaluable in leading to this concept in vascular biology.

Recently we have constructed an adenoviral vector that expresses iNOS. This virus was far more difficult to construct than the other viruses that we have made, for reasons that are not entirely clear. As expected, we found that gene transfer of iNOS, with generation of large amounts of NO, impaired contraction of the carotid artery in vitro. To our surprise, however, gene transfer of iNOS produced profound impairment of NO-mediated relaxation. Endothelium-dependent relaxation was greatly improved by inhibitors of iNOS, which indicates that the impairment was, in fact, due to expression of iNOS. We also found that tiron, a scavenger of

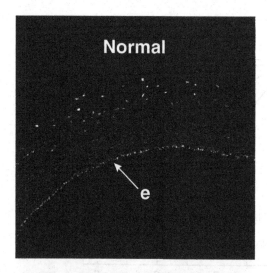

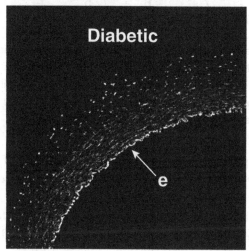

Figure 24.3 Detection of superoxide in situ in carotid artery. Confocal fluorescent photomicrographs of carotid artery from normal and diabetic rabbit incubated with hydroethidine. Carotid artery from the normal rabbit has minimal fluorescence in the endothelium (e) and adventitia. In contrast, carotid artery from the diabetic rabbit has increased ethidium bromide fluorescence reflecting increased superoxide anion levels throughout the vessel wall, which was greatest in the endothelium. (Reproduced from ref. 18. Lund DD, Faraci FM, Miller FJ Jr & Heistad DD (2000) Gene transfer of endothelial nitric oxide synthase improves relaxation of carotid arteries from diabetic rabbits. *Circulation*, **101**, 1027–33.)

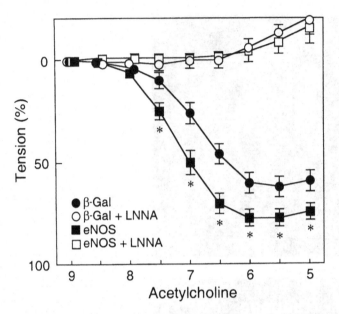

Figure 24.4 Effect of gene transfer on the response of carotid arteries to acetylcholine without (●) and with (○) pretreatment with N$^\omega$-nitro-L-arginine in diabetic rabbits. Vessels were treated with β-gal (●) or eNOS (■). (Reproduced from ref. 18. Lund DD, Faraci FM, Miller FJ Jr & Heistad DD (2000) Gene transfer of endothelial nitric oxide synthase improves relaxation of carotid arteries from diabetic rabbits. *Circulation*, **101**, 1027–33.)

superoxide, improved responses to acetylcholine after gene transfer of iNOS. We concluded from this study that iNOS produces superoxide in blood vessels, thereby impairing NO-dependent relaxation [20].

We expect that the ability to study vascular responses after gene transfer of iNOS will prove to be valuable. When iNOS is expressed after endotoxin or inflammatory stimuli, the response is complex, and it is difficult to determine the aspects of the response that are mediated by iNOS. Thus the ability to express iNOS per se should allow us to examine a variety of mechanisms.

Gene transfer of SOD in vivo

ECSOD, in contrast to CuZnSOD and manganese SOD, is the only isoform of SOD that is released into the extracellular space. Thus ECSOD is the primary extracellular antioxidant enzyme and it is also highly expressed in blood vessels [21].

We have constructed a recombinant adenovirus that expresses ECSOD, and are comparing the effects of intracranial gene transfer of CuZnSOD and ECSOD [12]. We have found that after gene transfer of CuZnSOD, there was a pronounced increase in total SOD activity in the basilar artery and meninges, but little increase in CSF. In striking contrast, gene transfer of ECSOD produced only a minimal increase in total SOD activity in the basilar artery and meninges, but a three-fold increase in SOD activity in CSF. One can therefore use this approach to increase SOD activity in blood vessels and tissues that line the subarachnoid space by injecting a virus that expresses CuZnSOD. Alternatively, one can produce a large increase in SOD activity in CSF by injecting a virus that expresses ECSOD.

A previous study described gene transfer of ECSOD to the liver, and then release of ECSOD into plasma by intravenous injection of heparin [22]. This approach was used because ECSOD can be displaced from heparan sulfate proteoglycan on cell surfaces by either dextran sulfate or heparin. We therefore examined effects of injection of dextran sulfate or heparin into the CSF after transduction with ECSOD. We found that injection of dextran sulfate or heparin into the cisterna magna increased total SOD activity in CSF to about 30 times basal levels. In contrast, after gene transfer of CuZnSOD, there was only a minimal increase in SOD activity in CSF after injection of dextran sulfate or heparin.

Thus we can inject Ad-CuZnSOD into the cisterna magna and produce an increase in SOD activity in tissues, and alternatively we can inject Ad-ECSOD into the cisterna magna and produce an enormous increase in ECSOD in CSF. We expect that this approach may be useful in studies of cerebral vascular pathophysiology.

Gene therapy for cerebrovascular disease and stroke

It is likely that gene therapy will be useful only for clinical conditions in which alternative approaches are not useful. If a vasoactive drug or peptide proves to be useful for a clinical condition, it seems unlikely that the risk : benefit ratio for gene therapy will be more appropriate. Despite this caution, however, because there are a variety of neurological diseases and stroke that are currently resistant to standard treatment, it seems important to explore the potential role of gene therapy for those conditions.

We are particularly optimistic that gene therapy may prove to be useful in prevention of vasospasm and stroke after SAH. We anticipate that, when an aneurysm is clipped after SAH, it will be possible to simultaneously administer a vector in the CSF to prevent vasospasm.

To work toward using gene therapy to prevent vasospasm after SAH, we have addressed several problems. First, we demonstrated that the vector can be delivered to vessels at the base of the brain [5], which are vessels that commonly develop spasm after SAH. Second, we have used a promoter (respiratory sincytial virus (RSV) promoter) that provides expression of the transgene product during the 2 to 3 weeks after SAH when there is risk of cerebral vasospasm [23]. Third, we have demonstrated that gene transfer can be successful after SAH [24].

Recently we have focused on the possibility that gene transfer of CGRP may be appropriate in preventing vasospasm after SAH. This rationale is based on the findings that CGRP is an extremely potent cerebral vasodilator, CGRP appears to be depleted from perivascular nerve terminals after SAH [25] and responsiveness of cerebral vessels to CGRP appears to be augmented after SAH.

Therefore, we constructed an adenovirus that encodes prepro-CGRP, and have examined the effects of gene transfer using a variety of approaches [26]. In tissue culture, transfection with Ad-CGRP produces an increase in CGRP in the culture medium, with an increase in cyclic AMP (cAMP) in recipient cells. After injection of Ad-CGRP into the cisterna magna of rabbits, the concentration of CGRP increased by almost 100-fold in CSF. The increase in CGRP produced a large increase in cAMP in the basilar artery. Gene transfer of CGRP inhibited contraction of the basilar artery in response to several stimuli, and altered vascular responses were restored to normal by pretreatment with a CGRP-1 receptor antagonist.

In very recent studies, we have examined effects of gene transfer of CGRP in rabbits after simulated SAH [27]. We injected blood into the CSF, and using digital subtraction angiography, we demonstrated approximately 30% constriction of the basilar artery in control rabbits. In contrast, after gene transfer of CGRP, there was no constrictor response to SAH. In those initial studies, we used an RSV promoter, which does not produce peak expression until approximately 3 to 5 days after gene transfer. It was therefore necessary to give the CGRP virus before SAH to prevent vasospasm. Because this would not be clinically useful, we have constructed another virus with a cytomegalovirus (CMV) promoter to see whether Ad-CMVCGRP could be given after SAH to prevent vasoconstriction. In preliminary recent experiments, we are finding that gene transfer of CGRP after SAH prevents vasoconstriction after SAH. On the basis of these studies, we are very optimistic that it will be possible to prevent vasospasm after SAH, using gene transfer approaches.

Where do we go from here?

It seems unlikely that gene therapy by the methods that we currently use will be clinically useful until a better vector is developed. The major problem with the adenoviral vector is that it produces an inflammatory response when large doses of the virus are given.

One approach to reduction of the inflammatory response to adenoviral vectors would be to give a far lower dose of the virus. We have used several approaches to enhance gene transfer to cerebral vessels [28–30]. Our hope is that, by enhancing gene transfer and expression of the transgene product, we will be able to reduce the dose of virus sufficiently that there will be little or no inflammatory response. To date, the most promising approach is to coprecipitate the virus with calcium phosphate [30].

An alternative would be to administer the adenovirus with a substance that would attenuate the inflammatory response. A variety of approaches have been tried in other organs, and it is possible that eventually this will prove to be useful in the brain as well.

In our opinion, however, it seems most likely that a new, safer vector will need to be developed before the approach can be used safely in patients. For example, the "gutted" or "gutless" adenoviral vector [2] appears to have a markedly reduced inflammatory response. In the meantime, while we eagerly await the development of new, safe and effective vectors, we suggest that gene transfer approaches are useful in allowing novel approaches to study cerebral vessels. We also suggest that gene transfer is attractive because it has potential for unique therapeutic approaches for clinical conditions that we cannot effectively treat at the present time.

Acknowledgments

We thank Arlinda LaRose for typing the manuscript. We also thank Drs. Kazunori Toyoda, Hiroaki Ooboshi, Hiroshi Nakane, Yi Chu, Kristy Lake-Bruse, Michael Muhonen, C. David Rios, Donald Lund, Michael Welsh and Beverly Davidson for invaluable assistance with studies described in this manuscript. Original studies by the authors were supported by National Institutes of Health grants HL-16066, NS-24621, HL-14388, HL-62984, DK-54759, and funds provided by the Veterans Affairs Medical Service.

REFERENCES

1 Heistad DD & Faraci FM (1996) Gene therapy for cerebral vascular disease. *Stroke*, 27, 1688–93.

2 Schiedner G, Morral N, Parks RJ, Wu Y, Koopmans SC, Langston C, Graham FL, Beaudet AL & Kochanek S (1998) Genomic DNA transfer with a high-capacity adenovirus vector results in improved in vivo gene expression and decreased toxicity. *Nature Genetics*, 18, 180–3.

3 Rios CD, Chu Y, Davidson BL & Heistad DD (1998) Ten steps to gene therapy for cardiovascular diseases. *Journal of Laboratory and Clinical Medicine*, 132, 104–11.

4 Ooboshi H, Toyoda K, Faraci FM, Lang MG & Heistad DD (1998) Improvement of relaxation in an atherosclerotic artery by gene transfer of endothelial nitric oxide synthase. *Arteriosclerosis, Thrombosis, and Vascular Biology*, 18, 1752–8.

5 Ooboshi H, Welsh MJ, Rios CD, Davidson BL & Heistad DD (1995) Adenovirus-mediated gene transfer in vivo to cerebral blood vessels and perivascular tissue. *Circulation Research*, **77**, 7–13.

6 Ríos CD, Ooboshi H, Piegors DJ, Davidson BL & Heistad DD (1995) Adenovirus-mediated gene transfer to normal and atherosclerotic arteries: a novel approach. *Arteriosclerosis, Thrombosis, and Vascular Biology*, **15**, 2241–5.

7 Ooboshi H, Chu Y, Ríos CD, Faraci FM, Davidson BL & Heistad DD (1997) Altered vascular function after adenovirus-mediated overexpression of endothelial nitric oxide synthase. *American Journal of Physiology: Heart and Circulatory Physiology*, **273**, H265–70.

8 Tsutsui M, Chen AFY, O'Brien T, Crotty TB & Katusic ZS (1998) Adventitial expression of recombinant eNOS gene restores NO production in arteries without endothelium. *Arteriosclerosis, Thrombosis, and Vascular Biology*, **18**, 1231–41.

9 Chen AFY, Jiang S-W, Crotty TB, Tsutsui M, Smith LA, O'Brien T & Katusic ZS (1997) Effects of in vivo adventitial expression of recombinant endothelial nitric oxide synthase gene in cerebral arteries. *Proceedings of the National Academy of Science USA*, **94**, 12568–73.

10 Meyrelles SS, Mao HZ, Heistad DD & Chapleau MW (1997) Gene transfer to carotid sinus in vivo: a novel approach to investigation of baroreceptors. *Hypertension*, **30**, 708–13.

11 Betz AL, Yang G-Y & Davidson BL (1995) Attenuation of stroke size in rats using an adenoviral vector to induce overexpression of interleukin-1 receptor antagonist in brain. *Journal of Cerebral Blood Flow & Metabolism*, **15**, 547–51.

12 Nakane H, Chu, Y., Faraci FM, Oberley LW & Heistad DD (2001) Gene transfer of ECSOD increases SOD activity in cerebrospinal fluid. *Stroke*, **32**, 184–9.

13 Stevenson SC, Marshall-Neff J, Teng B, Lee CB, Roy S & McClelland A (1995) Phenotypic correction of hypercholesterolemia in ApoE-deficient mice by adenovirus-mediated in vivo gene transfer. *Arteriosclerosis, Thrombosis, and Vascular Biology*, **15**, 479–84.

14 Kobayashi K, Oka K, Forte T, Ishida B, Teng B, Ishimura-Oka K, Nakamuta M & Chan L (1996) Reversal of hypercholesterolemia in low density lipoprotein receptor knockout mice by adenovirus-mediated gene transfer of the very low density lipoprotein receptor. *Journal of Biological Chemistry*, **271**, 6852–60.

15 Lake-Bruse KD, Faraci FM, Shesely EG, Maeda N, Sigmund CD & Heistad DD (1999) Gene transfer of endothelial nitric oxide synthase (eNOS) in eNOS-deficient mice. *American Journal of Physiology*, **277**, H770–H776.

16 Miller FJ, Gutterman DD, Ríos CD, Heistad DD & Davidson BL (1998) Superoxide production in vascular smooth muscle contributes to oxidative stress and impaired relaxation in atherosclerosis. *Circulation Research*, **82**, 1298–305.

17 Ooboshi H, Ríos CD, Chu Y, Christenson SD, Faraci FM, Davidson BL & Heistad DD (1997) Augmented adenovirus-mediated gene transfer to atherosclerotic vessels. *Arteriosclerosis, Thrombosis, and Vascular Biology*, **17**, 1786–92.

18 Lund DD, Faraci FM, Miller FJ Jr & Heistad DD (2000) Gene transfer of endothelial nitric oxide synthase improves relaxation of carotid arteries from diabetic rabbits. *Circulation*, **101**, 1027–33.

19 Nakane H, Miller FJ Jr, Faraci FM, Toyoda K & Heistad DD (2000) Gene transfer of endothelial nitric oxide synthase reduces angiotensin II-induced endothelial dysfunction. *Hypertension*, **35**, 595–601.

20 Gunnett CA, Faraci FM, Chu Y, Brooks RM II & Heistad DD (2001) Nitric-oxide dependent vasorelaxation is impaired following gene transfer of inducible NO synthase. *Arteriosclerosis, Thrombosis, and Vascular Biology*, **21**, (in press).

21 Strålin P, Karlsson K, Johansson BO & Marklund SL (1995) The interstitium of the human arterial wall contains very large amounts of extracellular superoxide dismutase. *Arteriosclerosis, Thrombosis, and Vascular Biology*, **15**, 2032–6.

22 Li Q, Bolli R, Qiu Y, Tang X-L, Murphree SS & French BA (1998) Gene therapy with extra-cellular superoxide dismutase attenuates myocardial stunning in conscious rabbits. *Circulation*, **98**, 1438–48.

23 Christenson SD, Lake KD, Ooboshi H, Faraci FM, Davidson BL & Heistad DD (1998) Adenovirus-mediated gene transfer in vivo to cerebral blood vessels and perivascular tissue in mice. *Stroke*, **29**, 1411–16.

24 Muhonen MG, Ooboshi H, Welsh MJ, Davidson BL & Heistad DD (1997) Gene transfer to cerebral blood vessels after subarachnoid hemorrhage. *Stroke*, **28**, 822–9.

25 Edvinsson L, Ekman R, Jansen I, McCulloch J, Mortensen A & Uddman R (1991) Reduced levels of calcitonin gene-related peptide-like immunoreactivity in human brain vessels after subarachnoid haemorrhage. *Neuroscience Letters*, **121**, 151–4.

26 Toyoda K, Faraci FM, Russo AF, Davidson BL & Heistad DD (2000) Gene transfer of calcito-nin gene-related peptide to cerebral arteries. *American Journal of Physiology: Heart and Circulatory Physiology*, **278**, H586–H594.

27 Toyoda K, Faraci FM, Watanabe Y, Ueda T, Andresen JJ, Chu Y, Otake S & Heistad DD (2000) Gene transfer of calcitonin gene-related peptide prevents vasoconstriction after subarachnoid hemorrhage. *Circulation Research*, **87**, 818–24.

28 Toyoda K, Ooboshi H, Chu Y, Fasbender A, Davidson BL, Welsh MJ & Heistad DD (1998) Cationic polymer and lipids enhance adenovirus-mediated gene transfer to rabbit carotid artery. *Stroke*, **29**, 2181–8.

29 Christenson SD, Lund D, Ooboshi H, Faraci FM, Davidson BL & Heistad DD (1999) Approaches to enhance expression after adenovirus-mediated gene transfer to the carotid artery. *Endothelium*, **7**, 75–82.

30 Toyoda K, Andresen JJ, Zabner J, Faraci FM & Heistad DD (2000) Calcium phosphate pre-cipitates augment adenovirus-mediated gene transfer to blood vessel in vitro and in vivo. *Gene Therapy*, **7**, 1284–91.

Part VIII

Neurogenesis and plasticity

Co-Chairs: Frank R. Sharp & Justin A. Zivin

25

Transplantation of neural stem cells: cellular and gene therapy in pediatric hypoxic–ischemic brain injury

Kook In Park[1], Philip E. Stieg[2] & Evan Y. Snyder[3]

[1] Department of Pediatrics and Pharmacology, Yonsei University College of Medicine, Seoul, Korea and
   Departments of Pediatrics, Neurosurgery, & Neurology, Children's Hospital, Boston, MA
[2] Department of Neurosurgery, Brigham & Women's Hospital, Harvard Medical School, Boston, MA
[3] Department of Pediatrics, Neurosurgery, & Neurology, Children's Hospital, Boston, MA

Introduction

Stroke is the third most common cause of death, and being among the most common causes of severe disability in adults of developed countries [1] accounts for a large proportion of health care costs. Its impact on individual patients, their families and society as a whole is immense. Approximately 200 per 100 000 adults per year will have their first stroke. Because the incidence of stroke increases with age, the absolute number of patients with stroke is likely to increase even more, given that the population of aged adults is also increasing [2,3]. However, brain injury from ischemia does not affect only the adult population. It is a major cause of mortality and severe neurodevelopmental disability (cerebral palsy, mental retardation, epilepsy and learning disabilities) in the pediatric – especially the newborn – population [4,5]. The drain on resources to support such children (often long into adulthood or an entire lifetime) is also quite significant. Although the etiologies for ischemic brain injury in adults and children may differ, much of the pathophysiology underlying neural cell death and dysfunction is quite similar. In the case of newborn infants, despite advances in technology allowing better obstetric and neonatal care and a deeper understanding of the pathophysiology of perinatal asphyxia, the incidence of hypoxic–ischemic encephalopathy (HIE) in neonates has remained essentially unchanged over the last few decades. Except for thrombolysis therapy for acute stroke in the adult, current clinical management of both adult stroke and HIE has been limited to supportive measures; it is not directed toward preventing or interrupting the processes underlying brain injury or promoting regeneration [1,4,5]. Given the absence of effective therapies for stroke and perinatal HIE, it is important to derive new strategies. Unfortunately, despite recent substantial research into neuroprotection, no neuroprotective agents have been shown conclusively to be clinically effective [1,5–7].

There has been a growing interest in the therapeutic potential of neural stem cells (NSCs) progenitors for therapy in stroke, HIE and other central nervous system (CNS) dysfunctions. NSCs are the primordial, multipotent, self-renewing cells that, during the earliest stages of development, are believed to give rise to the vast array of specialized cells of the nervous system. They are thought to persist throughout life, not only in a few discrete regions but probably throughout the brain, serving homeostatic and perhaps self-repair functions. The growing interest in NSC biology, as it might apply to HIE and stroke, represents a somewhat different focus on CNS injury. While most strategies under investigation seek to short circuit cell death and/or promote neuroprotection, i.e., to combat progression of neuropathological processes, stem cell biology shines the spotlight instead on a non-pathological process, on reinvoking developmental processes for purposes of regeneration. In other words, a putative stem cell-mediated strategy would be rooted not so much in "combating" pathology as in abetting natural self-repair processes postulated – at least based on data emerging from our laboratory – to exist in the CNS in response to a wide range of injuries and degenerative processes.

In this context, therefore, the interest in NSCs derives from the realization that these cells are not simply a substitute for fetal tissue in transplantation paradigms or simply a "better" vehicle for gene delivery. We in the field of developmental neuroscience believe that the basic biology of these cells endows them with a potential that other vehicles for gene therapy and repair may not possess [8–10].

This biological potential endows NSCs with the ability to integrate into the neural circuitry after transplantation. This property, in turn, may allow for the regulated release of various gene products. It may also allow for literal neural cell replacement. While presently available, gene transfer vectors usually depend on relaying new genetic information through established neural circuits, which may, in fact, have already degenerated and become dysfunctional. NSCs may actually participate in the reconstitution of these pathways. The replacement of enzymes and of cells may be targeted not only to specific, anatomically circumscribed regions of the CNS [11–15], but also, if desired, by simple modifications in technique, to actual large areas of the CNS in a widespread manner [16–22]. This ability is important because most neurological diseases are not localized to specific sites, as is Parkinson's disease. Rather, their neuropathology is often extensive, multifocal or even global; stroke and HIE provide ideal examples of just how broad the regions of degeneration may be. Intriguingly, NSCs may actually be uniquely responsive to neurodegenerative environments [23–25]. This type of responsiveness of NSCs may optimize cell replacement and therapeutic gene expression within the damaged CNS.

The neural stem cell response to ischemic injury

Little is actually known about the response of NSCs to CNS injury in general, let alone HI brain injury in particular. Is it possible to repopulate an "ablated" CNS with neural stem cells in the way hematopoietic stem cells reconstitute lethally irradiated bone marrow? HI was initially viewed by us as an injury that is not only of importance in its own right but also might serve as a prototype for other large, acquired brain injuries [26]. It occurred to us that to help to answer this question we might be able to use one of our prototypical NSC clones, clone C17.2 [27–29], as "reporter cells". This well-characterized clone is just one of several with stem cell features that exist in the literature: multipotent, self-renewing, self-maintaining, nestin positive and responsive to various stem cell trophins. As one would demand of a putative stem cell, NSCs from clone C17.2 are able to participate in the development of the CNS throughout the neuraxis and across developmental periods, from fetus to adult [16,17,22,24,25,28,29]. Engrafted and integrated NSCs are visible because they have also been transduced with a reporter gene, *lacZ*, that allows the cells to stain blue when processed with 5-bromo-4-chloro-3-indolyl β-D-galactoside (X-Gal) histochemistry, or to appear brown after reaction with an antibody against *Escherichia coli* β-galactosidase (β-gal) (in immunoperoxidase and immunofluorescence protocols, respectively) [24,27]. This ability to identify progeny of a donor NSC is important because, by their nature, NSCs integrate and intermingle seamlessly into the host after transplantation, do not form a discernible graft–host border (as in traditional neural transplantation paradigms) and actually come to resemble host neural cells of the same phenotype. When we talk about using clone C17.2 NSCs as "reporter" cells, we mean using well-characterized, indelibly marked cells with a known ancestry, with potential and clonal relationships that are traceable, that are abundant and homogeneous, that intermingle imperceptibly with host cells in vivo and that can, therefore, be used as a tool for mirroring, probing and tracking, i.e., "reporting" on the behaviors of neighboring endogenous progenitors that are otherwise invisible to such monitoring and whose own clonal relationships and degree of homogeneity are much less certain. Such cells would also allow well-controlled experiments to proceed with minimal variability in cell population under study from experiment to experiment, animal to animal and condition to condition. The type of injury in which NSCs were investigated in these preliminary experiments was focal HIE engendered by permanent ligation of the right common carotid artery of a week-old mouse followed by exposure of the animal to 8% ambient oxygen. This combination of ischemia and hypoxia resulted in extensive injury to the hemisphere ipsilateral to the carotid ligation while leaving the contralateral hemisphere as an intact control.

In the first set of pilot experiments [26], we wondered what might be observed if we took a normal animal in which "reporter" NSCs had become stably integrated throughout the brain during a critical period of its development (creating virtually a chimeric brain of host and reporter cells) and then exposed that animal to unilateral HI injury. The experimental paradigm, therefore, was as follows: clone C17.2 NSCs were transplanted into the cerebral ventricles of mice on the day of birth (P0), allowing the NSCs access to the subventricular germinal zone (SVZ) that lines the ventricular system running the length of the neuraxis; this results in widespread migration, stable integration and intermixture of donor NSCs with host cells throughout the parenchyma [16]. The right hemisphere was subjected to HI injury at 1 week of age (P7). The brains were analyzed 2 to 5 weeks later. The resulting picture in these preliminary studies was complex but intriguing. In contrast to the intact side where the reporter NSCs remained widely and evenly interspersed throughout the intact parenchyma, the reporter NSCs in the HI-injured hemisphere appeared to be densely and preferentially clustered around the infarction cavity. The heavy accumulation and number of cells in that location suggested either that many NSCs had migrated to that particular area, or that the cells near there had proliferated, or both. In addition, in the penumbra of the infarction, an increased number of donor-derived cells was identified immunocytochemically as oligodendrocytes and neurons. Neurons and oligodendrocytes are the two neural cell types that are most susceptible to HI injury and that are least likely to regenerate spontaneously in the "postdevelopmental" mammalian cortex. Furthermore, in the intact hemisphere, as might be expected from NSCs implanted after the completion of embryonic cortical neurogenesis, no donor-derived neurons and many fewer oligodendrocytes were noted. Therefore, following HI brain injury, NSCs appeared to evince components of altered proliferation, migration and differentiation. This is precisely the type of behavior one might expect of a stem cell; it certainly mirrors the behavior of the hematopoietic stem cell, a cell with a much older literature. We decided to start examining each of these components in a systematic fashion [26].

First we asked whether there was new transient proliferation by quiescent NSCs, both reporter and host. To answer this question, a transplant of reporter NSCs was performed at P0 into the cerebral ventricles; unilateral HI injury was induced at P7 (after the cells had stably integrated, differentiated and become quiescent); the mice were then pulsed with bromodeoxyuridine (BrdU), a nucleotide analogue, at various post-HI injury time points. The preliminary analysis revealed that before injury, donor-derived cells were completely quiescent (as previously known); however, after HI injury, the percentage of reporter ($lacZ^+$) cells that became mitotic (i.e., incorporated BrdU) increased rapidly, peaked at about 3 days after induction of HI and then fell back to 0 by 1 week after HI. The host cells did precisely the same thing; their pattern of proliferation was virtually superimposable upon that of donor cells, peaking approximately 3 days after HI and then returning to 0, also suggesting an induction of transient proliferation.

That there were so many changes peaking 3 days after injury is intriguing. The literature on stroke, and in fact, on other injuries, has suggested that the interval of 3 to 7 days after insult is a very metabolically, biochemically and molecularly active temporal "window" during which a variety of mitogens, trophins, extracellular matrix molecules and other factors are uniquely elaborated. We shall return to this "window" and its impact on neural stem cell biology later in the review.

Next, we began to approach the question of whether reporter NSCs (and by extension, host NSCs) in fact migrated to the areas of neurodegeneration. NSCs (clone C17.2) were transplanted into only the left intracerebroventricular space at P0. At 1 week of age, unilateral HI injury was induced in the contralateral right hemisphere in some animals, while in others the right hemisphere was left intact. In animals with an intact right hemisphere, engrafted stem cells simply remained stably distributed and densely integrated throughout the parenchyma of only the transplanted left hemisphere. But in animals in which the right hemisphere had been infarcted, cells at multiple levels throughout the cerebrum dramatically appeared to migrate across the corpus callosum and any available interhemispheric commissure to the infarcted region (Figure 25.1). With high magnification under light and electron microscopy, one could appreciate the leading processes of NSCs migrating along interhemispheric connections toward the damaged areas. Even within the infarct, one could see reporter cells migrating into the heart of the necrotic area.

Therefore there seems to be evidence that NSCs already integrated into the CNS will migrate to an area of subsequent infarction. Will reporter NSCs implanted *after* HI injury also be drawn to areas of damage? To investigate this question, the following paradigm was followed: unilateral (right) HI injury was induced at P7, and reporter NSCs were transplanted into the contralateral (left) cerebral ventricle 3 days later (at P10). As a control, some animals not subjected to right HI were also transplanted on the left at P10. As before, in the intact animals, the NSCs remained nicely but stably integrated on the transplanted left side. However, in the animals that were infarcted on the right before transplantation on the left, reporter NSCs avidly migrated across the corpus callosum and other interhemispheric commissures to the area of infarction throughout the length of the cerebrum. Furthermore, they integrated into those infarcted areas as if drawn or directed by a tropism for the region. When reporter NSCs were injected directly into the infarcted area on the right, they never migrated in the other direction to the contralateral intact side in these pilot studies.

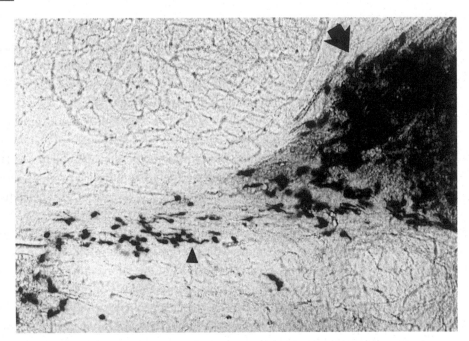

Figure 25.1   Migration by transplanted "reporter" stem cells to the ischemic area of a mouse brain subjected to unilateral, focal hypoxic–ischemic brain injury. Clone C17.2 neural stem cells were injected into the left cerebral ventricle of a mouse on the day of birth (postnatal day 0). At 1 week of age, the animal was subjected to contralateral right-sided hypoxic–ischemic injury. The animal was analyzed at maturity with X-Gal histochemistry to identify LacZ-expressing donor-derived cells (which stain blue). Some cells appeared to migrate along the corpus callosum (arrowhead) throughout the cerebrum toward the highly ischemic area (arrow). (Reproduced from ref. 52.)

This last manipulation, that of injecting NSCs directly into the infarct, suggests what our next set of experiments entailed. NSCs (clone C17.2) were transplanted directly into the degenerating infarcted region at various time points after the induction of unilateral HI. When implantation was performed shortly after HI (e.g., the following day), robust engraftment was seen throughout the infarcted area. If transplantation was postponed until 5 weeks after HI, virtually no, if any, engraftment was achieved. Engraftment was most exuberant 3 to 7 days after HI (Figure 25.2).

Is there indeed a change in differentiation fate by the reporter NSCs in these areas of degeneration compared with what might be seen in the intact brain? Immunocytochemical and ultrastructural examination of the engrafted regions, particularly in the penumbra of the infarct, suggests that indeed there is. Donor-derived cells (recognized by an anti-β-gal antibody) were assessed for the expression of neural cell type-specific antibodies (e.g., NeuN, neurofilament,

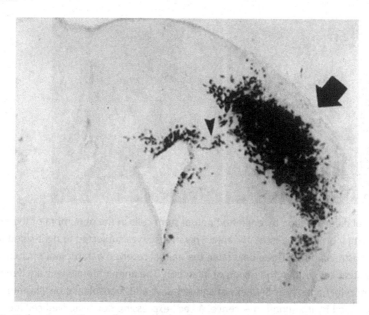

Figure 25.2 Robust engraftment by transplanted neural stem cells within the ischemic region of a
mouse brain subjected to unilateral focal hypoxic–ischemic (HI) injury. This mouse was
subjected to right HI injury on postnatal day 7. Three days later, the animal received a
transplant of clone C17.2 neural stem cells within the region of infarction. The animal was
analyzed at maturity with X-Gal histochemistry. A representative coronal section is shown.
Robust engraftment was evident within the ischemic area (arrow). A similar engraftment
was evident throughout the hemisphere. Even cells implanted outside the region of
infarction appeared to migrate along the corpus callosum toward the ischemic area
(arrowhead) (see also Figure 25.1). The most exuberant engraftment was evident 3 to 7
days after HI. Immunocytochemical and ultrastructural analysis revealed that a
subpopulation of donor-derived cells, especially those in the penumbra, differentiated
into neurons (see Figure 25.3) and oligodendroglia, the two neural cell types most
characteristically damaged by HI and the cell types least likely to regenerate
spontaneously in the postnatal brain. (Reproduced from ref. 52.)

microtubule-associated protein-2 (MAP-2) for neurons (Figure 25.3), 2′,3′-cyclic
nucleotide 3′-phosphodiesterase for oligodendrocytes, glial fibrillary acidic protein
for astrocytes, nestin for immature, undifferentiated progenitors). A subpopulation of donor NSCs in the injured postnatal neocortex differentiated into neurons
(~5%) and oligodendrocytes (~4%). Other cell types were astroglial, though no
scarring seemed apparent, and undifferentiated progenitors. As noted below, these
numbers contrast significantly with what one finds in an intact age-matched recipient neocortex. The presence of donor-derived neurons was detected as much as
1 mm away from the heart of the infarction cavity on the side of the lesion, suggesting a relatively large "sphere of influence" exerted by the injured tissue.

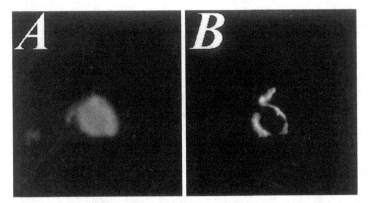

Figure 25.3. Neuronal differentiation by engrafted neural stem cells in the penumbra of the infarct after transplantation into the ischemic area. This mouse was subjected to right-sided focal HI injury postnatal day 7. Three days later, the animal received a transplant of clone C17.2 neural stem cells within the region of infarction. The animal's brain was analyzed with immunocytochemistry at 5 weeks of age (25 days after transplantation). Immunolabeling was revealed by immunofluorescence. A LacZ-expressing donor-derived cell identified by an anti-β-gal antibody (A) also reacted to an anti-MAP-2 antibody (B), suggesting the mature neuronal differentiation of a donor-derived cell. (Reproduced from ref. 52.)

(Interestingly, occasionally we would note host-derived neurons in an otherwise severely destroyed cortex; this type of finding is consistent with our belief that some host NSCs, like the reporter NSCs, do try to shift their differentiation toward compensation for neural cell death, a phenomenon that we are perhaps augmenting with our transplants. More on this phenomenon later.) Examination of the penumbra under the electron microscope in these preliminary studies supported the immunocytochemical assessments. A significant number of donor-derived oligodendrocytes and neurons were appreciated. Some donor-derived pyramidal neurons received synaptic input from the host.

Quantification of the differentiation pattern by transplanted reporter NSCs in the injured neocortex compared with that in the intact neocortex is dramatic and illuminating. Whereas 5% of engrafted NSCs on the injured side differentiated into neurons, no neuronal differentiation by NSCs was seen at all in the intact neocortex, consistent with both the normal absence of neurogenesis in the postnatal mammalian cortex and with our own prior findings [24,30]. There was a five-fold increase in the number of donor-derived oligodendrocytes in the injured neocortex compared with the intact neocortex. The number of astrocytes did not significantly differ between the two sides. Also, there was an upregulation of nestin in donor NSCs in response to injury (almost three times as many donor cells were nestin positive in the injured cortex as compared with the intact cortex, suggesting that they may become activated or primed to make a differentiation choice).

These preliminary quantitative data are presented to make a qualitative point. On the intact side of the infarcted animal, there was no neuronal differentiation at all; on the injured side, 5% of donor-derived cells were now neurons. The magnitude of that number is less significant than the phenomenon of qualitatively going from consistently no neurons to neurons of any number at a stage in development when no cortical neurons should normally be born. As mentioned previously, oligodendrocytes and neurons are the two neural cell types most damaged by HI injury. It appears from these preliminary data that the NSCs may have been attempting to repopulate and reconstitute that area of injury, particularly within a certain temporal window, by "shifting" their normal differentiation fate to compensate for the loss of those particular cell types, especially neurons. It seems indeed likely that as a consequence of this type of neurodegeneration, signals are elaborated to which NSCs (donor and probably host) are able to respond in a reparative fashion. Precisely what those signals are is an area of ongoing investigation. They no doubt are a complex mix of various mitogens, neurotrophins, adhesion molecules, cytokines, etc.

Although the preliminary numerical data cited above are presented principally to illustrate the "shift" toward neuronal differentiation by NSCs in response to injury, it is instructive to note that, given the vast number of NSCs that engrafted into the infarcted region, a differentiation of even 5% of such cells into neurons translated into tens of thousands of replacement neurons supplied to that degenerating region. We do not actually know how many neurons and how much circuitry is required to functionally reconstruct a damaged mammalian system. We do know that, fortunately, 100% restoration is not needed; older lesion data would suggest that as little as 10% may be sufficient.

Combining cell replacement with gene therapy via the NSC

Despite the fact that neuronal differentiation of 5% of transplanted NSCs may be sufficient to repair an HI-injured region of the brain, we nevertheless wondered whether that percentage could be increased. Neurotrophin-3 (NT-3) is known to play a role in inducing neuronal differentiation [31,32]. It appeared feasible that neuronal differentiation of both host and donor NSCs might be enhanced if the latter were engineered before transplantation to (over)express NT-3. A subclone of NSCs was transduced with a retrovirus encoding rat NT-3 [33,34]. The engineered NSCs successfully produced large amounts of NT-3 in vitro and in vivo. We have determined that both the parent NSCs and the NT-3-overexpressing NSC subclones, express TrkC receptors (the receptor for NT-3) [34]. These receptors are appropriately tyrosine-phosphorylated in response to exogenous NT-3; this phosphorylation can be blocked by K252a, an inhibitor of neurotrophin-induced tyrosine kinase activity. Therefore, it appeared that these engineered NSC clones not only could secrete excess amounts of NT-3 but also could probably respond to NT-3 in an autocrine or paracrine fashion, a very appealing scenario.

In tissue culture, these NT-3-overexpressing NSCs, like the parent NSC clone, still differentiated into all three neural cell types (neurons, astrocytes and oligodendrocytes). However, unlike the parent clone, whose percentage of neurons fell in serum-containing medium as new cells were born, the proportion of this NT-3-expressing subclone that continued to express neuronal markers in culture for prolonged periods (>3 weeks) remained quite high (~90%) [34].

In an experimental paradigm identical to that described previously, cells from the NT-3-expressing NSC subclone were implanted into the infarct of a unilaterally asphyxiated postnatal mouse brain 3 days after induction of HI injury [34]. The brains were analyzed 2 to 4 weeks later as described above. Indeed, on preliminary analysis, the percentage of donor-derived neurons was dramatically increased to 20% in the infarction cavity and to as high as 80% in the penumbra. Many of the neurons were calbindin-positive; they were also variously GABAergic (GABA is γ-aminobutyric acid), glutamatergic or cholinergic. Donor-derived glia were rare. It appears, therefore, that, when NSCs are transplanted within regions of HI injury, a greater percentage of them engineered ex vivo to express NT-3, differentiate into neurons. NT-3 probably does act on donor cells (as well as host cells) in an autocrine/paracrine fashion to enhance that neuronal differentiation. Interestingly, this pilot experiment enunciates the feasibility of using NSCs for simultaneous combined gene therapy and cell replacement in the same transplant procedure using the same clone of cells in the same transplant recipient – an appealing stem cell property with implications for therapies in other degenerative conditions.

Does the injured mammalian brain attempt self-repair?

In the transplant studies described above, the grafted and stably integrated NSC clones, whose response to focal HI cerebral degeneration was tracked, were viewed as "reporter cells", mirroring the behavior of the brain's own NSCs, which putatively alter their fate – their proliferation, migration and differentiation – in an effort to repopulate damaged areas. The thinking would be that, if the brain's inclinations are toward self-repair via the NSCs, then that response might be augmented. Is this truly what endogenous progenitors "attempt" to do? We launched a series of *non-transplant*-based experiments to explore whether the "reporter cells" were indeed reporting on a true phenomenon.

It has been recognized for decades [35–37] that two highly circumscribed regions of the mammalian cerebrum continue to generate neurons throughout life. These "privileged" areas are designated "neurogenic regions" and exist lifelong in the olfactory bulb (OB) by way of the SVZ and in the hippocampal dentate gyrus [38–42], including in humans [43,44]. (The reason for their persistence, quite frankly, still remains a mystery.) The remainder of the CNS is termed "non-neurogenic"; in other words, neuronal generation does not take place beyond fetal life, the normal period of neuron birth. Consequently, neuronal *regeneration* does not occur in the vast majority of the "postdevelopmental" CNS after injury or disease [45]. However, the fact that the cerebrum does retain a capacity for neurogenesis from proliferating cells in the SVZ and dentate gyrus throughout life suggests that these neural progenitor cells may provide an endogenous population with significant neuroregenerative potential (either constitutively or after manipulation).

The findings in the previous sections postulated that after brain injury and during phases of neurodegeneration, signals might be transiently elaborated, even in "non-neurogenic" regions, to which progenitor and stem cells can respond in a reparative fashion. Were an intrinsic capacity for producing new neural cells (including neurons) in classically non-neurogenic regions to be apparent, even at low, ostensibly clinically silent levels, this might attest to a degree of inherent CNS plasticity not previously appreciated, might explain certain observed levels of unanticipated recovery often seen by clinicians after adult and pediatric stroke and might lend insight into the teleological significance of persistent neurogenic zones while offering a substrate from which better strategies for brain repair might be launched.

After unilateral HI brain injury in preliminary studies, the migration and differentiation of mitotic neural progenitor cells (NPCs) in the SVZ of both hemispheres were assessed using two methods [46]. First, we tracked the behavior of newly proliferative endogenous NPCs by intraperitoneally injecting the proliferation marker BrdU, which is selectively and permanently incorporated into the nuclear genomic material of all cells entering S-phase, hence labeling dividing cells. Starting 2 hours after induction of unilateral HI, mice were pulsed with BrdU every 4 hours for the subsequent 12 hours. As an additional independent marker of newly mitotic cells, in parallel experiments a replication-incompetent, help virus-free retroviral vector encoding the *lacZ* reporter transgene [47] was also used to directly label such cells. A retroviral provirus becomes permanently integrated into the genome and passes stably to the progeny of only those cells progressing through S-phase. Successful infection (as indicated by *lacZ* expression) is, therefore, another unambiguous marker of mitotic cells. In order to label proliferating SVZ cells, the *lacZ*-encoding vector was injected into both lateral ventricles of the mice being subjected to unilateral HI.

HI brain injury induced a significantly increased proliferation of the SVZ progenitor population ipsilateral to the lesioned right side compared with the grossly intact contralateral left side and uninjured control group. Expansion of BrdU-positive cells was most pronounced in the dorsolateral wall of the lateral ventricles adjacent to the infarction cavity, and a relatively dense stream of "newly born" cells oriented toward and into the injured cerebral cortex was apparent. The normal fate of most of the cells born in the SVZ (particularly the anterior portion) is to migrate rostrally along the rostral migratory stream (RMS) into the OB, where they differentiate into neurons [38–41]. Certainly, that typical developmental program was evident in the intact left hemisphere. Intriguingly, although more cells were actually born in the right SVZ ipsilateral to the lesion in response to HI, significantly fewer BrdU-positive cells were present in the RMS, and the number of newly born cells that actually reached the right OB was significantly reduced, as if the newly born cells on the damaged side were "shunted" or "drawn" *away* from their normal migratory route *toward* the site of injury. Interestingly, the number of newborn cells that reached the RMS and OB from the SVZ *contralateral* to the lesion, though certainly much greater than that ipsilateral, was also significantly reduced as compared with the non-injured control group, suggesting that injury has a broad effect throughout the brain and may draw cells even from distant regions. In other words, the CNS environment appears to change radically after injury, particularly that induced by HI.

To help to determine the differentiation fate in vivo of injury-generated BrdU-labeled cells, particularly in non-neurogenic regions, they were analyzed for their coexpression of neural cell type-specific antigens. Over a 3 week period after the final BrdU pulse, many of the cells induced to proliferate yielded new oligodendrocytes, astrocytes, and intriguingly, neurons (4.0%, 1.2%, and 1.2% at 1, 2, and 3 weeks, respectively). These new neurons (probably an underrepresentation, given the time course of the BrdU pulses) were evident not only in the compromised hemisphere, but in the contralateral hemisphere as well, suggesting again the widespread "ripple" effect of signals emanating from even an ostensibly localized lesion. (No BrdU$^+$ neurons were seen in the cortices of uninjured control mice.) That these newly born neurons in non-neurogenic regions might persist permanently was suggested by their continued detection essentially undiminished for at least 2 months after injury.

As a complement to BrdU labeling and to track more rigorously the fate of these newly proliferative, injury-responsive periventricular NPCs, a retroviral vector encoding *lacZ* was injected into both lateral ventricles of the mice subjected to unilateral HI. In response to HI, *lacZ*-expressing (i.e., β-gal$^+$) periventricular cells migrated into the adjacent striatum and hippocampus, into the cortex ipsilateral to the lesion and into the cortical penumbra. Confirming the observation previously noted, a subpopulation of the newly proliferative and migratory β-gal$^+$ cells now expressed the mature neuronal marker, NeuN, in all of these "non-neurogenic" regions, suggesting de novo neurogenesis. (Interestingly, even in the grossly intact contralateral hemisphere, some β-gal⁺ periventricular cells (often in groups) also migrated into the cortex and overlying hippocampal CA1 area, becoming neurons.)

Translating progenitor and stem cell biology into therapy

The findings in the previous section suggest (as did the transplant studies described previously) that, after CNS injury and during acute phases of the resultant neuro-degeneration, factors are elaborated to which donor-derived and endogenous neural progenitor and stem cells may respond in a reparative fashion and which can promote the establishment of new neurons even within non-neurogenic regions of the "post-developmental" CNS. Neural stem and progenitor cells appear to be capable of responding to neurogenic signals not only during their normal develop-mental expression but also when induced in later stages during critical periods after injury. Stem cells seem to have a tropism for and a trophism within degenerating CNS regions. They seem to be able to "shift" their differentiation fate. This phe-nomenon seems to be magnified at the peak of active neurodegeneration. Given these observations, we further speculate that the CNS may "attempt" to repair itself with its own endogenous pool of progenitors and stem cells, but that supply may simply be insufficient either in number or in factors regulating mobilization, recruitment, migration, differentiation, survival, neurite extension and synapto-genesis in the context of HI injury. Therefore, the net impact of the production of new nerve cells may be limited. If this is the case, perhaps we can augment that stem cell population with exogenous stem cells and/or exogenous trophic factors to enable more significant recovery. Such a strategy would certainly benefit from iden-tifying those transiently expressed signals. Such identification may permit them to be supplied exogenously in order to recruit the host's own internal stem cell reser-voir more effectively. In fact, donor stem cells genetically engineered ex vivo (as we did with the NT-3-expressing stem cells) may be one method for supplying some of those tropic and trophic factors. Under certain circumstances, in fact, one clone of transplanted stem cells may be able to serve multiple therapeutic functions: both gene delivery and cell replacement.

Therefore one strategy that can take its place in the repertoire with other valu-able repair strategies may be stem cell based: using the host's own appropriately activated reserve of stem cells augmented by an exogenous supply of stem cells introduced during or shortly after injury or neurodegeneration (apparent "windows of opportunity"). It may, in fact, be possible to treat chronic lesions by re-expressing certain "signals" (e.g., certain cytokines) that emulate the more acute phase, to which stem cells may then respond in a reparative fashion. All these speculations are absolutely predicated on exploring the dynamic processes by which multipotent stem cells make their phenotypic choices in developing and degenerating the CNS.

[It should be added that the observations described above in pediatric stroke appear to apply as well to adult stroke. In pilot studies performed collaboratively with the laboratory of Seth Finkelstein, the combined administration of NSCs and the neurotrophic fibroblast growth factor 2 (FGF-2) appears to promote significant behavioral recovery in adult rats subjected to experimental middle cerebral artery occlusion. While space does not allow a detailed description of these studies, these observations suggest that the biology of stem cell-based self-repair may apply throughout the life of a mammal.]

The abiding faith in "translational neuroscience" is, of course, that the biology that endows rodent neural stem cells with their therapeutic potential is conserved in the human CNS. Progress in this regard is, gratifyingly, being made. Several neural stem cell clones and populations have been isolated from human fetal brains and these cells appear to emulate many of the appealing properties of their rodent counterparts [21,44,48–50]: they differentiate, in vitro and in vivo, into all three neural cell types; they vouchsafe conservation of neurodevelopmental principles after engraftment into the developing mouse brain; they express foreign genes in vivo in a widely disseminated manner; and they can replace missing neural cell types when grafted into various mutant mice.

In order to determine whether findings with rodent NSCs in response to injury might extend to cells from the human CNS and to explore their therapeutic potential in the treatment of HI in infants, human NSCs (in pilot studies) were injected into the infarction cavity of mice, using the same experimental paradigm described above [51]. Human NSCs showed robust engraftment within the ischemic region and its penumbra, migrated extensively and preferentially toward the site of injury and differentiated into all three neural cell types. A subpopulation of donor-derived neurons expressed glutamate, GABA, tyrosine hydroxylase and choline acetyltransferase in various CNS regions. Preliminary data suggest that human NSCs grafted into the HI-injured brain sites in mice partially restored some motor and cognitive functions, as demonstrated by rotarod performance, the step-through type passive avoidance test and the habituation of exploratory behavior test. These findings suggest that human NSCs might be capable of replacing some neural cell populations lost to experimental HI injury in mice and could provide a rationale for ultimate stem cell-based therapy for human ischemic and other degenerative CNS diseases.

Acknowledgments

K.I. Park was partly supported by grant no. 981–0713–097–2 from the Basic Research Program and BDRC of the Korean Science and Engineering Foundation and grant no. HMP-98–N-1–0003 of the Ministry of Health & Welfare, R.O. Korea. E.Y. Snyder was partly supported by grants from the March of Dimes and from the NINDS (nos. NS34247 and NS33852).

REFERENCES

1 Davenport R & Dennis M (2000) Neurological emergencies: acute stroke. *Journal of Neurology, Neurosurgery & Psychiatry*, **68**, 277–88.

2 Sudlow CL & Warlow CP (1996) Comparing stroke incidence worldwide: what makes studies comparable? *Stroke*, **27**, 550–8.

3 Warlow CP, Dennis MS, Van Gijn J, Hankey GJ, Sandercock PAG, Bamgard JM, et al. (1996) The Organization of Stroke Services. In *Stroke. A Practical Guide to Management*, eds. C P Warlow, MS Dennis, J Van Gijn, Hankey GJ, Sandercock PAG, Bamgard JM, et al. pp. 598–631. Oxford: Blackwell Science.

4 Volpe JJ (ed.) (1995) *Neurology of the Newborn*, 3rd edn. Philadelphia: WB Saunders.

5 Vannucci RC & Perlman JM (1997) Interventions for perinatal hypoxic–ischemic encephalopathy. *Pediatrics*, **100**, 1004–14.

6 du Plessis AJ & Johnston MV (1997) Hypoxic–ischemic brain injury in the newborn. Cellular mechanisms and potential strategies for neuroprotection. *Clinics in Perinatology*, **24**, 627–54.

7 del Zoppo G, Ginis I, Hallenbeck JM, Iadecola C, Wang X & Feuerstein GZ (2000) Inflammation and stroke: putative role for cytokines, adhesion molecules and iNOS in brain response to ischemia. *Brain Pathology*, **10**, 95–112.

8 Snyder EY & Wolfe JH (1996) Central nervous system cell transplantation: a novel therapy for storage diseases? *Current Opinion in Neurology*, **9**, 126–36.

9 Snyder EY & Fisher LJ (1996) Gene therapy in neurology. *Current Opinion in Pediatrics*, **8**, 558–68.

10 Snyder EY & Senut MC (1997) The use of nonneuronal cells for gene delivery. *Neurobiology of Disease*, **4**, 69–102.

11 Martinez-Serrano A, Lundberg C, Horellou P, Fischer W, Bentlage C, Campbell K, McKay RD, Mallet J & Björklund A (1995) CNS-derived neural progenitor cells for gene transfer of nerve growth factor to the adult rat brain: complete rescue of axotomized cholinergic neurons after transplantation into the septum. *Journal of Neuroscience*, **15**, 5668–80.

12 Martinez-Serrano A, Fischer W & Björklund A (1995) Reversal of age-dependent cognitive impairments and cholinergic neuron atrophy by NGF-secreting neural progenitors grafted to the basal forebrain. *Neuron*, **15**, 473–84.

13 Martinez-Serrano A, Fischer W, Söderström S, Ebendal T & Björklund A (1996) Long-term functional recovery from age-induced spatial memory impairments by nerve growth factor gene transfer to the rat basal forebrain. *Proceedings of the National Academy of Sciences, USA*, **93**, 6355–60.

14 Martinez-Serrano A & Björklund A (1996) Protection of the neostriatum against excitotoxic damage by neurotrophin-producing, genetically modified neural stem cells. *Journal of Neuroscience*, **16**, 4604–16.

15 Martinez-Serrano A & Snyder EY (1999) Neural stem cell lines for CNS regeneration: basic science and clinical applications. In *CNS Regeneration*, eds. M Tuszynski & J Kordower, pp. 203–50. San Diego: Academic Press.

16 Snyder EY, Taylor RM & Wolfe JH (1995) Neural progenitor cell engraftment corrects lysosomal storage throughout the MPS VII mouse brain. *Nature*, **374**, 367–70.

17 Lacorazza HD, Flax JD, Snyder EY & Jendoubi M (1996) Expression of human β-hexosaminidase α-subunit gene (the gene defect of Tay–Sachs disease) in mouse brains upon engraftment of transduced progenitor cells. *Nature Medicine*, **2**, 424–9.

18 Lynch WP, Snyder EY, Qualtiere L, Portis JL & Sharpe AH (1996) Late virus replication events in microglia are required for neurovirulent retrovirus-induced spongiform neurodegeneration: evidence from neural progenitor-derived chimeric mouse brains. *Journal of Virology*, **70**, 8896–907.

19 Lynch WP, Sharpe AH & Snyder EY (1999) Neural stem cells as engraftable packaging lines can mediate gene delivery to microglia: evidence from studying retroviral env-related neurodegeneration. *Journal of Virology*, **73**, 6841–51.

20 Billinghurst LL, Taylor RM & Snyder EY (1998) Remyelination: cellular and gene therapy. *Seminars in Pediatric Neurology*, **5**, 211–28.

21 Flax JD, Aurora S, Yang C, Simonin C, Wills AM, Billinghurst LL, Jendoubi M, Sidman RL, Wolfe JH, Kim SU & Snyder EY (1998) Engraftable human neural stem cells respond to developmental cues, replace neurons, and express foreign genes. *Nature Biotechnology*, **16**, 1033–9.

22 Yandava BD, Billinghurst LL & Snyder EY (1999) "Global" cell replacement is feasible via neural stem cell transplantation: evidence from the dysmyelinated shiverer mouse brain. *Proceedings of the National Academy of Sciences, USA*, **96**, 7029–34.

23 Snyder EY & Macklis JD (1996) Multipotent neural progenitor or stem-like cells may be uniquely suited for therapy for some neurodegenerative conditions. *Clinical Neuroscience*, **3**, 310–16.

24 Snyder EY, Yoon C, Flax JD & Macklis JD (1997) Multipotent neural precursors can differentiate toward replacement of neurons undergoing targeted apoptotic degeneration in adult mouse neocortex. *Proceedings of the National Academy of Sciences, USA*, **94**, 11663–8.

25 Rosario CM, Yandava BD, Kosaras B, Zurakowski D, Sidman RL & Snyder EY (1997) Differentiation of engrafted multipotent neural progenitors toward replacement of missing granule neurons in meander tail cerebellum may help determine the locus of mutant gene action. *Development*, **124**, 4213–24.

26 Park KI, Jensen FE & Snyder EY (1995) Neural progenitor transplantation for hypoxic–ischemic brain injury in immature mice. *Society for Neuroscience Abstract*, **21**, 2027.

27 Snyder EY, Deitcher DL, Walsh C, Arnold-Aldea S, Hartwieg EA & Cepko CL (1992) Multipotent neural cell lines can engraft and participate in development of mouse cerebellum. *Cell*, **68**, 33–51.

28 Snyder EY, Flax JD, Yandava BD, Park KI, Liu S, Rosario CM et al. (1997) Transplantation and differentiation of neural "stem-like" cells: possible insights into development and therapeutic potential. In *Research and Perspectives in Neurosciences: Isolation, Characterization, and Utilization of CNS Stem Cells*, eds. FH Gage & Y Christen, pp. 173–96. New York: Springer-Verlag.

29 Snyder EY (1998) Neural stem-like cells: developmental lessons with therapeutic potential. *The Neuroscientist*, **4**, 408–25.

30 Gage FH, Coates PW, Palmer TD, Kuhn HG, Fisher LJ, Suhonen JO, Peterson DA, Suhr ST & Ray J (1995) Survival and differentiation of adult neuronal progenitor cells transplanted to the adult brain. *Proceedings of the National Academy of Sciences, USA*, **92**, 11879–83.

31 Ghosh A & Greenberg ME (1995) Distinct roles for bFGF and NT-3 in the regulation of cortical neurogenesis. *Neuron*, **15**, 89–103.

32 Johe KK, Hazel TG, Muller T, Dugich-Djordjevic MM & McKay RDG (1996) Single factors direct the differentiation of stem cells from the fetal and adult central nervous system. *Genes & Development*, **10**, 3129–40.

33 Liu Y, Himes BT, Solowska J, Moul J, Chow SY, Park KI, Tessler A, Murray M, Snyder EY & Fischer I (1999) Intraspinal delivery of neurotrophin-3 using neural stem cells genetically modified by recombinant retrovirus. *Experimental Neurology*, **158**, 9–26.

34 Park KI, Jensen FE, Stieg PE, Himes T, Fischer I & Snyder EY (1997) Transplantation of neurotrophin-3 (NT-3) expressing neural stem-like cells into hypoxic-ischemic brain injury. *Society for Neuroscience Abstract*, **23**, 346.

35 Sidman RL, Miale IL & Feder N (1959) Cell proliferation and migration in the primitive ependymal zone: an autoradiographic study of histogenesis in the nervous system. *Experimental Neurology*, **1**, 322–33.

36 Altman J & Das GD (1965) Autoradiographic and histological evidence of postnatal hippocampal neurogenesis in rats. *Journal of Comparative Neurology*, **124**, 319–35.

37 Altman J (1969) Autoradiographic and histological studies of postnatal neurogenesis. IV. Cell proliferation and migration in the anterior forebrain, with special reference to persisting neurogenesis in the olfactory bulb. *Journal of Comparative Neurology*, **137**, 433–57.

38 Lois C & Alvarez-Buylla A (1994) Long-distance neuronal migration in the adult mammalian brain. *Science*, **264**, 1145–8.

39 Lois C, García-Verdugo JM & Alvarez-Buylla A (1996) Chain migration of neuronal precursors. *Science*, **271**, 978–81.

40 Goldman SA & Luskin MB (1998) Strategies utilized by migrating neurons of the postnatal vertebrate forebrain. *Trends in Neurosciences*, **21**, 107–14.

41 Kakita A & Goldman JE (1999) Patterns and dynamics of SVZ cell migration in the postnatal forebrain: monitoring living progenitors in slice preparations. *Neuron*, **23**, 461–72.

42 Wu W, Wong K, Chen J-h, Jiang Z-h, Dupuis S, Wu JY & Rao Y (1999) Directional guidance of neuronal migration in the olfactory system by the protein Slit. *Nature*, **400**, 331–6.

43 Eriksson PS, Perfilieva E, Bjork-Eriksson T, Alborn AM, Nordborg C, Peterson DA & Gage FH (1998) Neurogenesis in the adult human hippocampus. *Nature Medicine*, **4**, 1313–17.

44 Pincus DW, Keyoung HM, Harrison-Restelli C, Goodman RR, Fraser RA, Edgar M, Sakakibara S, Okano H, Nedergaard M & Goldman SA (1998) Fibroblast growth factor-2/brain-derived neurotrophic factor-associated maturation of new neurons generated from adult human subependymal cells. *Annals of Neurology*, **43**, 576–85.

45 Ramon y Cajal S (1928) *Degeneration and Regeneration of the Nervous System*. London: Oxford University Press.

46 Park KI, Jensen FE, Stieg PE & Snyder EY (1998) Hypoxic–ischemic (HI) brain injury may direct the proliferation, migration, and differentiation of endogenous neural progenitors. *Society for Neuroscience Abstract*, **24**, 1310.

47 Price J, Turner D & Cepko C (1987) Lineage analysis in the vertebrate nervous system by retrovirus-mediated gene transfer. *Proceedings of the National Academy of Sciences, USA*, **84**, 156–60.

48 Svendsen CN, Caldwell MA, Shen J, ter Borg MG, Rosser AE, Tyers P, Karmiol S & Dunnett SB (1997) Long-term survival of human central nervous system progenitor cells transplanted into a rat model of Parkinson's disease. *Experimental Neurology*, **148**, 135–46.

49 Vescovi AL, Parati EA, Gritti A, Poulin P, Ferrario M, Wanke E, Frolichsthal-Schoeller P, Cova L, Arcellana-Panlilio M, Colombo A & Galli R (1999) Isolation and cloning of multipotential stem cells from the embryonic human CNS and establishment of transplantable human neural stem cell lines by epigenetic stimulation. *Experimental Neurology*, **156**, 71–83.

50 Fricker RA, Carpenter MK, Winkler C, Greco C, Gates MA & Björklund A (1999) Site-specific migration and neuronal differentiation of human neural progenitor cells after transplantation in the adult rat brain. *Journal of Neuroscience*, **19**, 5990–6005.

51 Park KI & Snyder EY (1999) Transplantation of human neural stem cells, propagated by either genetic or epigenetic means, into hypoxic–ischemic (HI) brain injury. *Society for Neuroscience Abstract*, **25**, 212.

52 Park KI, Liu S, Flax JD, Nissim S, Stieg PE & Snyder EY (1999) Transplantation of neural progenitor and stem cells: developmental insights may suggest new therapies for spinal cord and other CNS dysfunction. *Journal of Neurotrauma*, **16**, 675–87.

26

Neural plasticity after cerebral ischemia

Jialing Liu[1], Toshiaki Nagafuji[2], Philip R. Weinstein[3] & Frank R. Sharp[4]

[1,3] Department of Neurological Surgery, University of California at San Francisco and San Francisco Veterans Affairs Medical Center, San Francisco, CA
[2] Shionogi & Co., Osaka, Japan
[4] Department of Neurology, University of Cincinnati, Cincinnati, OH

Introduction

Neural stem cells that fulfill all the classic criteria for stem cells, including (i) multipotency, (ii) highly proliferative potential and self-renewal and (iii) a limited capacity to regenerate after injury or disease, continue to exist in the adult central nervous system (CNS). This chapter describes how cerebral global ischemia increases the proliferation of neural stem cells in the dentate gyrus, producing new neurons and glia in two separate compartments, namely the granule cell layer and the dentate hilus. Our recent data show that focal ischemia, though it rarely damages hippocampal neurons, increases the proliferation of dentate gyrus stem cells. Regeneration in the dentate gyrus after cerebral ischemia represents an injury-induced neural plasticity.

Neural stem cells in the adult CNS

Locations of adult neural stem cells

There are only two types of neuron normally generated in the adult brain, i.e., dentate granule cells and olfactory bulb interneurons. The sources of neural stem cells for generating these neurons are located at the subventricular zone (SVZ) of the lateral ventricles and at the subgranular zone (SGZ) of the dentate gyrus [1], both believed to be developmental remnants of the embryonic germinal zone. Recent evidence suggests that a group of glial fibrillary acidic protein-expressing cells in the SVZ are the precursor cells for generating neuroblasts in the rostral migratory stream, and eventually neurons in the olfactory bulb [2]. Proliferating SVZ cells form a chain and migrate longitudinally through the SVZ to join the rostral migratory stream into the olfactory bulb. These cells then move radially into the granule and glomerular layers and differentiate into local interneurons [3].

There is no evidence that under normal conditions the stem cells in the SVZ form neurons in locations other than olfactory [4,5]. In contrast to the long-distance migration of SVZ-derived neurons, newborn neurons in the adult hippocampus are produced locally. Adult hippocampal progenitor cells divide at the dentate gyrus SGZ and form neurons in the granule cell layer [6,7]. Transplantation studies show that stem cells from the adult hippocampus are capable of developing into neurons of destined phenotypes by responding to local environmental cues [8], suggesting that these stem cells retain the plasticity to differentiate into various types of neuron.

Regulation of proliferation and differentiation of adult neural stem cells

In the subependyma

Evidence from in vitro and/or in vivo systems indicates that basic fibroblast growth factor (bFGF), epidermal growth factor (EGF) and transforming growth factor-alpha (TGF-α) increase the proliferation of neural stem cells. Both EGF and bFGF expand the SVZ progenitor population after infusion into the lateral ventricle of the adult rat brain [9]. bFGF increases the number of neurons reaching the olfactory bulb, and EGF enhances the differentiation of astrocytes. Ablation of the olfactory bulb also increases the proliferation of stem cells in the SVZ [10], suggesting that a tight censorship regulates the production of neurons in the target area of the SVZ stem cells.

In the dentate gyrus

Hormones, neurotransmitters, environmental stimuli and growth factors are among the mediators involved in the regulation of adult hippocampal neurogenesis. Glutamatergic deafferentation and N-methyl-D-aspartate (NMDA) receptor antagonists induce dentate gyrus progenitor proliferation with increased newborn neurons in the granule cell layer [11]. Adrenal steroids and stress result in the opposite effect [12,13]. Differentiation of neurons within the adult rat dentate gyrus is reduced in animals with hypothyroidism [14]. Enriched environments result in more total granule cell neurons by increasing the survival rate of the progeny of the dividing progenitor cells [15,16]. Voluntary wheel running increases both the proliferation of dentate gyrus stem cells and the survival of their progeny [16]. Cerebral ischemia [17], seizures [18] and mechanical injury of granule cells [19] also increase dentate gyrus neurogenesis. The finding that production of new neurons in the adult dentate gyrus is tightly regulated by physiological cues and injury further suggests that neurogenesis is a functionally significant process.

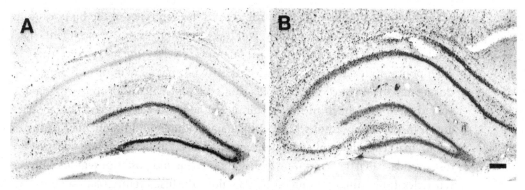

Figure 26.1 Neurogenesis in the pyramidal cell layer and the dentate gyrus takes place during different stages of development. BrdU was given intraperitoneally (100 mg/kg) to newborn rats at postnatal day 1 or to timed-pregnant rats on embryonic day 17. Injected animals were sacrificed 1 month later and BrdU incorporation was assayed by immunohistochemistry. Note that BrdU-immunoreactive nuclei were present throughout all cell layers in the hippocampus of animals that received the labeling on embryonic day 17 (B). However, BrdU incorporation was seen only in the dentate gyrus granule cell layer and sporadically in the molecular layer of animals injected on postnatal day 1 (A), suggesting that proliferation and migration of CA1 pyramidal neurons occur during the late embryonic period. Bar = 200 μm.

The origin of neural stem cells in the hippocampus

Results from thymidine labeling suggest that migration of proliferating cells from the embryonic ventricular zone to the hippocampus takes place in waves during development [20]. The primary dentate neuroepithelium, which is located around a ventricular indentation named the dentate notch, contains the stem cells for the development of dentate gyrus. By embryonic day 18, aggregates of proliferative cells migrate toward the dentate gyrus and form the multiple germinal matrix, which becomes highly active during the perinatal and early postnatal period. The great increase in the granule cell population during the infantile period is principally due to cells derived from this matrix. Between postnatal days 20 and 30 the germinal matrix disappears in the basal polymorphic layer and henceforth proliferative cells become largely confined to the SGZ [21].

Proliferative cells located at the amnionic neuroepithelium start migrating toward the stratum pyramidale from embryonic day 17, and later form the neurons in regions CA1 to CA3. Pyramidal neurons are postmitotic once formed, and there appear to be no stem cells for them in adulthood. Our results with bromodeoxyuridine (BrdU) labeling further confirm that neurogenesis in the pyramidal layer and the dentate gyrus takes place during different stages of development (Figure 26.1).

Migration of proliferating cells from the lateral ventricles to the hippocampus takes place only within a narrow window of time during development. This window precedes the retraction of the lateral ventricles, which extend dorsally to the hippocampus during embryonic and early postnatal life in rats. A zipper-like closure and fusion of ependymal cells along the ventricular wall occurs within the second week after birth in rats, resulting in the closure of the ventricular space dorsal to the hippocampus [22]. Only a small lumen and fragmented seams of ependymal cells remain at each lateral ventricle in adult rats. This lumen forms the rostrocaudal canal that communicates at its anterior and posterior regions with the ventricles. Interestingly, proliferating cells along the fused ventricular wall dorsal to the hippocampus in adult rodents also appear as fragmented clusters and in much lower frequency than those situated at the SVZ lining (Figure 26.2). It is unclear whether the diminished BrdU labeling in this region is associated with the age-dependent decline of the proliferative potential of neural stem cells in general, or is related to the fusion of ependymal cells and the disappearance of SVZ cells after early postnatal life.

Injury-induced stem cell proliferation and neurogenesis

Injury-induced neurogenesis in the adult CNS was first shown to occur in phylo-genetically "lower" species such as fish and lizards. Fish are able to regenerate neurons and axons in the CNS after injuries and experimentally induced lesions [23–25]. In addition to increased proliferation of neurons, mechanical lesions of the corpus cerebelli in gymnotiform fish could also induce migration and neuro-nal differentiation of cells along the lesion path born prior to the application of the injury [26]. 3-Acetylpyridine injected peritoneally leads to a specific lesion in the lizard medial cortex. A period of maximal proliferative activity was detected from the third day after 3-acetylpyridine injection until day 7. Electron microscopy revealed that the newborn cells were neuroblasts or immature neurons; they grad-ually replaced the dead neurons in the lesion site [27,28]. An electrolytic lesion of the nucleus ectostriatum in adult ring doves increased the number of newborn neurons in the forebrain by 2.38 times [29]. The ability of mammals to replace injured neurons in the CNS appears to be more limited, especially in adult animals. Neurogenesis in the murine olfactory system is both physiological and injury ini-tiated. After bulbectomy, neuronal progenitor cells in the ipsilateral olfactory epi-thelium respond to the injury by increasing proliferation [30–32]. In the taste system, sensory cells are disposable and are completely replaced within less than 2 weeks [33]. In the auditory and vestibular systems, replacement is not physiologi-cal and, when it does occur, appears to be injury induced [34]. There is currently no evidence for a neural stem cell in the adult mammalian retina, and the retina of

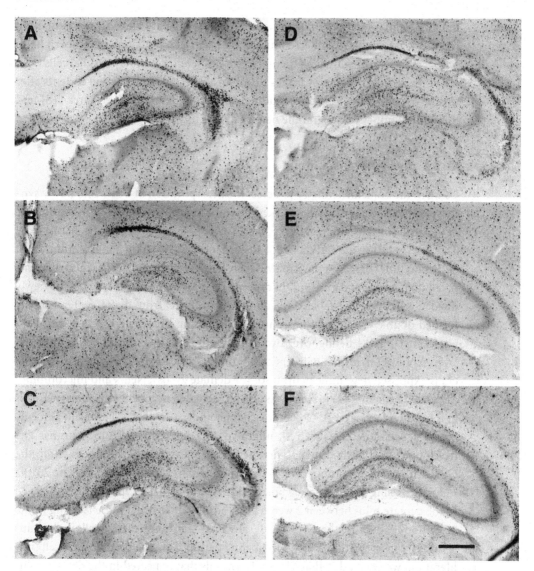

Figure 26.2 Reduction of proliferative activity in the ependyma above the hippocampus during the first few days of postnatal life in rats. BrdU was given intraperitoneally (100 mg/kg) to newborn rats from postnatal day 1 (A), 2 (B), 3 (C), 4 (D), 6 (E) and 8 (F), 6 hours prior to sacrifice. Note that progressively reduced numbers of BrdU-incorporated nuclei appear in the ventricle lining from postnatal days 1 to 8. Within the hippocampus, BrdU-labeled nuclei also gradually dissolve and become restricted to the granule cell layer after postnatal day 8. Bar = 500 μm (F).

the mature mammal does not show regenerative capacity after damage, although there is a possibility for the reinitiation of stem cell potential at the peripheral retinal margin from retinal pigmented epithelium or from müllerian glial cells [35]. However, recent evidence indicates that neurogenesis occurs in adult rodents after various types of brain injury including cerebral ischemia [17], seizures [18] and mechanical injury of the granule neurons [19].

Neuroplasticity after global ischemia

Using immunohistochemistry to detect the incorporation of BrdU into newly synthesized DNA, we observed a marked increase in cellular proliferation in the SGZ of the dentate gyrus between 1 and 2 weeks after 10 minutes of global ischemia [17]. The threshold for the induction of neurogenesis is between 2 and 4 minutes of occlusion time. Based on in vitro evidence, dentate gyrus stem cells could differentiate into neurons and glia [36]. In order to determine the phenotypes of the newly divided cells, we pulse-labeled the animals with BrdU from days 9 to 12 and performed double immunofluorescence labeling using BrdU and cell markers. By 4 weeks after BrdU labeling, over two thirds of the dividing cells in the granule cell layer expressed neuronal markers calbindin D_{28k} (a calcium-binding protein generally expressed in granule neurons of the dentate gyrus), NeuN and microtubule-associated protein-2 [17]. There was also an increased number of newborn neurons in the granule cell layer (GCL) after ischemia, indicating that a significant percentage of progenitor cells survived, migrated and differentiated into neurons. The development of newly differentiated neurons appeared to be confined within the GCL, with a few migrating toward the molecular layer, as indicated in Plate 26.1C.

An increasing number of newborn cells with a glial phenotype was also observed in the dentate hilus between 2 weeks and 1 month after BrdU pulse labeling (Plate 26.1E and F). Because there was hardly any BrdU-immunoreactive cells in the hilus at any given time within a 24 hour labeling period since the peak of stem cell proliferation, we concluded that the newborn cells that appeared in the dentate hilus were derived from the migration and differentiation of dividing stem cells. Similar to the survival rate of newly divided cells in the normal mouse SGZ [16], more than 50% of the newborn cells died within the first 2 weeks after global ischemia in gerbil SGZ. Approximately 60% of the surviving BrdU-immunoreactive cells turned into neurons in the GCL 1 month later [17].

Focal cerebral ischemia also increases the proliferation of dentate gyrus neural stem cells

Focal cerebral ischemia is associated with NMDA receptor modulation that plays an important role in the regulation of dentate gyrus neural stem cells. To

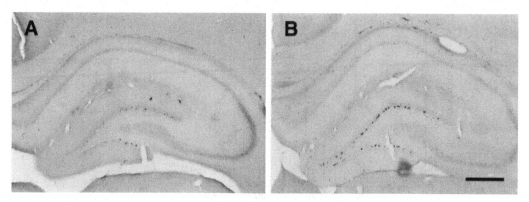

Figure 26.3 Increased cell proliferation in the SGZ after Tamura's permanent MCAO. BrdU immunohistochemistry from control (A) and ischemic (B) (11 days after ischemia) brains. BrdU was administered 1 day before sacrifice. Bar = 500 μm (B).

investigate whether focal cerebral ischemia affects the proliferation of dentate gyrus stem cells, we performed permanent middle cerebral artery occlusion (MCAO) using Tamura's model [37]. With Tamura's method, the animals tend to survive MCAO better than with permanent MCAO produced by the suture model, since the strokes are less severe.

Tamura's permanent MCAO and BrdU labeling

Adult male Sprague–Dawley rats (300 to 380 g) were anesthetized with 3% isoflurane and maintained with 1% isoflurane in a mixture of 30% O_2 / 70% N_2. A tiny craniectomy was made around the foramen ovale. The left MCA trunk proximal to the lenticulostriate artery (arteries) was exposed and electrocoagulated as previously described [37,38]. In sham-operated animals, the surgical manipulations were carried out in the same manner as described above except for the electrocauterization of the MCA. Throughout the surgical operations, both the temperature of the right temporal muscle and the rectum were maintained at 37 ± 0.5 °C with a heating blanket until the animals recovered from surgery. After recovery the animals was monitored for an additional 2 hours to prevent hypothermia. BrdU was administered intraperitoneally (100 mg/kg) 24 hours prior to sacrifice.

Increased stem cell proliferation in the SGZ 11 days after focal ischemia

A 3.5-fold increase in BrdU incorporation at the dentate gyrus SGZ occurred in 40% of the rats that were subjected to permanent MCAO on day 11 (Figure 26.3). The number of BrdU-immunoreactive nuclei gradually returned to base line level 5 weeks after ischemic surgery (Figure 26.4). Histological examination indicated that the rats with increased BrdU incorporation in the dentate gyrus SGZ after focal ischemia also had various degrees of injury to the entorhinal cortex [39]. This is in

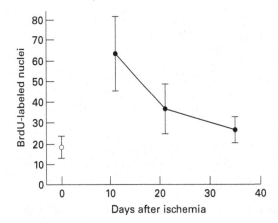

Figure 26.4 Time course of cell proliferation in the SGZ of dentate gyrus after Tamura's permanent
MCAO. The number of BrdU-immunoreactive nuclei in the SGZ from various time points
after ischemia (●) and in untreated animals (○) were plotted against days after ischemia.
BrdU was given 1 day before sacrifice.

contrast to our findings after global ischemia in gerbils, where entorhinal lesions
did not occur in the animals with ischemia-induced neurogenesis.

Distinct pathways are involved in regulating the growth of dentate gyrus stem cells after different types of ischemia

Layer II of the entorhinal cortex projects to the dentate gyrus [40]. Lesions of the
entorhinal cortex removed afferent input to granule neurons that have been shown
to increase neurogenesis in the dentate gyrus [11]. The neurons in the perforant
path are most likely to be glutamatergic [41]. Comparing results from two different ischemic models brings out some interesting observations. (i) Multiple mechanisms contribute to ischemia-induced neurogenesis. Granule cell loss and lesions
of the entorhinal cortex can both stimulate the proliferation of dentate gyrus stem
cells. (ii) The degree of neurogenesis resulting at least partially from granule cell
death appears to be more rigorous than that from perforant deafferentation.

The signal for neurogenesis in the dentate gyrus is likely to come from mature
granule cells, which have been to shown to play a role in regulating production of
new neurons [19]. In the case of global ischemia, granule cell death is a direct and
potent stimulus for regulating stem cell proliferation, reflected by high levels of
BrdU incorporation. Since the terminals of the perforant path fibers from the
entorhinal cortex project on the dendritic spines of granule neurons [42], it is reasonable to speculate that cell death in the perforant path after MCAO stimulates
dentate gyrus stem cells to divide, perhaps via a reduction of glutamatergic input.

This is further supported by the similar level of increased stem cell proliferation observed between cerebral focal ischemia and administration of NMDA receptor antagonists [11]. Our data also suggest that CA1 neuronal death is not necessary nor sufficient to upregulate dentate stem cell proliferation, since Tamura's MCAO does not produce CA neuronal loss, and focal occlusion of the MCA using the suture model rarely increases BrdU incorporation in the SGZ, despite occasional CA1 cell death.

REFERENCES

1 Weiss S & van der Kooy D (1998) CNS stem cells: where's the biology (a.k.a. beef)? *Journal of Neurobiology*, **36**, 307–14.

2 Doetsch F, Caille I, Lim DA, García-Verdugo JM & Alvarez-Buylla A (1999) Subventricular zone astrocytes are neural stem cells in the adult mammalian brain. *Cell*, **97**, 703–16.

3 Doetsch F, García-Verdugo JM & Alvarez-Buylla A (1997) Cellular composition and three-dimensional organization of the subventricular germinal zone in the adult mammalian brain. *Journal of Neuroscience*, **17**, 5046–61.

4 Kirschenbaum B, Doetsch F, Lois C & Alvarez-Buylla A (1999) Adult subventricular zone neuronal precursors continue to proliferate and migrate in the absence of the olfactory bulb. *Journal of Neuroscience*, **19**, 2171–80.

5 Luskin MB (1998) Neuroblasts of the postnatal mammalian forebrain: their phenotype and fate. *Journal of Neurobiology*, **36**, 221–33.

6 Gage FH, Kempermann G, Palmer TD, Peterson DA & Ray J (1998) Multipotent progenitor cells in the adult dentate gyrus. *Journal of Neurobiology*, **36**, 249–66.

7 Kuhn HG, Dickinson-Anson H & Gage FH (1996) Neurogenesis in the dentate gyrus of the adult rat: age-related decrease of neuronal progenitor proliferation. *Journal of Neuroscience*, **16**, 2027–33.

8 Suhonen JO, Peterson DA, Ray J, & Gage FH (1996) Differentiation of adult hippocampus-derived progenitors into olfactory neurons in vivo. *Nature*, **383**, 624–7.

9 Kuhn HG, Winkler J, Kempermann G, Thal LJ & Gage FH (1997) Epidermal growth factor and fibroblast growth factor-2 have different effects on neural progenitors in the adult rat brain. *Journal of Neuroscience*, **17**, 5820–9.

10 Carr VM & Farbman AI (1992) Ablation of the olfactory bulb up-regulates the rate of neurogenesis and induces precocious cell death in olfactory epithelium. *Experimental Neurology*, **115**, 55–9.

11 Cameron HA, McEwen BS & Gould E (1995) Regulation of adult neurogenesis by excitatory input and NMDA receptor activation in the dentate gyrus. *Journal of Neuroscience*, **15**, 4687–92.

12 Cameron HA & Gould E (1994) Adult neurogenesis is regulated by adrenal steroids in the dentate gyrus. *Neuroscience*, **61**, 203–9.

13 Gould E, Cameron HA, Daniels DC, Woolley CS & McEwen BS (1992) Adrenal hormones suppress cell division in the adult rat dentate gyrus. *Journal of Neuroscience,* 12, 3642–50.

14 Madeira MD, Cadete-Leite A, Andrade JP & Paula-Barbosa MM (1991) Effects of hypothyroidism upon the granular layer of the dentate gyrus in male and female adult rats: a morphometric study. *Journal of Comparative Neurology,* 314, 171–86.

15 Kempermann G, Kuhn HG & Gage FH (1997) More hippocampal neurons in adult mice living in an enriched environment. *Nature,* 386, 493–5.

16 van Praag H, Kempermann G & Gage FH (1999) Running increases cell proliferation and neurogenesis in the adult mouse dentate gyrus. *Nature Neuroscience,* 2, 266–70.

17 Liu J, Solway K, Messing RO & Sharp FR (1998) Increased neurogenesis in the dentate gyrus after transient global ischemia in gerbils. *Journal of Neuroscience,* 18, 7768–78.

18 Parent JM, Yu TW, Leibowitz RT, Geschwind DH, Sloviter R & Lowenstein DH (1997) Dentate granule cell neurogenesis is increased by seizures and contributes to aberrant network reorganization in the adult rat hippocampus. *Journal of Neuroscience,* 17, 3727–38.

19 Gould E & Tanapat P (1997) Lesion-induced proliferation of neuronal progenitors in the dentate gyrus of the adult rat. *Neuroscience,* 80, 427–36.

20 Altman J & Bayer SA (1990) Mosaic organization of the hippocampal neuroepithelium and the multiple germinal sources of dentate granule cells. *Journal of Comparative Neurology,* 301, 325–42.

21 Altman J & Bayer SA (1990) Migration and distribution of two populations of hippocampal granule cell precursors during the perinatal and postnatal periods. *Journal of Comparative Neurology,* 301, 365–81.

22 Kawamata S, Stumpf WE & Bidmon HJ (1995) Adhesion and fusion of ependyma in rat brain. *Acta Anatomica,* 152, 205–14.

23 Anderson MJ & Waxman SG (1985) Neurogenesis in adult vertebrate spinal cord in situ and in vitro: a new model system. *Annals of the New York Academy of Sciences,* 457, 213–33.

24 Meyer RL, Sakurai K & Schauwecker E (1985) Topography of regenerating optic fibers in goldfish traced with local wheat germ injections into retina: evidence for discontinuous microtopography in the retinotectal projection. *Journal of Comparative Neurology,* 239, 27–43.

25 Stuermer CA, Bastmeyer M, Bahr M, Strobel G & Paschke K (1992) Trying to understand axonal regeneration in the CNS of fish. *Journal of Neurobiology,* 23, 537–50.

26 Zupanc GKH (1999) Neurogenesis, cell death and regeneration in the adult gymnotiform brain. *Journal of Experimental Biology,* 202, 1435–46.

27 Font E, Desfilis E, Pérez-Cañellas M, Alcántara S & García-Verdugo JM (1997) 3–Acetylpyridine-induced degeneration and regeneration in the adult lizard brain: a qualitative and quantitative analysis. *Brain Research,* 754, 245–59.

28 Molowny A, Nacher J & Lopez-Garcia C (1995) Reactive neurogenesis during regeneration of the lesioned medial cerebral cortex of lizards. *Neuroscience,* 68, 823–36.

29 Zuo MX (1998) The studies on neurogenesis induced by brain injury in adult ring dove. *Cell Research,* 8, 151–8.

30 Farbman AI, Brunjes PC, Rentfro L, Michas J & Ritz S (1988) The effect of unilateral naris occlusion on cell dynamics in the developing rat olfactory epithelium. *Journal of Neuroscience,* 8, 3290–5.

31 Gordon MK, Mumm JS, Davis RA, Holcomb JD & Calof AL (1995) Dynamics of MASH1 expression in vitro and in vivo suggest a non-stem cell site of MASH1 action in the olfactory receptor neuron lineage. *Molecular & Cellular Neurosciences*, **6**, 363–79.

32 Schwartz Levey M, Chikaraishi DM & Kauer JS (1991) Characterization of potential precursor populations in the mouse olfactory epithelium using immunocytochemistry and autoradiography. *Journal of Neuroscience*, **11**, 3556–64.

33 Farbman AI (1980) Renewal of taste bud cells in rat circumvallate papillae. *Cell & Tissue Kinetics*, **13**, 349–57.

34 Farbman AI (1997) Injury-stimulated neurogenesis in sensory systems. *Advances in Neurology*, **72**, 157–61.

35 Reh TA & Levine EM (1998) Multipotential stem cells and progenitors in the vertebrate retina. *Journal of Neurobiology*, **36**, 206–20.

36 Reynolds BA & Weiss S (1992) Generation of neurons and astrocytes from isolated cells of the adult mammalian central nervous system. *Science*, **255**, 1707–10.

37 Tamura A, Graham DI, McCulloch J & Teasdale GM (1981) Focal cerebral ischaemia in the rat. 1. Description of technique and early neuropathological consequences following middle cerebral artery occlusion. *Journal of Cerebral Blood Flow & Metabolism*, **1**, 53–60.

38 Nagafuji T, Matsui T, Koide T & Asano T (1992) Blockade of nitric oxide formation by N-omega-nitro-L-arginine mitigates ischemic brain edema and subsequent cerebral infarction in rats. *Neuroscience Letters*, **147**, 159–62.

39 Liu J, Nagafuji T & Sharp FR (1999) Focal cerebral ischemia increases the proliferation of the hippocampal neural stem cells in adult rats. *Neuroscience Abstract*.

40 Steward O & Scoville SA. (1976) Cells of origin of entorhinal cortical afferents to the hippocampus and fascia dentata of the rat. *Journal of Comparative Neurology*, **169**, 347–70.

41 Fonnum F (1970) Topographical and subcellular localization of choline acetyltransferase in rat hippocampal region. *Journal of Neurochemistry*, **17**, 1029–37.

42 Nafstad PHJ (1967) An electron microscope study on the termination of the perforant path fibres in the hippocampus and the fascia dentata. *Zeitschrift für Zellforschung und Mikroskopische Anatomie*, **76**, 532–42.

27

Environmental effects on recovery after stroke

Barbro B. Johansson

Wallenberg Neuroscience Center, Lund, Sweden

Introduction

There is increasing evidence that functional improvement after permanent brain lesions is related to lesion-induced plasticity in the intact brain [1–6]. An important question is to what extent postischemic interventions can influence plasticity and functional outcome after brain infarction. We have shown previously that sensorimotor functions improve significantly more in rats that are postoperatively housed in an enriched environment than in rats housed in standard laboratory cages [7–9]. In a comparison among different kinds of activities, social interaction was superior to wheel running, and an enriched environment allowing free physical activity combined with social interaction resulted in the best performance [10]. We have also shown that enriched housing can improve outcome after neural grafting to a neocortical infarct [11,12]. I will discuss some studies on potential mechanisms behind the environmental stimulation of outcome after focal brain ischemia.

In the studies quoted below, cortical infarct was induced by ligation of the middle cerebral artery (MCA) distal to the striatal branches in 3- to 4-month-old male spontaneously hypertensive rats [7]. Before the operation all rats were housed in standard cages, four rats in each cage. During the first 24 to 30 postoperative hours they were housed in individual cages, then either returned to standard cages or transferred to larger cages, furnished with horizontal and inclined boards and equipped with various items [8]. Twice or three times a week the space between the boards was changed and some objects were replaced with new ones. For details see the references given in connection with each study. Our design differs from that in most studies on enriched environment because the standard rats were not socially deprived. Usually control rats are housed in individual cages, which enhances differences between control and enriched animals.

Environmental effects on postischemic gene expression

Ischemia is a strong inducer of gene expression in the brain. Many genes are induced within minutes or hours after ligation of the MCA, often returning to normal levels within the first 24 hours [13–15]. It has been proposed that the early gene activation is, at least in part, caused by spreading depression [16]. Little is known about late postischemic events. We have tested the hypothesis that postischemic housing in an enriched environment might increase brain-derived neurotrophic factor (BDNF) gene expression. Contrary to our hypothesis, higher values were seen in rats housed in a standard environment [17]. Significant differences were observed between standard rats above and enriched rats below the baseline in the peri-infarct region, contralateral cortex and hippocampus 2 to 12 days after induction of ischemia. Unpublished data on BDNF protein levels 12 days after MCA occlusion have indicated a significant difference corresponding to BDNF mRNA in the peri-infarct region. A similar dampening of postischemic gene expression in rats housed in an enriched environment was seen for nerve growth factor-induced gene A mRNA. With this gene, however, a late significant increase in the enriched group was observed 30 days after the lesion [18].

Cortical networks adjacent to a focal brain infarct are hyperexcitable because of an imbalance between excitatory and inhibitory synaptic function due to increased N-methyl-D-aspartate receptor-mediated excitation and reduced GABAergic inhibition (GABA is γ-aminobutyric acid) [19]. Hyperexcitability has also been recorded in the contralateral hemisphere 1 week after MCA occlusion [20]. Both a detrimental and a beneficial plasticity-promoting role for lesion-induced hyperexcitability have been proposed [21]. One possible interpretation of our data is that early postischemic dampening of the peri-infarct neuronal hyperactivity might be beneficial. Another possibility is that there is no causality between BDNF mRNA and functional outcome. Interactions between trophic and growth inhibitory factors, which were shown to be increased in the postischemic phase [22], have to be considered. For further discussion see Zhao et al. [17].

Environmental effects on dendritic spines

Dendritic spines are the primary postsynaptic targets of excitatory glutaminergic synapses in the mature brain and have been proposed as the primary sites of synaptic plasticity [23–25]. Video recordings from hippocampal neurons expressing actin tagged with green fluorescent protein have shown that the dendritic spine shape in mature neurons may change within seconds, suggesting that anatomical plasticity at synapses can be very rapid [26]. Highly localized dendritic Ca^{2+} signals, limited to a small dendritic segment and even to single dendritic spines, have been demonstrated under in vivo conditions [27]. Those signals can be blocked by NMDA receptor antagonists and are thought to be caused primarily by the entry of extracellular Ca^{2+} [28]. Current data indicate that the dendritic tree is covered with a variety of excitable synaptic channels operating on different time scales and with activity-dependent sensitivity enabling a sophisticated neuronal plastic capability [29].

It is known that environmental enrichment can enhance dendritic branching and increase the number of dendritic spines and synapses [30–33]. Rearing animals in social isolation has the opposite effect [34]. Measurement of the dendritic spines has been shown to be a more sensitive method for detecting environmental influence than measurement of dendritic branching [34].

Most studies on environmental influence on dendritic morphology have been performed with modifications of the Golgi technique or electron microscopy. Due to the small size, large number and highly variable shapes of dendritic spines, standard light microscopy of Golgi impregnation and electron microscopy of single thin sections are less adequate for identifying individual spines. A three-dimensional approach is essential [35]. Furthermore, with the Golgi method neurons are stained sporadically and there is no control over which neurons will be stained. Confocal microscopy after microinjection of Lucifer yellow into individual neurons allows a three-dimensional visualization of dendritic spines, a more detailed analysis of spine morphology and more exact quantification of the number of dendritic spines than standard light microscopy [36]. Neurons can be selected for injection on the basis of their spacing, to avoid dendritic overlap. With this technique we have studied whether postischemic placement in an enriched environment after focal brain ischemia influences dendritic spine morphology and number in layers II and III and V and VI in the somatosensory cortex contralateral to a cortical infarct [37].

Basal, apical and oblique apical dendrites of pyramidal neurons in control nonlesioned rats housed in an enriched environment had significantly more (20% to 40%) branches than rats housed in standard environments ($P<0.05$). Individual spine morphology was significantly changed, with more branched spines and an increase in spine head and neck diameter (Figure 27.1). Pyramidal neurons in infarcted rats postoperatively housed in an enriched environment had more oblique, apical dendritic branches in layers II and III and significantly more spines in all types of dendrites than those in rats in standard cages ($P<05$). However, in pyramidal neurons in layers V and VI the number of spines was reduced in both groups, with the largest decrease in apical dendrites and no difference between enriched and standard rats [37].

Dendritic spines disappear after deafferentation but dendrites can be reinnervated by sprouting from axonal terminals in the vicinity. Accordingly, cortical

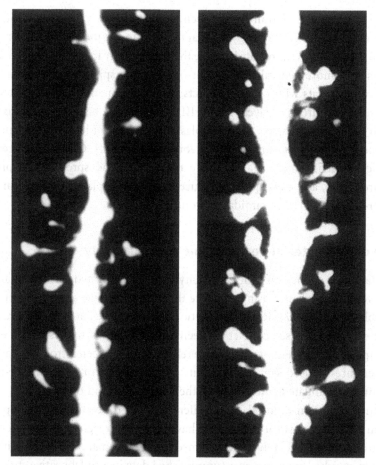

Figure 27.1   Spine morphology and distribution on basal dendrites in layer V pyramidal neurons in the somatosensory cortex of rats housed in standard cages (left) or in an enriched environment for 3 weeks (right). Confocal imaging after microinjection of Lucifer yellow.

lesions in the mouse result in a progressive and transient spine loss of striatal neurons 3 to 10 days after the lesion, with regrowth and recovery of 80% of unlesioned control spines 20 days postlesion [38].

The cortex contralateral to the lesion loses its callosal projections. Callosal projections have been extensively studied in the motor cortex and were shown to be present in layers II, III and V to about the same extent, although cells in layer V formed fewer callosal synapses [39]. In the somatosensory cortex the density of interhemispheric connections in those layers varies with the subfield [40,41]. Cutting cortical connections in adult rats caused a biphasic degeneration of the axonal terminals with one maximum after 2 to 7 days and a second peak after 10 to 20 days [42].

In intact rats, reach training has been shown to selectively alter dendritic branching in layer-II and layer-III pyramidal neurons in the motor-somatosensory forelimb cortex [43]. Our results indicate that free activity in an enriched environment leads to a more general stimulation of dendritic spines in pyramidal neurons. However, in rats with cortical infarcts the environmental enrichment selectively stimulated neurons in layers II and III, neurons that have extensive connections with other cortical areas. Synaptic plasticity in cortical horizontal connections is proposed to underlie cortical map reorganization [44]. Our data suggest that an enriched environment may enhance the growth and sprouting of presynaptic neurons and, as a consequence, induce postsynaptic plastic changes on spines in layer-II and layer-III pyramidal neurons.

Possible role of astrocytes in postischemic brain plasticity

So far most studies on brain plasticity have concentrated on neuronal changes. However, there is increasing evidence that astrocytes take an active part in synaptic plasticity [45–47]. Rapid astrocytic changes in the cortex and ultrastructural evidence for increased contact between astrocytes and synapses in rats reared in a complex environment suggest a close relationship between astrocytic plasticity and experience-induced synaptic plasticity [48]. In intact rats, an enriched environment can stimulate neurogenesis in the hippocampus in mice and rats [49,50]. In a study on lesion-induced cell proliferation and differentiation of hippocampal stem cells after cortical infarcts we have observed a significant difference in the neuron to glia ratio in the newly formed cells between animals housed in standard and in enriched environments (unpublished data in a collaborative study with Dr. Peter Eriksson, Göteborg University).

Conclusion

The patient's own attitude, activity and social interaction [51] influence functional outcome and quality of life after stroke. The experimental evidence that postischemic environmental enrichment, without specific interventions or forced training, can significantly influence molecular events and improve functional outcome emphasizes the importance of general stimulation and activation in stroke rehabilitation, clearly in addition to and not as a substitute for specific required interventions. The fact that an enriched environment can interact with neocortical grafting supports this view [11,12].

REFERENCES

1 Jenkins WM & Merzenich MM (1987) Reorganization of neocortical representations after brain injury: a neurophysiological model of the bases of recovery from stroke. *Progress in Brain Research,* **71**, 249–66.

2 Pons TP, Garraghty PE & Mishkin M (1988) Lesion-induced plasticity in the second somatosensory cortex of adult macaques. *Proceedings of the National Academy of Sciences, USA,* **85**, 5279–81.

3 Kaas JH (1991) Plasticity of sensory and motor maps in adult mammals. *Annual Review of Neuroscience,* **14**, 137–67.

4 Nudo RJ, Wise BM, SiFuentes F & Milliken GW (1996) Neural substrates for the effects of rehabilitative training on motor recovery after ischemic infarct. *Science,* **272**, 1791–4.

5 Xerri C, Merzenich MM, Peterson BE & Jenkins W (1998) Plasticity of primary somatosensory cortex paralleling sensorimotor skill recovery from stroke in adult monkeys. *Journal of Neurophysiology,* **79**, 2119–48.

6 Johansson BB (2000) Brain plasticity and stroke rehabilitation. The Willis lecture. *Stroke,* **31**, 223–30.

7 Grabowski M, Sørensen JC, Mattsson B, Zimmer J & Johansson BB (1995) Influence of an enriched environment and cortical grafting on functional outcome in brain infarcts of adult rats. *Experimental Neurology,* **133**, 96–102.

8 Ohlsson A-L & Johansson BB (1995) Environment influences functional outcome of cerebral infarction in rats. *Stroke,* **26**, 644–9.

9 Johansson BB (1996) Functional outcome in rats transferred to an enriched environment 15 days after focal brain ischemia. *Stroke,* **27**, 324–6.

10 Johansson BB & Ohlsson A-L (1996) Environment, social interaction, and physical activity as determinants of functional outcome after cerebral infarction in the rat. *Experimental Neurology,* **139**, 322–7.

11 Mattsson B, Sørensen JC, Zimmer J & Johansson BB (1997) Neural grafting to experimental neocortical infarcts improves behavioral outcome and reduces thalamic atrophy in rats housed in an enriched but not in standard environments. *Stroke,* **28**, 1225–31.

12 Zeng J, Mattsson B, Schulz MK, Johansson BB & Sørensen JC (2000) Expression of zinc-positive cells and terminals in fetal neocortical homografts to adult rat depends on lesion type and rearing conditions. *Experimental Neurology,* **164**, 176–83.

13 Kinouchi H, Sharp FR, Chan PH, Koistinaho J, Sagar SM & Yoshimoto T (1994) Induction of c-*fos, junB,* c-*jun,* and *hsp70* mRNA in cortex, thalamus, basal ganglia, and hippocampus following middle cerebral artery occlusion. *Journal of Cerebral Blood Flow & Metabolism,* **14**, 808–17.

14 Akins PT, Liu PK & Hsu CY (1996) Immediate early gene expression in response to cerebral ischemia. Friend or foe? *Stroke,* **27**, 1682–7.

15 Koistinaho J & Hökfelt T (1997) Altered gene expression in brain ischemia. *Neuroreport,* **8**, i–viii.

16 Kinouchi H, Sharp FR, Chan PH, Mikawa S, Kamii H, Arai S & Yoshimoto T (1994) MK-801 inhibits the induction of immediate early genes in cerebral cortex, thalamus, and hippocampus, but not in substantia nigra following middle cerebral artery occlusion. *Neuroscience Letters*, **179**, 111–14.

17 Zhao LR, Mattsson B & Johansson BB (2000) Environmental influence on brain-derived neurotrophic factor messenger RNA expression after middle cerebral artery occlusion in spontaneously hypertensive rats. *Neuroscience*, **97**, 177–84.

18 Dahlqvist P, Zhao L, Johansson I-M, Mattsson B, Johansson BB, Seckl JR & Olsson T (1999) Environmental enrichment alters nerve growth factor-induced gene A and glucocorticoid receptor messenger RNA expression after middle cerebral artery occlusion in rats. *Neuroscience*, **93**, 527–35.

19 Qu M, Mittmann T, Luhmann HJ, Schleicher A & Zilles K (1998) Long-term changes of ionotropic glutamate and GABA receptors after unilateral permanent focal cerebral ischemia in the mouse brain. *Neuroscience*, **85**, 29–43.

20 Reinecke S, Lutzenburg M, Hagemann G, Bruehl C, Neumann-Haefelin T & Witte OW (1999) Electrophysiological transcortical diaschisis after middle cerebral artery occlusion (MCAO) in rats. *Neuroscience Letters*, **261**, 85–8.

21 Buchkremer-Ratzmann I, August M, Hagemann G & Witte OW (1996) Electrophysiological transcortical diaschisis after cortical photothrombosis in rat brain. *Stroke*, **27**, 1105–19.

22 Yuguchi T, Kohmura E, Sakaki T, Nonaka M, Yamada K, Yamashita T, Kishiguchi T, Sakaguchi T & Hayakawa T (1997) Expression of growth inhibitory factor mRNA after focal ischemia in rat brain. *Journal of Cerebral Blood Flow & Metabolism*, **17**, 745–52.

23 Calverley RK & Jones DG (1990) Contributions of dendritic spines and perforated synapses to synaptic plasticity. *Brain Research Reviews*, **15**, 215–49.

24 Eilers J & Konnerth A (1997) Dendritic signal integration. *Current Opinion in Neurobiology*, **7**, 385–90.

25 Harris KM (1999) Structure, development, and plasticity of dendritic spines. *Current Opinion in Neurobiology*, **9**, 343–8.

26 Fischer M, Kaech S, Knutti D & Matus A (1998) Rapid actin-based plasticity in dendritic spines. *Neuron*, **20**, 847–54.

27 Svoboda K, Denk W, Kleinfeld D & Tank DW (1997) In vivo dendritic calcium dynamics in neocortical pyramidal neurons. *Nature*, **385**, 161–5.

28 Kovalchuk Y, Eilers J, Lisman J & Konnerth A (2000) NMDA receptor-mediated subthreshold $Ca(2+)$ signals in spines of hippocampal neurons. *Journal of Neuroscience*, **20**, 1791–9.

29 Segev I & Rall W (1998) Excitable dendrites and spines: earlier theoretical insights elucidate recent direct observations. *Trends in Neurosciences*, **21**, 453–60.

30 Bennett EL, Diamond MC, Krech D & Rosenzweig MR (1964) Chemical and anatomical plasticity of brain. *Science*, **146**, 610–19.

31 Globus A, Rosenzweig MR, Bennett EL & Diamond MC (1973) Effects of differential experience on dendritic spine counts in rat cerebral cortex. *Journal of Comparative & Physiological Psychology*, **82**, 175–81.

32 Kolb B (1995) *Brain Plasticity and Behavior*. Mahwah, NJ: Lawrence Erlbaum.

33 Comery TA, Stamoudis CX, Irwin SA & Greenough WT (1996) Increased density of multiple-head dendritic spines on medium-sized spiny neurons of the striatum in rats reared in a complex environment. *Neurobiology of Learning and Memory*, **66**, 93–6.

34 Bryan GK & Riesen AH (1989) Deprived somatosensory-motor experience in stumptailed monkey neocortex: dendritic spine density and dendritic branching of layer IIIB pyramidal cells. [erratum: *Journal of Comparative Neurology*, **289**, 709, 1989] *Journal of Comparative Neurology*, **286**, 208–17.

35 Harris KM, Jensen FE & Tsao B (1992) Three-dimensional structure of dendritic spines and synapses in rat hippocampus (CA1) at postnatal day 15 and adult ages: implications for the maturation of synaptic physiology and long-term potentiation. *Journal of Neuroscience*, **12**, 2685–705.

36 Belichenko PV & Dahlström A (1995) Mapping of the human brain in normal and pathological situations: the single cell and fiber level, employing Lucifer yellow microinjections, immunofluorescence, and 3D confocal laser scanning reconstruction. *Neurosci Protocols*, Elsevier Science, Amsterdam, 95–050–03–01–30.

37 Johansson BB & Belichenko P (2001) Environmental influence on neuronal and dendritic spine plasticity after permanent focal brain ischemia. In *Maturation Phenomenon in Cerebral Ischemia IV*, eds. U Ito & NG Bazan, pp. 77–83. Berlin: Springer-Verlag.

38 Cheng HW, Rafols JA, Goshgarian HG, Anavi Y, Tong J & McNeill TH (1997) Differential spine loss and regrowth of striatal neurons following multiple forms of deafferentation: a Golgi study. *Experimental Neurology*, **147**, 287–98.

39 Porter LL & White EL (1986) Synaptic connections of callosal projection neurons in the vibrissal region of mouse primary motor cortex: an electron microscopic/horseradish peroxidase study. *Journal of Comparative Neurology*, **248**, 573–87.

40 Jones EG & Powell TPS (1970) An electron microscopic study of the laminar pattern and mode of termination of afferent fibre pathways in the somatic sensory cortex of the cat. *Philosophical Transactions of the Royal Society of London. Series B: Biological Sciences*, **257**, 45–62.

41 Hayama T & Ogawa H (1997) Regional differences of callosal connections in the granular zones of the primary somatosensory cortex in rats. *Brain Research Bulletin*, **43**, 341–7.

42 Wolff JR, Eins S, Holzgraefe M & Záborszky L (1981) The temporo-spatial course of degeneration after cutting cortico-cortical connections in adult rats. *Cell and Tissue Research*, **214**, 303–21.

43 Withers GS & Greenough WT (1989) Reach training selectively alters dendritic branching in subpopulations of layer II–III pyramids in rat motor-somatosensory forelimb cortex. *Neuropsychologia*, **27**, 61–9.

44 Hess G, Aizenman CD & Donoghue JP (1996) Conditions for the induction of long-term potentiation in layer II/III horizontal connections of the rat motor cortex. *Journal of Neurophysiology*, **75**, 1765–78.

45 Vernadakis A (1996) Glia-neuron intercommunications and synaptic plasticity. *Progress in Neurobiology*, **49**, 185–214.

46 Pfrieger FW & Barres BA (1996) New views on synapse–glia interactions. *Current Opinion in Neurobiology*, **6**, 615–21.

47 Jones TA, Hawrylak N & Greenough WT (1996) Rapid laminar-dependent changes in GFAP immunoreactive astrocytes in the visual cortex of rats reared in a complex environment. *Psychoneuroendocrinology*, **21**, 189–201.

48 Jones TA & Greenough WT (1996) Ultrastructural evidence for increased contact between astrocytes and synapses in rats reared in a complex environment. *Neurobiology of Learning and Memory*, **65**, 48–56.

49 Kempermann G, Brandon EP & Gage FH (1998) Environmental stimulation of 129/SvJ mice causes increased cell proliferation and neurogenesis in the adult dentate gyrus. *Current Biology*, **8**, 939–42.

50 Nilsson M, Perfilieva E, Johansson U, Orwar O & Eriksson PS (1999) Enriched environment increases neurogenesis in the adult rat dentate gyrus and improves spatial memory. *Journal of Neurobiology*, **39**, 569–78.

51 Johansson BB, Jadbäck G, Norrving B, Widner H & Wiklund I (1992) Evaluation of long-term functional status in first-ever stroke patients in a defined population. *Scandinavian Journal of Rehabilitation Medicine Supplement*, **26**, 105–14.

Part IX

Magnetic resonance imaging in clinical stroke

Co-Chairs: Michael E. Moseley & Gregory W. Albers

28

Magnetic resonance imaging in stroke trials

Steven Warach

National Institute of Neurological Disorders & Stroke, Bethesda, MD

Introduction

The disappointingly slow progress in developing effective therapies for ischemic stroke has led to a re-evaluation of the strategies for stroke drug development and the methods used in clinical trials. Magnetic resonance imaging (MRI) techniques have been proposed and have begun to be used in stroke trials as a means of optimizing patient selection and as a direct measure of the effect of treatments on the brain.

One objective in all clinical trials is the selection of a sample sufficiently homogeneous to reduce the statistical variance of the data, thereby optimizing the sensitivity of the design to detecting a therapeutic response, while remaining representative of the population of interest. Ischemic stroke trials have traditionally sought to limit the range of disease studied according to one or more of several dimensions, such as clinical severity at the time of enrollment, exclusion of non-ischemic causes for the clinical syndrome, lesion location and vascular territory, stroke mechanism and comorbidities. In the modern era of stroke clinical trials these dimensions have been assessed by clinical criteria at the bedside usually aided by the exclusion of cerebral hemorrhage or other non-ischemic pathology by non-contrast computed tomography (CT) scan as the only imaging tool required. Except for the trials of intravenous recombinant tissue plasminogen activator in the treatment of ischemic stroke within the first 3 hours [1], this traditional approach has led to no approved therapies for stroke, a great degree of pessimism with regard to thrombolysis beyond 3 hours and to the concept of neuroprotection in stroke.

Since several imaging modalities may provide more accurate and specific information than a clinical assessment and a normal CT scan, it has been proposed that positive imaging diagnoses would improve patient selection toward the goal of a more optimal target sample for stroke clinical trials, a sample selected on the basis of an imaging diagnosis of a pathology that the drug is hypothesized to treat, e.g., an arterial occlusion or perfusion defect for thrombolytic drugs. This principle has been supported by the results of the intra-arterial pro-urokinase stroke study, PROACT II [2]. Prior attempts to prove the efficacy of thrombolysis initiated between 3 and 6 hours from onset without a positive diagnosis of arterial occlusion or perfusion defect have not been successful [3–5]. However, in PROACT II [2] patients were selected based on evidence of arterial occlusions at the M1 or M2 levels of the middle cerebral artery by conventional arteriography, and a significant clinical benefit was observed when thrombolysis was initiated up to 6 hours from symptom onset (median time to treat was 5.3 hours). Whereas, trials of intravenous thrombolysis between 3 and 6 hours in a general sample of ischemic stroke patients were not positive, selection of the optimal subgroup by imaging diagnosis of the appropriate arterial lesion was an effective strategy in this time period for PROACT II. This study contradicted the increasingly promoted hypothesis that treatment of stroke by thrombolysis (or any therapy) beyond 3 hours would not be successful. Selection of the optimal target population by angiography led to slower recruitment and a more expensive trial, but to a successful result. The results of that trial suggested that a more prolonged study duration, increased expense and potential delay in treatment to complete a screening test may be justified by the greater chance of demonstrating therapeutic success using a more homogeneous and rational selection of patients.

The appeal of MRI methods is that, whereas the standard CT scan examination of acute ischemic stroke will typically appear normal in the first hours after stroke onset, the methods of magnetic resonance angiography, perfusion-weighted imaging (PWI) and diffusion-weighted imaging (DWI) provide information on arterial patency, tissue blood flow and parenchymal injury from the earliest times after onset of ischemic symptoms in a brief, non-invasive examination. DWI detects tissue injury within minutes of ischemia, has high sensitivity and specificity for the diagnosis of ischemic stroke and permits measurement of lesion volumes that correlate with clinical severity and prognosis [6–12]. Untreated, the lesion seen with DWI typically enlarges over hours to days and will progress to infarction. PWI depicts focal cerebral ischemia. In the majority of cases the volume of ischemic tissue seen with PWI is greater than the region of parenchymal injury evident on DWI and this diffusion–perfusion mismatch is considered to be a marker of the ischemic penumbra, the tissue at greatest risk for infarct progression [13–21]. Furthermore, increasing theoretical, experimental and clinical evidence suggests that MRI using magnetic susceptibility-weighted pulse sequences may be sensitive to the early detection of hemorrhage [22–24]. Although prospective comparisons of MRI and CT for sensitivity to hemorrhage detection have yet to be reported, the proper acquisition and interpretation of MRI can eliminate the need for a screening CT scan and regain some of the time spent on adding an MRI examination to a screening evaluation. The target pathology revealed by MRI also represents the

Table 28.1. Proposed uses of MRI (DWI, PWI, MRA) as a selection tool in stroke trials

Positive radiological diagnosis of ischemic lesion by DWI
Select by location (e.g., cortical, MCA territory, etc.)
Select by size (DWI)
Select by perfusion defect (PWI, MRA) for reperfusion therapies
Select by diffusion–perfusion mismatch (DWI, PWI) for neuroprotective drugs
Exclude if confounding subacute or chronic lesions

Notes:
MRI, magnetic resonance imaging; DWI, diffusion-weighted imaging; PWI, perfusion-weighted imaging; MRA, magnetic resonance angiography; MCA, middle cerebral artery.

biological marker of the disease that can serve as a surrogate measure for assessing the effects of a therapy. Three potential uses of MRI in clinical trials have been proposed: patient selection, proof of pharmacological principle and outcome measure.

Patient selection

In proposing MRI as a selection criterion (Table 28.1), the goal would be a sample based upon a positive imaging diagnosis of a pathology rationally linked to the drug's mechanisms of action. Requiring a positive diagnosis of acute ischemic injury by DWI would ideally assure that no patients with diagnoses mimicking stroke are included in the sample, a desirable objective unachievable in trials using bedside impression and normal CT scans as the basis of inclusion. The goal of image-based patient selection is to narrow the range of patient's characteristics, leading to a more homogeneous sample, reducing within-group variance and increasing the statistical power of the experimental design to demonstrate efficacy. Optimal patient selection would be based on positive imaging evidence of the ischemic pathology that the therapy has been developed to treat. The simplest use as an inclusion criterion would include the presence of a lesion on DWI to increase the diagnostic certainty of ischemic stroke (Figure 28.1). For reperfusion therapies, the optimal target of therapy would be patients with evidence of an arterial occlusion or hypoperfusion (Figure 28.2) [17,25]. For neuroprotective drugs, optimal selection of patients would be acute lesions involving the cerebral cortex and with a larger region of hypoperfusion, the diffusion–perfusion mismatch indicative of tissue at risk for infarction (Figure 28.3, Table 28.2). Patients might also be excluded from the trial during screening if subacute or chronic lesions are found that may confound measurements of lesion volumes or clinical severity as outcome variables. Because of a relatively, large error of measurement associated with small lesions [26], lesions larger than a minimum volume (e.g., $5\,cm^3$) may be desirable.

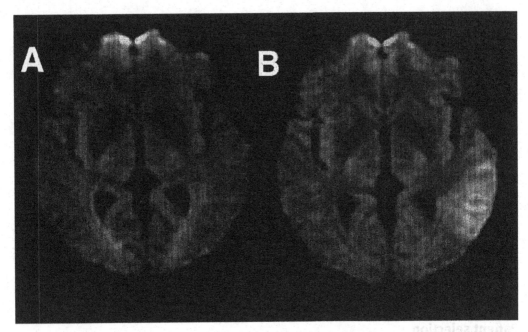

Figure 28.1 DWI of a 3 hour stroke. (A) Fluid-attenuated inversion recovery image without diffusion-weighting shows no acute lesion. (B) DWI demonstrates the acute lesion as a region of hyperintensity (brightness) in the left temporal lobe.

Furthermore, an upper limit of lesion volume at enrollment would permit an opportunity for lesion growth and may better differentiate the effect on lesion size of an effective treatment from a placebo. Selection of patients by DWI is also optimally suited for using the change in lesion volume as a direct measure of the neuroprotective effect of the drug.

Proof of pharmacological principle using MRI as a marker of response to therapy: replicating the preclinical experiment in patients

Before an experimental stroke therapy is brought from the laboratory to clinical trial it is necessary to demonstrate that the treatment causes reduction in lesion volume in experimental models. The fundamental premise of drug discovery and development in acute stroke is that treatments that reduce lesion size are those most likely to lead to clinical benefit. In clinical trial programs that depend solely on clinical end-points as indices of benefit, drugs may be brought to phase III testing, costing several years and tens of millions of dollars, without the slightest evidence that the drug will have the therapeutic effect observed in the experimental model. Only a safe and acceptable dose must be demonstrated by the end of phase II. However, the question of whether the treatment causes reduction of lesion volume

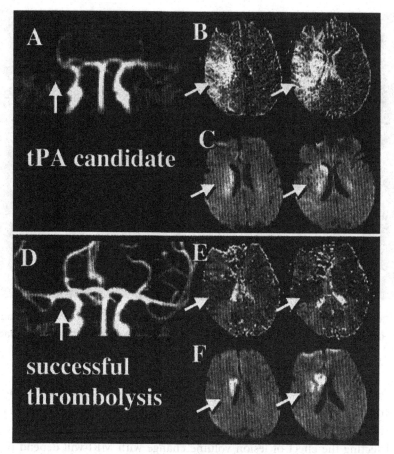

Figure 28.2 Example of MRI-based selection for thrombolysis. (A) Magnetic resonance angiography demonstrates right middle cerebral artery occlusion (arrow). (B) Two representative PWI slices demonstrate delayed relative mean transit time in the entire right middle cerebral artery territory. (C) Two corresponding DWI slices demonstrate parenchymal injury only in the deeper parts of the right middle cerebral artery territory (arrows), a diffusion–perfusion mismatch. After recombinant tissue plasminogen activator (tPA) therapy, recanalization of the right middle cerebral artery is seen (D), with normalization of perfusion (E, arrows) and limitation of the parenchymal damage (F, arrows).

may be answerable in the study of 100 to 200 patients in phase II, whereas five to ten times as many patients are typically tested in phase III studies in order to evaluate the treatment with clinical end-points. Thus a phase II MRI end-point trial to replicate the preclinical experiment in a patient population may be a rational and cost-effective basis for deciding whether to proceed with phase III testing. A positive lesion outcome study in late phase II would be supportive of the decision to proceed with phase III trials.

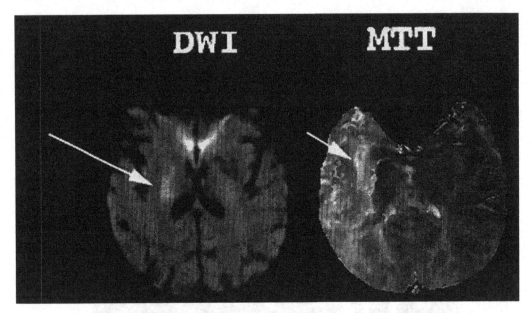

Figure 28.3 The diffusion–perfusion mismatch. A small lesion (arrow) on the DWI in a 3 hour stroke relative to the larger PWI abnormality on a relative mean transit time (MTT) image.

MRI measurements have proven to be markers of clinical severity measured by stroke scales [11,15,27,28], and changes in lesion volume over time are associated with change in clinical severity (Table 28.3) [29]. The exact sample size required for detecting the effect of lesion volume change with MRI will depend upon many factors in the design of a trial. The citicoline MRI trial [29], with approximately 40 evaluable patients per group, approached but did not reach significance. Estimates based on that study are that 58 patients per treatment arm would have been sufficient to demonstrate a neuroprotective effect, a sample size compatible with typical phase II sample sizes. That study and natural history samples suggest that sample sizes of 50 to 100 should be sufficient to demonstrate a neuroprotective effect on lesion volume in patients.

Surrogate end-point in phase III trials to support drug registration

It is proposed that a treatment emergent advantage on a measure of lesion volume is a surrogate of clinical benefit for stroke trials (Table 28.4). The rationale for the use of lesion volume as a surrogate measure in stroke trials may be summarized as follows. In animal models, lesion volume reduction is both necessary and sufficient evidence of neuroprotection. The clinical benefit for neuroprotective drugs is mediated through a reduction in cell death and brain tissue loss. Drugs that reduce infarct volume are the ones most likely to cause clinical benefit.

Table 28.2. The diffusion–perfusion mismatch

MRI marker of the ischemic penumbra
The strongest predictor of lesion growth from baseline
Present in approximately 80% of MCA territory strokes out to 6 hours poststroke
Distinction of benign hypoperfusion from true tissue at risk not yet possible prospectively

Notes:
MRI, magnetic resonance imaging; MCA, middle cerebral artery.

Table 28.3. MRI as a biomarker of clinical status

Improved?	% patients with lesion decrease**	Median change* (cm³)	Mean change (SE)** (cm³)
Yes	74	−2.8	3.8 (3.8)
No	36	3.7	25.5 (6.8)

Notes:
* $P<0.01$; ** $P<0.001$; SE, standard error.
Acute lesion volumes correlated with clinical scales and with final lesion volumes. Strong association of reduction in lesion volume with clinical improvement: week 12 minus baseline lesion volume change related to clinical improvement ($n=81$). (From ref. 29).

Table 28.4. Magnetic resonance imaging as outcome measure

Necessary but not sufficient evidence of protective effect
Protective effect may be attenuation of expected lesion growth or partial DWI lesion reversal
Clinical benefit unlikely if no protective effect on lesion volume (go/no go decision at phase II)
Smaller sample size requirements than for typical clinical end-points (~50 to 100 per arm)
May be confirmatory evidence supporting positive clinical end-point trial for regulatory
   approval

The factors required for validation of MRI as a surrogate marker are summarized in Table 28.5. The first four of these requirements have been met (see discussion and references above). Confirmation of the validity of many of these features of DWI and PWI in acute stroke has recently come from the first prospective multicenter stroke trial using MRI as an inclusion and primary outcome measure, the citicoline MRI stroke trial [29]. In that study identical MRI hardware and software were used in 17 centers across the USA to study 100 patients with ischemic stroke within 24 hours from onset. The patients were randomly assigned to citicoline (500 mg/day) or placebo. Diffusion and perfusion MRI were obtained prior to treatment, at 1 week and at 12 weeks. Image data processing and volumetric

Table 28.5. Requirements of a validated surrogate for DWI and PWI

To fully establish diffusion and perfusion MRI as a useful tool and validate surrogate in stroke trials several conditions need to be satisfied (the first four have been met, see text):

1. DWI and PWI as biological markers of the disease process in ischemic stroke
2. The tests are sensitive and specific for the diagnosis of stroke in patients
3. Lesion volumes correlate with clinical function as measured by clinical rating scales, predict outcome and covary over time with clinical severity
4. Rational covariates affecting lesion volumes identified
5. Proven utility in identifying effective treatments in trials

Notes:
DWI, diffusion-weighted imaging; PWI, perfusion-weighted imaging; MRI, magnetic resonance imaging.

analysis were performed at a single central laboratory using a single expert reader blinded to each patient's clinical severity and treatment assignment. The primary MRI inclusion criterion was a lesion volume of 1 to $120\,cm^3$ in the middle cerebral artery territory gray matter. The primary efficacy end-point was a change in the lesion volume from pretreatment to week 12. Although the primary efficacy end-point of an effect of citicoline on lesion growth was numerically different (181% increase in lesion volume in patients given the placebo vs. 34% increase for citicoline-treated patients), it was not statistically significant. However, the study replicated the findings of other investigations regarding the relationship of MRI-derived lesion volumes to patients' clinical status. Acute lesion volumes by DWI in 100 patients significantly correlated with acute clinical severity on the NIH Stroke Scale (NIHSS) scores ($r=0.64$) and with chronic lesion volume ($r=0.79$); the chronic lesion volume by T_2-weighted MRI significantly correlated with the chronic NIHSS score ($r=0.63$). The strongest predictor of change in lesion size from baseline in the 81 patients who completed their week 12 assessment was the size of the perfusion abnormality ($P<0.0001$ by covariance analysis). The volume change over the 12 weeks of observation was significantly related to the patient's clinical improvement. Patients meeting the protocol-specified criterion of clinical improvement (improvement on the NIHSS score of seven points or more) had a significantly more favorable response on the lesion volume change outcome variable than those who did not improve. The differentiation of improved from not improved was present whether the lesion volume change was assessed as an absolute decrease (74% vs. 36%), median change ($-2.8\,cm^3$ vs. $3.7\,cm^3$) or mean (standard error) change (3.8 (3.8) cm^3 vs. 25.5 (6.8) cm^3) (Table 28.5). This prospective multicenter, centrally analyzed trial confirmed the value of MRI as a marker of disease severity

Table 28.6. Validation of MRI lesion volumes as a surrogate outcome: explanations of possible discordance between clinical and surrogate lesion volume measures

---

If clinical end-point shows a benefit but lesion volume does not:
    Imaging methods are insensitive to neuroprotection
    Clinical benefit not mediated by neuroprotection

If lesion volume shows a benefit but the clinical end-point does not:
    Trial design or clinical measures are insensitive to detecting a clinical effect
    Toxicity offsets neuroprotective effect

Notes:
MRI, magnetic resonance imaging.

and progression in stroke trials and indicated that the change in MRI lesion size is likely to predict clinical improvement in clinical trials.

The fifth criterion of validation, the concordance of effects on clinical outcomes and surrogate outcomes, remains to be demonstrated. Effective drugs will show benefit on both clinical and imaging outcome measures. The citicoline trials provide support for this, wherein trends on both clinical and imaging outcome measures have been observed [29–32]. Ineffective drugs will show benefit on neither clinical nor imaging outcome measures. The latter has been found for the GAIN neuroprotective trials, which showed no effect on clinical or MRI surrogate outcomes [33,34]. This comparison is only meaningful if studies are optimally designed and equally powered to show the effect on their respective outcome measures, i.e., the optimal sample size for imaging studies may be too small to show clinical effects. Possible explanations for discordant clinical vs. surrogate marker results are listed in Table 28.6.

The concept that improvement on a measure of brain lesion volume is a proper surrogate outcome for destructive central nervous system diseases has been already accepted by academic and regulatory communities alike. Approval of β-interferon for the treatment of multiple sclerosis was based in part upon lesion volume as a surrogate marker of disease activity even though the surrogate was not considered to be fully validated. A surrogate outcome measure in clinical trials does not need to be fully validated as a condition of drug approval. Recent changes to the Federal Food Drug and Cosmetic Act, which regulates the Food and Drug Administration (FDA) approval process, have specified a fast track drug designation to expedite review for drugs that have "the potential to address unmet medical needs for serious and life-threatening conditions" [35]. Drugs to treat stroke have fallen under this designation. Ordinarily a drug must have a beneficial effect on a clinical end-point or on a validated surrogate end-point to demonstrate effectiveness. The new regulations state that a drug "may be approved if it has an effect on a surrogate end-point that is *reasonably likely to predict clinical benefit*. Such surrogate end-points are considered *not to be validated* because, while suggestive of clinical benefit, their relationship to clinical outcomes, such as morbidity and mortality, is not proven" (italics added) [35]. The issue with regard to MRI as a surrogate in stroke trials is whether it is *reasonably likely to predict clinical benefit*. The hypothesis that neuroprotection, the restriction of infarct volume, is reasonably likely to be clinically beneficial to patients is the premise of virtually all acute stroke drugs being developed. The clinical data discussed above support its value as a surrogate.

Strict validation must eventually be proven, but as we see from FDA regulations it is no longer required in order to use lesion volume by MRI as a surrogate outcome in stroke trials. A benefit on the surrogate may be acceptable as an independent source of confirmatory data in support of a clinical benefit seen in a single trial. The question, therefore, is no longer *whether* MRI surrogates should be used in trials, but *how* they should be used.

Industry-sponsored MRI-based stroke trials

The pharmaceutical industry has taken the initiative in investigating this final step in validation. The results of several industry-sponsored drug trials using MRI as a surrogate will be known over the next several years, and those studies should provide the most decisive information regarding the utility of MRI as a surrogate outcome measure in stroke trials. Three multicenter randomized clinical trials using MRI as a key selection and outcome variable have been completed and reported. Several others are in progress or being planned.

Conclusion

There have been concerns raised in the past that the use of MRI in stroke clinical trails is impractical for technical and logistical reasons (e.g., scan duration and availability). The practical limitations have disappeared with the widespread availability of ultrafast echoplanar imaging with diffusion and perfusion capability on commercial MRI scanners. A highly motivated, well-coordinated center can perform emergency diffusion and perfusion MRI with a latency to scan and a scanning session duration comparable to that of emergency head CT. There are now over 100 centers worldwide capable of and experienced in performing these types of acute MRI examinations. Key design issues with regard to the use of diffusion and perfusion MRI in stroke trials are proposed in Table 28.7. MRI-based recruitment into trials with a time window of 6 hours have proven feasible, as has specific selection based on lesion size, location and the diffusion–perfusion mismatch. As

Table 28.7. Proposed features of clinical trials

Imaging methods
    DWI, PWI, MRA, T_2/FLAIR

Selection criteria
    Cortical DWI lesion >5 cm^3
    Diffusion–perfusion mismatch
    No pre-existing lesions in same vascular territory

Outcome variable
    Change in lesion volume, pretreatment to chronic (3 months)

Data analysis
    Transformed lesion volume (percentage change, log, cube root)
    Covariance analysis on baseline variables:
        NIHSS score, volume of hypoperfusion, initial lesion volume

---

Notes:
DWI, diffusion-weighted imaging; PWI, perfusion-weighted imaging; MRA, magnetic resonance angiography; FLAIR, fluid-attenuated inversion recovery; NIHSS, National Institutes of Health Stroke Scale.

the field of stroke clinical trials examines opportunities for improving trial design, positive imaging diagnoses in patient selection and use of imaging as treatment assessments are likely to assume increasingly useful roles. Patient selection and outcomes based exclusively on clinical assessment and non-hemorrhagic CT scans may no longer be appropriate for all trials.

REFERENCES

1 The National Institute of Neurological Disorders; Stroke rtPA Stroke Study Group (1995) Tissue plasminogen activator for acute ischemic stroke. *New England Journal of Medicine*, 333, 1581–7.

2 Furlan A, Higashida R, Wechsler L, Gent M, Rowley H, Kase C, Pessin M, Ahuja A, Callahan F, Clark WM, Silver F & Rivera F (1999) Intra-arterial prourokinase for acute ischemic stroke. The PROACT II study: a randomized controlled trial. *Journal of the American Medical Association*, 282, 2003–11.

3 Hacke W, Kaste M, Fieschi C, von Kummer R, Davalos A, Meier D, Larrue V, Bluhmki E, Davis S, Donnan G, Schneider D, Diez-Tejedor E & Trouillas P (1998) Randomised double-blind placebo-controlled trial of thrombolytic therapy with intravenous alteplase in acute ischaemic stroke (ECASS II). *Lancet*, 352, 1245–51.

4 Hacke W, Kaste M, Fieschi C, Toni D, Lesaffre E, von Kummer R, et al. (1995) Intravenous thrombolysis with recombinant tissue plasminogen activator for acute hemispheric stroke. The European Cooperative Acute Stroke Study (ECASS). *Journal of the American Medical Association*, **274**, 1017–25.

5 Clark WM, Wissman S, Albers GW, Jhamandas JH, Madden KP & Hamilton S (1999) Recombinant tissue-type plasminogen activator (alteplase) for ischemic stroke 3 to 5 hours after symptom onset. The ATLANTIS Study: a randomized controlled trial. *Journal of the American Medical Association*, **282**, 2019–26.

6 Moseley ME, Cohen Y, Mintorovitch J, Chileuitt L, Shimizu H, Kucharczyk J, Wendland MF & Weinstein PR (1990) Early detection of regional cerebral ischemia in cats: comparison of diffusion- and T2-weighted MRI and spectroscopy. *Magnetic Resonance in Medicine*, **14**, 330–46.

7 Lovblad KO, Laubach HJ, Baird AE, Curtin F, Schlaug G, Edelman RR & Warach S (1998) Clinical experience with diffusion-weighted MR in patients with acute stroke. *AJNR. American Journal of Neuroradiology*, **19**, 1061–6.

8 Warach S, Chien D, Li W, Ronthal M & Edelman RR (1992) Fast magnetic resonance diffusion-weighted imaging of acute human stroke. [erratum: *Neurology*, **42**, 2192, 1992] *Neurology*, **42**, 1717–23.

9 Warach S, Gaa J, Siewert B, Wielopolski P & Edelman RR (1995) Acute human stroke studied by whole brain echo planar diffusion-weighted magnetic resonance imaging. *Annals of Neurology*, **37**, 231–41.

10 Baird AE & Warach S (1998) Magnetic resonance imaging of acute stroke. [erratum: *Journal of Cerebral Blood Flow & Metabolism*, **18**, 1046, 1998] *Journal of Cerebral Blood Flow & Metabolism*, **18**, 583–609.

11 Lovblad KO, Baird AE, Schlaug G, Benfield A, Siewert B, Voetsch B, Connor A. Burzynski C, Edelman RR & Warach S (1997) Ischemic lesion volumes in acute stroke by diffusion-weighted magnetic resonance imaging correlate with clinical outcome. *Annals of Neurology*, **42**, 164–70.

12 Warach S, Dashe JF & Edelman RR (1996) Clinical outcome in ischemic stroke predicted by early diffusion-weighted and perfusion magnetic resonance imaging: a preliminary analysis. *Journal of Cerebral Blood Flow & Metabolism*, **16**, 53–9.

13 Barber PA, Darby DG, Desmond PM, Yang Q, Gerraty RP, Jolley D, Donnan GA, Tress BM & Davis SM (1998) Prediction of stroke outcome with echoplanar perfusion- and diffusion-weighted MRI. *Neurology*, **51**, 418–26.

14 Barber PA, Davis SM, Darby DG, Desmond PM, Gerraty RP, Yang Q, Jolley D, Donnan GA & Tress BM (1999) Absent middle cerebral artery flow predicts the presence and evolution of the ischemic penumbra. *Neurology*, **52**, 1125–32.

15 Beaulieu C, de Crespigny A, Tong DC, Moseley ME, Albers GW & Marks MP (1999) Longitudinal magnetic resonance imaging study of perfusion and diffusion in stroke: evolution of lesion volume and correlation with clinical outcome. *Annals of Neurology*, **46**, 568–78.

16 Darby DG, Barber PA, Gerraty RP, Desmond PM, Yang Q, Parsons M, Li T, Tress BM & Davis SM (1999) Pathophysiological topography of acute ischemia by combined diffusion-weighted and perfusion MRI. *Stroke*, **30**, 2043–52.

17 Marks MP, Tong DC, Beaulieu C, Albers GW, de Crespigny A & Moseley ME (1999) Evaluation of early reperfusion and i.v. tPA therapy using diffusion- and perfusion-weighted MRI. *Neurology*, **52**, 1792–8.

18 Warach S, Li W, Ronthal M & Edelman RR (1992) Acute cerebral ischemia: evaluation with dynamic contrast-enhanced MR imaging and MR angiography. *Radiology*, **182**, 41–7.

19 Schlaug G, Benfield A, Baird AE, Siewert B, Lovblad KO, Parker RA, Edelman RR & Warach S (1999) The ischemic penumbra: operationally defined by diffusion and perfusion MRI. *Neurology*, **53**, 1528–37.

20 Baird AE, Benfield A, Schlaug G, Siewert B, Lovblad KO, Edelman RR & Warach S (1997) Enlargement of human cerebral ischemic lesion volumes measured by diffusion-weighted magnetic resonance imaging. *Annals of Neurology*, **41**, 581–9.

21 Tong DC, Yenari MA, Albers GW, O'Brien M, Marks MP & Moseley ME (1998) Correlation of perfusion- and diffusion-weighted MRI with NIHSS score in acute (<6.5 hour) ischemic stroke. *Neurology*, **50**, 864–70.

22 Linfante I, Llinas RH, Caplan LR & Warach S (1999) MRI features of intracerebral hemorrhage within 2 hours from symptom onset. *Stroke*, **30**, 2263–7.

23 Schellinger PD, Jansen O, Fiebach JB, Hacke W & Sartor K (1999) A standardized MRI stroke protocol: comparison with CT in hyperacute intracerebral hemorrhage. *Stroke*, **30**, 765–8.

24 Patel MR, Edelman RR & Warach S (1996) Detection of hyperacute primary intraparenchymal hemorrhage by magnetic resonance imaging. *Stroke*, **27**, 2321–4.

25 Schellinger PD, Jansen O, Fiebach JB, Heiland S, Steiner T, Schwab S, Pohlers O, Ryssel H, Sartor K & Hacke W (2000) Monitoring intravenous recombinant tissue plasminogen activator thrombolysis for acute ischemic stroke with diffusion and perfusion MRI. *Stroke*, **31**, 1318–28.

26 Laubach HJ, Jakob PM, Loevblad KO, Baird AE, Bovo MP, Edelman RR & Warach S (1998) A phantom for diffusion-weighted imaging of acute stroke. *Journal of Magnetic Resonance Imaging*, **8**, 1349–54.

27 Baird AE, Lovblad KO, Dashe JF, Connor A, Burzynski C, Schlaug G, et al. (2000) Clinical correlations of diffusion and perfusion lesion volumes in acute ischemic stroke. *Cerebrovascular Diseases*, **10**, 441–8.

28 van Everdingen KJ, van der Grond J, Kappelle LJ, Ramos LM & Mali WP (1998) Diffusion-weighted magnetic resonance imaging in acute stroke. *Stroke*, **29**, 1783–90.

29 Warach S, Pettigrew LC, Dashe JF, Pullicino P, Lefkowitz DM, Sabounjian L, et al. (2000) Effect of citicoline on ischemic lesions as measured by diffusion-weighted magnetic resonance imaging. *Annals of Neurology*, **48**, 713–22.

30 Clark WM, Williams BJ, Selzer KA, Zweifler RM, Sabounjian LA & Gammans RE (1999) A randomized efficacy trial of citicoline in patients with acute ischemic stroke. *Stroke*, **30**, 2592–7.

31 Clark W, Gunion-Rinker L, Lessov N & Hazel K (1998) Citicoline treatment for experimental intracerebral hemorrhage in mice. *Stroke*, **29**, 2136–40.

32 Warach S & Sabounjian LA (2000) ECCO 2000 study of citicoline for treatment of acute ischemic stroke: effects on infarct volumes measured by MRI. *Stroke*, **31**, 42.

33 Lees KR, Asplund K, Carolei A, Davis SM, Diener H-C, Kaste M, Orgogozo J-M, Whitehead J, for the GAIN International Investigators (2000) Glycine antagonist (gavestinel) in neuroprotection (GAIN International) in patients with acute stroke: a randomised controlled trial. *Lancet*, 355, 1949–54.

34 Warach S, Kaste M & Fisher M (2000) The effect of GV150526 on ischemic lesion volume: the GAIN Americas and GAIN international MRI substudy. *Neurology*, 54 Suppl 3, A87–A88.

35 US House of Representatives (1997) Prescription drug user fee reauthorization and drug regulatory modernization act of 1997. *House of Representatives Report*, 105th Congress, 1st Session, Report 105–310, Section 4, pp. 54–56. Washington, DC.

29

Disappearing deficits and disappearing lesions: diffusion/perfusion MRI in transient ischemic attack and intra-arterial thrombolysis

Jeffrey L. Saver[1] & Chelsea Kidwell[2]

[1,2] UCLA Stroke Center, Los Angeles, CA

Introduction

The brain responds dynamically to ischemic insult. A brief period of focal ischemia may disrupt synaptic transmission and produce transient neurological deficits without causing permanent tissue injury. A somewhat more severe ischemic insult may sufficiently disrupt the cellular energetic state to impair maintenance of ionic gradients across cell membranes, producing cytotoxic edema. Early restoration of blood flow may permit cellular re-energization and restoration of ionic gradients, with edema resolution. However, some cells that initially restore membrane integrity experience a late, secondary stage of injury and delayed cell death. These findings, previously elucidated in animal models, have now been demonstrated for the first time in acute human brain ischemia by diffusion magnetic resonance imaging (MRI).

Standard brain imaging techniques, computed tomography (CT) and conventional MRI, are insensitive to these dynamic and regionally varying neural parenchymal responses to tissue ischemia. In contrast, the novel MRI technique of diffusion imaging permits visualization of these critical tissue processes, affording new insights into the physiopathology of human cerebral ischemia. We will here review recent diffusion MRI findings in two settings of transient cerebral ischemic insult in human patients: spontaneous transient ischemic attacks and thrombolysis-induced cerebral reperfusion.

Transient ischemic attack

Transient ischemic attacks (TIAs) are defined as neurological symptoms due to focal cerebral ischemia that resolve completely within 24 hours [1]. The 24 hour cutoff employed in this definition was first promulgated in the 1950s, based on limited data [2]. Accumulating evidence suggests that this traditional 24 hour operational definition is imprecise, and at times misleading. Large-scale studies have altered our understanding of the typical duration of TIAs, showing that most resolve within 10 to 60 minutes rather than lasting several hours [3,4]. Imaging studies have challenged the simplistic assumption that because clinical symptoms of a TIA resolve, significant ischemic tissue injury must not occur. Several studies have shown that many patients meeting the clinical criteria for a TIA demonstrate neuroanatomically relevant infarcts on standard neuroimaging (2% to 48% using CT [5–10], 31% to 39% using conventional MRI [11,12]). The probability of finding an infarct on imaging appears to increase when the TIA persists longer than 1 hour.

Waxman and Toole [13] coined the phrase "cerebral infarction with transient signs" to describe patients who meet the clinical criteria for a TIA but show a relevant infarct on imaging. Rapid clinical resolution in these individuals reflects neuroplasticity, with rapid recruitment and utilization of alternative circuits to replace those injured by ischemia, not absence of any tissue injury. Conversely, the rare patient may be encountered who has clinical deficits lasting longer than 24 hours but without concurrent tissue infarction. These observations have called into question the utility of the 24 hour cutoff, and indeed of any definition of a TIA based solely on clinical manifestations and an arbitrarily assigned time window, rather than tissue changes and physiological processes.

We and others have hypothesized that diffusion MRI would provide a more sensitive and specific evaluation of ischemic insult in TIA patients compared with standard CT and MRI studies [14–16]. We studied consecutive TIA patients using diffusion MRI and compared them to a group of contemporary patients with completed stroke to determine: (i) the incidence of diffusion-weighted imaging (DWI) and apparent diffusion coefficient (ADC) abnormalities in TIA patients compared with standard T_2-weighted MRI sequences; (ii) whether the presence of an abnormality on diffusion MRI correlates with the duration, location or mechanism of symptoms; (iii) whether the diffusion MRI signature in a TIA differs from that in completed stroke; and (iv) the impact of diffusion imaging data on clinical diagnosis of TIA localization and mechanism [14].

UCLA study

Clinical, conventional MRI and diffusion MRI data were collected on consecutive patients presenting to the University of California at Los Angeles (UCLA) Medical Center over a 6 month period with symptoms of a transient ischemic attack. TIAs were defined as symptoms of presumed ischemic cerebrovascular etiology lasting less than 24 hours. Patients with brain stem and/or hemispheric symptoms were included while patients with isolated amaurosis fugax were excluded. All MRIs were obtained within 3 days of symptom onset. During the enrollment period, 61

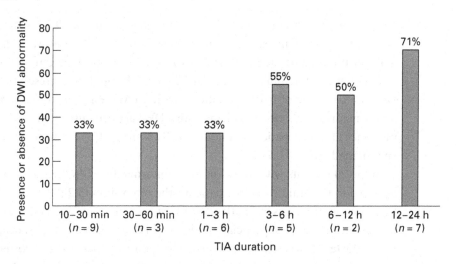

Figure 29.1   Relation of TIA symptom duration to presence or absence of DWI abnormality in the UCLA series.

patients were admitted to our university hospital with symptoms suggestive of a cerebral TIA. Forty-two had MRIs and 19 did not, due to metal implants (5), refusal/claustrophobia (6), MRI technical difficulty (3) and attending physician preference (5).

Among the 42 clinical TIA patients, 20 (48%) demonstrated a focal abnormality on DWI, consistent with acute neural bioenergetic compromise. In five (25%) of these 20 patients there was no lesion correlate on initial T_2-weighted (T2W) sequences. The remaining 15 patients did exhibit lesion abnormalities on the T2W sequences, in the same regions as the DWI alterations. Two patients with visible but very small DWI abnormalities did not have a measurable ADC volume. There was a strong correlation between ADC and DWI volumes ($r = 0.77$). There were no significant differences between patients who demonstrated DWI abnormalities and those who did not, in age, sex and presence of hypertension, diabetes, tobacco use, hypercholesterolemia or history of prior stroke or a TIA.

A precise estimation of the duration of a TIA (all were unequivocally less than 24 hours) was available for 15 of the 20 patients with DWI abnormalities and 17 of the 22 without DWI abnormalities. Duration of TIA symptoms for patients without a DWI abnormality was mean 3.2 hours (± 4.7 hours standard deviation (SD)), median 0.5 hours versus mean 7.3 hours (± 6 hours SD), median 4.0 hours for patients with a DWI abnormality (t test for difference in means, $P = 0.03$). The percentage of patients with a DWI abnormality within various symptom duration intervals increased as the total duration of symptoms increased (Figure 29.1).

The mean time from symptom onset to MRI study for all TIA patients was 17 hours (range 1.25 to 73 hours), and did not significantly differ between the two groups (mean 15.8 hours for DWI-negative patients, mean 19.5 hours for DWI-positive patients). One patient in the group without DWI lesions was still symptomatic at the time of the MRI, while two in the DWI-positive category were still symptomatic at the time of MR imaging. Interval from time of resolution of TIA symptoms to time of MRI for patients with a DWI abnormality was mean 12.7 hours, median 8.8 hours in patients with a DWI abnormality vs. mean 12.9 hours, median 5.1 hours in patients without a DWI abnormality (rank sums test for difference in medians, $P = 0.7$).

In the 20 patients with diffusion MRI abnormalities, DWI signal changes were localized to the brain stem in 4 patients, the cerebellum in 2 patients, subcortical hemispheric structures in 7 patients and cortical regions in 7 patients. Vascular territories affected were superficial middle cerebral artery in 6 patients, deep middle cerebral artery in 6 patients, brain stem perforators in 4 patients and posterior cerebral arteries in 2 patients. In these 20 patients, the final etiological mechanism was felt to be small vessel lacunar in 9 patients, large vessel atherothrombotic in 4 patients, and cardioembolic in 7 patients.

DWI results altered the attending physician's opinion regarding vascular localization in 7/20 patients, anatomical localization in 8/20 patients and probable TIA mechanism in 6/20 patients. The types of alteration in the diagnosis were quite varied and no single pattern predominated. For example, among etiological diagnoses, of 4 patients initially suspected of having large artery atherothrombotic mechanisms, 1 diagnosis was changed post-DWI to probable cardioembolic and 1 was changed to probable small vessel; of 7 initial cardioembolic diagnoses, 1 was changed to probable large vessel atherothrombotic and 1 was changed to probable small vessel; and of 9 initial small vessel diagnoses, 1 was changed to probable large vessel atherothrombotic and 1 was changed to probable cardioembolic.

There were significant differences in the DWI and ADC MR signature between the TIA patients with DWI abnormalities and the patients with completed stroke (Table 29.1). Patients with completed stroke had larger volumes and greater intensities of ADC and DWI alteration than TIA patients.

All 20 TIA patients demonstrating DWI abnormalities were contacted for a follow-up MRI, and 9 of these patients agreed to return for repeat neuroimaging. Three patients were studied with head CT and 6 with brain MRI 2 to 7 months postevent. Of these 9 patients, 5 (3 MRI, 2 CT) demonstrated a subsequent infarct in the region corresponding to the original DWI abnormality while 4 (3 MRI, 1 CT) did not. Five of the 22 patients without a DWI abnormality underwent follow-up imaging (3 MRI, 2 CT) 2 weeks to 15 months post-event. None demonstrated a subsequent relevant infarct.

Table 29.1. Comparison of DWI signature between TIA patients with diffusion MR abnormality and patients with completed stroke

	TIA patients (n=20) Mean (±SEM)	Patients with completed stroke (n=23), mean (±SEM)	P value
DWI lesion volume (cm³)	2.9 (8.4)	22.2 (7.8)	0.0002[a]
ADC volume (cm³)	0.7 (3.4)	10.5 (3.2)	0.0001[a]
DWI intensity	35% (5%)	62% (5%)	0.001[b]
Mean ADC value (μm²/s)	442 (6.7)	409 (6.1)	0.009[b]

Notes:
DWI, diffusion-weighted imaging; TIA, transient ischemic attack; MR, magnetic resonance; SEM, standard error of the mean; ADC, apparent diffusion coefficient.
[a] Rank sum test; [b] *t* test. (Modified from ref. 14 with permission)

Table 29.2. Time intervals and yield of diffusion MRI in transient ischemia attack (TIA) patients: three series

Series	TIA duration (mean) (hours)	Time from TIA onset to MRI (mean) (hours)	Frequency of positive DWI findings on MRI (%)
UCLA (n=42)	3.2[a]	17	48
Duke (n=40)	4.8	37	35
MGH (n=57)	1.9	39	46

Notes:
MRI, magnetic resonance imaging; DWI, diffusion-weighted imaging; UCLA, University of California at Los Angeles; Duke, Duke University, North Carolina; MGH, Massachusetts General Hospital, Boston, MA.
[a] Median duration was 2.0 hours.

Duke and Massachusetts General Hospital studies

Studies of diffusion MRI in TIA patients performed by investigators at Duke University and Massachusetts General Hospital (MGH) have confirmed and extended our findings [15,16]. Though differing somewhat in cohort characteristics and timing of MRIs, the three series show convergent results regarding the frequency of positive findings on DWIs among TIA patients, ranging from 35% in the Duke cohort, to 46% in the MGH cohort and 48% in the UCLA cohort (Table 29.2). Aggregating the three series, among 139 TIA patients studied, 43% exhibited diffusion MRI abnormalities. The Duke investigators found that in their cohort, as in ours, TIAs of longer clinical duration were more likely to be DWI-positive. Among DWI-positive patients, the mean TIA duration was 7.1 hours in the Duke cohort and

7.3 hours in the UCLA cohort; in DWI-negative patients the mean TIA duration was 3.2 hours in both cohorts. In contrast, TIA duration was not a predictor of DWI positivity in the MGH series. In part, this discrepancy may be due to the briefer average duration of TIAs and the longer interval from the onset of the TIA to the MRI in the MGH study. The MGH investigators did find that prior, non-stereotyped TIAs, identified stroke etiology and cortical symptoms were independent clinical predictors of DWI positivity. These clinical factors seem to index larger, more severe ischemic episodes, as does longer duration of clinical deficits, and this underlying physiological factor is likely to be the most critical for the appearance of DWI abnormality.

Discussion of TIA findings

These studies of diffusion MRI findings in TIA provide important new insights into the pathophysiology of TIAs and the clinical utility of new MRI sequences in TIA patients. Across all series, more than 2 of every 5 cerebral TIA patients demonstrated diffusion MRI evidence of acute bioenergetic compromise. In the UCLA study, among TIA patients with early DWI abnormalities who had follow-up imaging, approximately one half exhibited late CT or MRI evidence of established infarction. Together, these data suggest that approximately one quarter of cerebral TIA patients actually have cerebral infarction with transient signs. We also identified a distinct subset of TIA patients, representing about one fifth of TIA cases, who had early DWI abnormalities but no late evidence of established infarction. This finding in TIA patients suggests that DWI abnormalities may be reversible in humans if early restoration of blood flow is obtained. This observation is confirmed, with important additional complexities, by the MRI studies in patients undergoing reperfusion after thrombolytic stroke therapy that are discussed below.

In TIA patients, the ADC volume, mean ADC value, DWI volume and DWI signal intensity were all significantly less abnormal than in acute stroke patients. These differences support the concept that the cerebral ischemia experienced by patients with TIAs is lesser in volume and severity than that experienced by patients with clinically completed stroke syndromes.

Both the UCLA and Duke series found a strong statistical correlation between duration of TIA symptoms and presence of a lesion on DWI. This correlation, however, was not absolute. DWI lesions appeared in patients with clinical episodes as brief as 10 minutes, while some patients in the DWI-negative group had symptoms lasting more than 12 hours. DWI abnormalities do appear to be uncommon, if present at all, in patients with clinical symptoms lasting less than 5 minutes.

In addition to improving our understanding of the underlying pathophysiological processes that occur with TIAs, these data add to a growing body of evidence demonstrating the clinical utility of DWI [17,18]. A variety of studies have demonstrated that the diagnosis of a TIA is often difficult, especially for the non-neurologist [19,20]. Kraaijeveld and colleagues [21] found kappa measures of inter-rater agreement of only 0.65 among eight experienced neurologists diagnosing 56 TIA patients, and of only 0.31 for determination of the vascular territory involved. The size, appearance and location of DWI lesion(s) in a TIA may help to guide physicians in determining the underlying etiological mechanism and in choosing the optimal therapeutic regimen to reduce the probability of recurrent TIAs or completed stroke in the future.

In the UCLA study, information obtained from the DWI study led to a change in the suspected anatomical localization, vascular localization, and TIA mechanism in over one third of patients. In addition to clarifying the site and source of ischemia in patients with clinically definite TIAs, diffusion imaging also can be quite helpful in patients with atypical transient neurological symptoms when it is unclear whether the event was a TIA versus migraine, hyperventilation, brief seizure or other event that mimics a TIA. Although DWI abnormalities have rarely been reported in TIA mimics, a visualized diffusion abnormality in these cases generally provides supportive evidence of the diagnosis of a TIA.

The observation that DWI alone was positive in 25% of patients, while 75% had correlative lesions identified retrospectively on T2W imaging, underestimates the diagnostic impact of DWI. Even in the patients with visible lesions on T2W imaging, the diffusion imaging provided added clinical utility. Many of the T_2-positive patients had multiple foci of increased T_2 signaling, and determining which, if any, T_2 foci were new and related to the recent TIA may not have been possible without the DWI sequences. Standard T2W sequences alone are generally incapable of differentiating between acute and chronic events.

Identifying which patients have a new infarct on imaging may have important prognostic value [22]. In the Dutch TIA trial, evidence of any cerebral infarct on CT was an independent risk factor for subsequent stroke, myocardial infarction or vascular death [23,24]. Evans and colleagues [7] reported that in TIA patients, CT-verified infarction increased the risk of death by 109% over a 10 year period after the TIA. However, this study did not correlate the risk with evidence of a new, appropriately located TIA-related infarct. Eliasziw and colleagues [25] did not find an increased risk of ipsilateral stroke in a group of TIA patients with severe carotid stenosis treated medically as part of the North American Symptomatic Carotid Endarterectomy Trial; however, these results cannot be generalized to all TIA patients. Only larger series with long-term follow-up will be able to distinguish whether there is a difference in prognosis in TIA patients without diffusion abnormalities, TIA patients with transient diffusion abnormalities but no eventual lesion on T2W imaging, and patients with diffusion abnormalities and a subsequent lesion seen on T2W imaging.

Several issues require further study. The clinical prognostic significance of finding an associated DWI abnormality in a patient with a TIA remains uncertain. We concur with the general view advanced by Caplan [26] that all TIA patients are at significant risk of subsequent vascular events and it is the underlying mechanism rather than the duration of symptoms that is most critical to determine. However, it may be that within each mechanism category, the longer duration of a TIA or presence of a DWI abnormality identifies a subgroup at increased risk. How often patients with DWI abnormalities are experiencing ongoing ischemia will need to be clarified by concurrent perfusion studies. The severity and size of the perfusion deficit might also be an indicator of the reversibility of the diffusion abnormality. Finally, the pathological correlates of DWI changes in a TIA require investigation, including how often signal abnormalities reflect, at the histopathological level, the absence of infarction, incomplete infarction or complete infarction [27].

Intra-arterial thrombolysis

Intravenous thrombolysis is of proven benefit for the treatment of acute ischemic stroke within 3 hours of symptom onset [28], and intra-arterial (IA) thrombolytic therapy shows promise up to 6 hours after symptom onset [29]. Treatment of the majority of patients, however, is limited by the narrow time window recommended for initiation of therapy [30,31]. There is a recognized need for objective neuroimaging methods to identify the best candidates for treatment and to monitor individual patient response to therapy [32,33]. Imaging characterization of an existing ischemic penumbra could extend the time window available for treatment in some patients by allowing physicians to treat a "tissue clock" rather than a "ticking clock."

Diffusion MRI is of established utility in evaluating patients with acute brain ischemia [18,34–36]. ADC values typically decease sharply shortly after stroke onset, remain low for at least 72 to 96 hours, then gradually increase, reaching or surpassing normal levels [37]. Serial studies have shown that the typical natural history of early acute ischemic diffusion lesion volumes is to grow over time [38,39]. In various series, between 62% and 88% of patients imaged initially under 6 hours exhibited lesion growth on follow-up imaging, with the percentage change in lesion volume ranging from 32% to 107% [38,40,41]. It is speculated that this lesion growth may be due to gradual failure of energy metabolism in the ischemic penumbra as it is recruited into the infarct core if early reperfusion does not occur [38].

Diffusion/perfusion MRI has been suggested as a means of identifying the ischemic penumbra [42]. A prevalent view posits that, in humans, the area of diffusion abnormality constitutes an already irreversible core infarction field and that the penumbra is the region showing the perfusion but not yet diffusion abnormality (diffusion/perfusion mismatch). However, animal studies suggest that this model of the ischemic penumbra may underestimate the volume of tissue that is salvageable early after ischemic onset. When reperfusion occurs within 2 to 3 hours in these animal models, the perfusion deficit resolves and is accompanied by partial reversal of the DWI and ADC abnormalities [43–47]. We hypothesized that in humans, as in animals, portions of the DWI and ADC lesions could be salvaged with early reperfusion.

In an ongoing study of the response of the human brain to reperfusion, we have been obtaining serial MRI studies before treatment, early after treatment (3 to 9 hours), and late after treatment (day 7) in ischemic stroke patients treated at UCLA Medical Center with IA thrombolysis. From a larger overall cohort, the findings reported herein are based on the first 11 patients in the series meeting the following inclusion criteria: symptom duration less than 6 hours, presence of a large artery occlusion in the anterior circulation at the time of catheter angiography and partial or complete vessel recanalization achieved post-thrombolysis.

Eligible patients were treated with combined intravenous (iv)/IA tissue-type plasminogen activator (tPA) if treatment was initiated within 3 hours, or only IA tPA or IA urokinase if treatment was initiated within more than 3 and less than 6 hours, or if a contraindication to iv therapy was present in patients treated under 3 hours. Combined iv/IA tPA was administered at a dose of 0.6 mg/kg iv, 10% bolus over 1 minute, remainder infused over 30 minutes, followed by a 10 mg IA/h infusion until recanalization was achieved or a maximum IA dose of 20 mg was reached [48]. Urokinase was infused at the site of the clot at the time of angiography until recanalization was achieved or a maximum of 1 000 000 units was reached. Gentle mechanical clot disruption was also performed at the time of IA thrombolytic infusion.

The clinical outcome was assessed using the National Institutes of Health Stroke Scale (NIHSS) at baseline, early post-thrombolysis at the time of repeat MRI and at days 1, 3, 7 and 90. The Barthel Index, Modified Rankin Scale and Glasgow Outcome Scale were assessed at baseline (pre-morbid) and day 90.

Among the 11 patients, the mean age was 72.5 (range 27 to 94), and the mean entry NIHSS was 13. Five patients were treated with combined iv/IA tPA and 6 solely with IA thrombolysis. Vessel occlusions on angiography were in the middle cerebral artery trunk or division in 5 patients, middle cerebral artery branch in 5 and in the anterior cerebral artery in 1. Two patients experienced asymptomatic hemorrhagic transformation following therapy.

Ten of 11 patients demonstrated a decrease in the ADC volume measure and 8 of 11 a decrease in the DWI volume measure from the pretreatment MRI to the early post-thrombolysis MRI. In the 10 patients with an early decline in the volume of ADC abnormality, the mean ADC volume decreased from 11.2 cm^3 to 2.5 cm^3, and in the 8 patients with early decline in DWI abnormality, the mean DWI volume decreased from 19.8 cm^3 pretreatment to 11.6 cm^3 early post-thrombolysis.

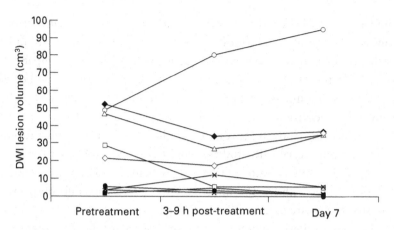

Figure 29.2 Evolution in individual DWI lesion volumes (cm³) from baseline MRI to early after thrombolysis MRI and day 7 MRI.

Among the patients displaying reversal of DWI abnormalities on early MRI, a varied pattern of further lesion evolution was noted at day 7. Four of seven patients with DWI reversal on early MRI and who underwent MRI on day 7 showed a secondary increase in the DWI lesion volume between the early post-thrombolysis and the day 7 MRI, while three patients showed stable reduction in DWI lesion volume on day 7 MRI (Figure 29.2). In the patients with a late reappearance of a signature of injury, secondary imaging abnormalities generally compromised some, but not all, of the regions of early normalization. Final infarct volume was defined as the larger of the DWI or T2W volumes on day 7 MRI. Overall, 6 of 11 patients had a net reduction in lesion volume from pretreatment DWI to final day 7 MRI. Examples from an illustrative case are shown in Figure 29.3.

Ten of the 11 patients had baseline perfusion studies. All had a significant diffusion–perfusion mismatch, with the perfusion volume exceeding the diffusion volume by a mean of 84% (range 53% to 98%). Nine of these patients had a follow-up perfusion study. In all, there was complete resolution of the initial perfusion deficit.

All 11 patients improved clinically after thrombolysis. The mean NIHSS decreased from 13 points at baseline to 9 points early after arterial recanalization to 5 points on day 7.

MRI findings in IA thrombolysis

Data from the first seven patients in this series formed the basis of the first report of reversibility of both diffusion and perfusion MRI abnormalities after thrombolytic therapy in human ischemic stroke patients [49]. These findings have since been confirmed by observations in subsequently treated patients in our series and

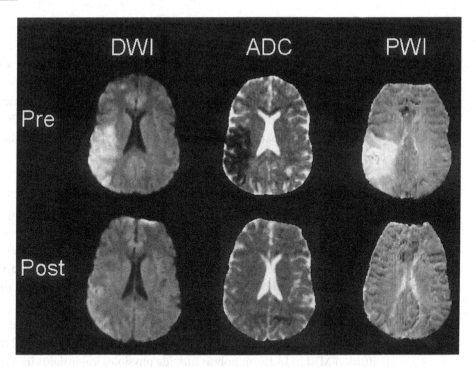

Figure 29.3 MRI scan showing reversal of diffusion and perfusion abnormalities in the right cerebral hemisphere after intra-arterial administration of tPA in a 27-year-old woman with left hemiparesis. Top row (Pre) shows DWI, ADC and PWI from a representative slice obtained 2.5 hours after symptom onset before thrombolytic therapy was begun. Vessel recanalization occurred 4 hours after symptom onset. Bottom row (Post) shows corresponding images obtained 3 hours after vessel recanalization, demonstrating a substantial decrease in the size of the DWI lesion and complete resolution of the perfusion and ADC deficits. The neurological deficit NIHSS score improved from 14 prethrombolysis to 3 at discharge from hospital.

from two other groups. Uno and colleagues [50] obtained diffusion and perfusion MRI scans before and after IA thrombolysis in 3 patients and found reversal of DWI abnormalities in 1. Lutsep and colleagues [51] reported a patient treated with IA thrombolysis 4 hours after onset in whom 82% of the volume of pretreatment DWI abnormalities was reversed on follow-up imaging. In addition to these observations with IA thrombolytic therapy, there have been occasional case reports of spontaneous reversal of ischemic diffusion abnormalities in humans [14,52].

Collectively, these findings mandate a fundamental revision of our understanding of MRI characterization of the ischemic penumbra. The results suggest that diffusion MRI lesions do not invariably represent irreversible injury and that the ischemic penumbra includes not only the areas of diffusion/perfusion mismatch but also portions within the diffusion abnormality itself.

While two groups have reported results of diffusion and perfusion imaging in patients undergoing intravenous thrombolysis, it is interesting to note that reversal of diffusion abnormalities has not, to date, been demonstrated in these patients. However, our findings are in accord with, and extend, their results. Marks and colleagues [53] found regions of higher ADC within the initial ischemic field on follow-up imaging of patients who had undergone reperfusion within 36 hours of onset compared with patients who did not undergo reperfusion. Schellinger and colleagues [54] found inhibition of lesion growth in patients who had undergone reperfusion compared with patients with persistent perfusion deficits. The ability of intravenous treatment studies to detect reversal of MRI diffusion abnormalities is limited by uncertainty in identifying which patients experience rapid versus delayed recanalization. Our study in patients treated with IA thrombolysis uniquely obtained pre- and postrecanalization diffusion and perfusion MRIs in all patients, and synchronized early post-treatment MRIs to recanalization time, providing a snapshot of post-thrombolysis pathophysiology obtained at a uniform time point across different patients.

The Prolyse in Acute Cerebral Thrombosis II (PROACT II) clinical trial suggested a beneficial effect of IA thrombolysis upon clinical end-points [29]. Studies of diffusion MRI in IA thrombolysis provide physiological insights into the mechanism by which IA therapy may confer benefit in select patients. The finding that recanalization achieved by IA thrombolysis leads not only to salvage of regions of diffusion/perfusion mismatch, but also to a dramatic reduction in the region of diffusion abnormality, delineates an anatomical mechanism by which IA therapy can improve clinical outcome.

We found that a late, secondary drop in ADC values occurred in approximately one half of patients. This delayed growth of the ADC volume generally compromised some, but not all of the region of ADC abnormality initially reversed by recanalization. These findings are the first demonstration of a late, secondary drop in the ADC in humans following successful recanalization. It is important for clinicians to be aware that some tissue that appears initially to be salvaged on early MRI when ADC normalizes may nonetheless proceed to late tissue infarction.

The phenomenon of late, secondary injury visualized on MRI has been described in several animal reperfusion models [55–59]. Potential mechanisms of this late secondary ADC decline include reperfusion injury [60], possibly related to inflammation or oxygen free radicals, ongoing excitotoxic injury emanating from the core infarct zone, and apoptosis. The physiological processes leading to secondary injury may be an appropriate, distinct target for neuroprotective therapy, using, for example, caspase inhibitors, newer anti-apoptotic agents, leukocyte adhesion inhibitors or other agents. Serial MRI studies to distinguish and quantify initial and secondary injury will probably be a critical element of future clinical trials of neuroprotective agents targeted specifically at these distinct stages of tissue damage.

Our findings have important implications for acute stroke management, since early assessment of the extent and reversibility of ischemia is needed to guide appropriate acute interventions. Prior studies have shown that the typical natural history of diffusion lesions in untreated patients is that they grow over the first few days after symptom onset, especially in patients with large artery occlusions that are imaged early after symptom onset [38,40,41,61]. Our demonstration that this growth can be arrested or even partially reversed with thrombolytic treatment illustrates that MRI offers a method to monitor treatment response in individual patients. It has been suggested that MRI screening may improve selection of the most appropriate candidates for treatment and possibly extend the therapeutic window beyond a rigid time frame in select patients. However, our results suggest that the use of DWI alone, or even the presence of a diffusion–perfusion mismatch, may not provide the optimal data with which to make thrombolytic treatment decisions.

A novel MRI approach to characterizing the ischemic penumbra in humans is to use the combined data from both the DWI and PWI sequences to identify pretreatment MRI signatures that predict tissue fate if vessel recanalization occurs. Both ADC and perfusion variables are important determinants of tissue progression to infarction or salvage. For example, in a preliminary analysis based on our first 13 patients who underwent vessel recanalization with IA thrombolysis, specific ADC thresholds could be identified to predict the likelihood of a voxel evolving infarction with various degrees of accuracy. Seventy-five percent of voxels with ADC values less than 380 and 67% of voxels with ADC values less than 420 were destined for infarction, despite recanalization. A multivariate model was derived that predicted tissue salvageability on a voxel-by-voxel basis with 73% accuracy in 13 patients undergoing vessel recanalization with IA thrombolysis [62]. In this model, the pretreatment ADC and perfusion measures were independent predictors of tissue fate, suggesting that imaging techniques that combine measures of both the tissue perfusion and tissue energetic state (such as MRI) have advantages over those that measure only tissue perfusion.

Conclusion

In conclusion, serial MRI studies have demonstrated reversibility of ischemic lesions visualized with diffusion–perfusion MRI in patients treated with IA thrombolysis. These findings indicate that the MRI definition of the ischemic penumbra needs to be refined to include regions of diffusion–perfusion mismatch and regions of the diffusion abnormality itself. Studies that include larger numbers of patients undergoing thrombolytic therapy should allow more precise delineation of MRI signatures of irreversible injury and of salvageability. Our studies have also demonstrated that MRI delineates a distinct, secondary stage of injury in the reperfused human brain. Further investigation is required to determine the precise time frame after reperfusion in which secondary injury evolves in humans, the clinical impact of MRI signals of secondary injury upon patients' functional recoveries and the ability of pharmacological agents to prevent the development of secondary injury in both animals and humans.

Acknowledgments

We are grateful to our collaborators in the UCLA Magnetic Resonance Imaging in Human Cerebral Reperfusion Study Group: Jeffrey R. Alger, Ph.D., Gary Duckwiler, M.D., Y. Pierre Gobin, M.D., Reza Jahan, M.D., James Mattiello, Ph.D., Sidney Starkman, M.D., Pablo Villablanca, M.D. and Fernando Vinuela, M.D.

REFERENCES

1 Special Report from the National Institute of Neurological Disorders and Stroke (1990) Classification of cerebrovascular diseases III. *Stroke*, 21, 637–76.

2 Ad Hoc Committee on Cerebrovascular Disease of the Advisory Council of the National Institute on Neurological Disease and Blindness (1958) A classification of and outline of cerebrovascular diseases. *Neurology*, 8, 395–434.

3 Levy DE (1988) How transient are transient ischemic attacks? *Neurology*, 38, 674–7.

4 Dyken ML, Conneally M, Haerer AF, Gotshall RA, Calanchini PR, Poskanzer DC, et al. (1977) Cooperative study of hospital frequency and character of transient ischemic attacks. I. Background, organization, and clinical survey. *Journal of the American Medical Association*, 237, 882–6.

5 Dennis M, Bamford J, Sandercock P, Molyneux A & Warlow C (1990) Computed tomography in patients with transient ischaemic attacks: when is a transient ischaemic attack not a transient ischaemic attack but a stroke? [see comments]. *Journal of Neurology*, 237, 257–61.

6 Koudstaal PJ, van Gijn J, Frenken CW, Hijdra A, Lodder J, Vermeulen M, et al. (1992) TIA, RIND, minor stroke: a continuum, or different subgroups? Dutch TIA Study Group. *Journal of Neurology, Neurosurgery & Psychiatry*, 55, 95–7.

7 Evans GW, Howard G, Murros KE, Rose LA & Toole JF (1991) Cerebral infarction verified by cranial computed tomography and prognosis for survival following transient ischemic attack. *Stroke*, 22, 431–6.

8 Bogousslavsky J & Regli F (1985) Cerebral infarct in apparent transient ischemic attack. *Neurology*, 35, 1501–3.

9 Awad I, Modic M, Little JR, Furlan AJ & Weinstein M (1986) Focal parenchymal lesions in transient ischemic attacks: correlation of computed tomography and magnetic resonance imaging. *Stroke*, **17**, 399–403.

10 Davalos A, Matias-Guiu J, Torrent O, Vilaseca J & Codina A (1988) Computed tomography in reversible ischaemic attacks: clinical and prognostic correlations in a prospective study. *Journal of Neurology*, **235**, 155–8.

11 Fazekas F, Fazekas G, Schmidt R, Kapeller P & Offenbacher H (1996) Magnetic resonance imaging correlates of transient cerebral ischemic attacks. *Stroke*, **27**, 607–11.

12 Kimura K, Minematsu K, Wada K, Yonemura K, Yasaka M & Yamaguchi T (2000) Lesions visualized by contrast-enhanced magnetic resonance imaging in transient ischemic attacks. *Journal of the Neurological Sciences*, **173**, 103–8.

13 Waxman SG & Toole JF (1983) Temporal profile resembling TIA in the setting of cerebral infarction. *Stroke*, **14**, 433–7.

14 Kidwell CS, Alger JR, Di Salle F, Starkman S, Villablanca P, Bentson J & Saver JL (1999) Diffusion MRI in patients with transient ischemic attacks. *Stroke*, **30**, 1174–80.

15 Engelter ST, Provenzale JM, Petrella JR & Alberts MJ (1999) Diffusion MR imaging and transient ischemic attacks. *Stroke*, **30**, 2762–3.

16 Ay H, Buonanno FS, Schaefer PW, Furie KL, Rordorf G, Gonzalez RG, Kistler JP & Koroshetz WJ (1999) Clinical and diffusion-weighted imaging characteristics of an identifiable subset of TIA patients with acute infarction. *Stroke*, **30**, 235.

17 Lee LJ, Kidwell CS, Alger J, Starkman S & Saver JL (2000) Impact on stroke subtype diagnosis of early diffusion-weighted magnetic resonance imaging and magnetic resonance angiography. *Stroke*, **31**, 1081–9.

18 Lutsep HL, Albers GW, DeCrespigny A, Kamat GN, Marks MP & Moseley ME (1997) Clinical utility of diffusion-weighted magnetic resonance imaging in the assessment of ischemic stroke. *Annals of Neurology*, **41**, 574–80.

19 Ferro JM, Falcao I, Rodrigues G, Canhao P, Melo TP, Oliveira V, et al. (1996) Diagnosis of transient ischemic attack by the nonneurologist. A validation study. *Stroke*, **27**, 2225–9.

20 Calanchini PR, Swanson PD, Gotshall RA, Haerer AF, Poskanzer DC, Price TR, et al. (1977) Cooperative study of hospital frequency and character of transient ischemic attacks. IV. The reliability of diagnosis. *Journal of the American Medical Association*, **238**, 2029–33.

21 Kraaijeveld CL, van Gijn J, Schouten HJ & Staal A (1984) Interobserver agreement for the diagnosis of transient ischemic attacks. *Stroke*, **15**, 723–5.

22 Toole JF (1991) The Willis lecture: transient ischemic attacks, scientific method, and new realities. *Stroke*, **22**, 99–104.

23 The Dutch TIA Trial Study Group (1993) Predictors of major vascular events in patients with a transient ischemic attack or nondisabling stroke. The Dutch TIA Trial Study Group. *Stroke*, **24**, 527–31.

24 van Swieten JC, Kappelle LJ, Algra A, van Latum JC, Koudstaal PJ & van Gijn J (1992) Hypodensity of the cerebral white matter in patients with transient ischemic attack or minor stroke: influence on the rate of subsequent stroke. Dutch TIA Trial Study Group. *Annals of Neurology*, **32**, 177–83.

25 Eliasziw M, Streifler JY, Spence JD, Fox AJ, Hachinski VC & Barnett HJ (1995) Prognosis for patients following a transient ischemic attack with and without a cerebral infarction on brain CT. North American Symptomatic Carotid Endarterectomy Trial (NASCET) Group. *Neurology*, **45** (3 Pt 1), 428–31.

26 Caplan LR (1983) Are terms such as completed stroke or RIND of continued usefulness? *Stroke*, **14**, 431–3.

27 Li F, Liu KF, Silva MD, Omae T, Sotak CH, Fenstermacher JD, et al. (2000) Transient and permanent resolution of ischemic lesions on diffusion-weighted imaging after brief periods of focal ischemia in rats: correlation with histopathology. *Stroke*, **31**, 946–54.

28 NINDS rtPA Stroke Group (1995) Tissue plasminogen activator for acute ischemic stroke. *New England Journal of Medicine*, **333**, 1581–7.

29 Furlan A, Higashida R, Wechsler L, Gent M, Rowley H, Kase C, et al. (1999) Intra-arterial prourokinase for acute ischemic stroke. The PROACT II study: a randomized controlled trial. Prolyse in acute cerebral thromboembolism. *Journal of the American Medical Association*, **282**, 2003–11.

30 Chiu D, Krieger D, Villar-Cordova C, Kasner SE, Morgenstern LB, Bratina PL, et al. (1998) Intravenous tissue plasminogen activator for acute ischemic stroke: feasibility, safety, and efficacy in the first year of clinical practice. *Stroke*, **29**, 18–22.

31 O'Connor RE, McGraw P & Edelsohn L (1999) Thrombolytic therapy for acute ischemic stroke: why the majority of patients remain ineligible for treatment. *Annals of Emergency Medicine*, **33**, 9–14.

32 Caplan LR, Mohr JP, Kistler JP & Koroshetz W (1997) Should thrombolytic therapy be the first-line treatment for acute ischemic stroke? Thrombolysis – not a panacea for ischemic stroke. *New England Journal of Medicine*, **337**, 1309–10.

33 Fisher M (1997) Characterizing the target of acute stroke therapy. *Stroke*, **28**, 866–72.

34 Warach S, Gaa J, Siewert B, Wielopolski P & Edelman RR (1995) Acute human stroke studied by whole brain echo planar diffusion-weighted magnetic resonance imaging. *Annals of Neurology*, **37**, 231–41.

35 Kidwell C, Villablanca P & Saver JL (2000) Advances in neuroimaging of acute stroke. *Current Atherosclerosis Reports*, **2**, 126–35.

36 Kalafut MA & Saver JL (2000) The acute stroke patient: the first six hours. In *Management of Ischemic Stroke*, ed. SN Cohen, pp. 17–52. New York: McGraw-Hill.

37 Schlaug G, Siewert B, Benfield A, Edelman RR & Warach S (1997) Time course of the apparent diffusion coefficient (ADC) abnormality in human stroke. *Neurology*, **49**, 113–19.

38 Baird AE, Benfield A, Schlaug G, Siewert B, Lovblad KO, Edelman RR, et al. (1997) Enlargement of human cerebral ischemic lesion volumes measured by diffusion-weighted magnetic resonance imaging [see comments]. *Annals of Neurology*, **41**, 581–9.

39 Albers GW, Lansberg MG, O'Brien MW, Ali J, Woolfenden AR, Tong DC, et al. (1999) Evolution of cerebral infarct volume assessed by diffusion-weighted MRI: implication for clinical stroke trials. *Neurology*, **52**, A453.

40 Barber PA, Darby DG, Desmond PM, Yang Q, Gerraty RP, Jolley D, et al. (1998) Prediction of stroke outcome with echoplanar perfusion- and diffusion-weighted MRI. *Neurology*, **51**, 418–26.

41 Tong DC, Yenari MA, Albers GW, M OB, Marks MP & Moseley ME (1998) Correlation of perfusion- and diffusion-weighted MRI with NIHSS score in acute (<6.5 hour) ischemic stroke [see comments]. *Neurology*, **50**, 864–70.

42 Fisher M & Garcia JH (1996) Evolving stroke and the ischemic penumbra. *Neurology*, **47**, 884–8.

43 Dijkhuizen RM, Berkelbach van der Sprenkel JW, Tulleken KA & Nicolay K (1997) Regional assessment of tissue oxygenation and the temporal evolution of hemodynamic parameters and water diffusion during acute focal ischemia in rat brain. *Brain Research*, **750**, 161–70.

44 Mintorovitch J, Moseley ME, Chileuitt L, Shimizu H, Cohen Y & Weinstein PR (1991) Comparison of diffusion- and T2-weighted MRI for the early detection of cerebral ischemia and reperfusion in rats. *Magnetic Resonance in Medicine*, **18**, 39–50.

45 Hossmann KA, Fischer M, Bockhorst K & Hoehn-Berlage M (1994) NMR imaging of the apparent diffusion coefficient (ADC) for the evaluation of metabolic suppression and recovery after prolonged cerebral ischemia. *Journal of Cerebral Blood Flow & Metabolism*, **14**, 723–31.

46 Hasegawa Y, Fisher M, Latour LL, Dardzinski BJ & Sotak CH (1994) MRI diffusion mapping of reversible and irreversible ischemic injury in focal brain ischemia. *Neurology*, **44**, 1484–90.

47 Minematsu K, Li L, Sotak CH, Davis MA & Fisher M (1992) Reversible focal ischemic injury demonstrated by diffusion-weighted magnetic resonance imaging in rats. *Stroke*, **23**, 1304–10; discussion 1310–11.

48 EMS Bridging Trial Investigators (1996) Combined intravenous and intra-arterial thrombolysis versus intra-arterial thrombolysis alone: preliminary safety and clot lysis. *Cerebrovascular Diseases*, **6**, 184.

49 Kidwell CS, Saver JL, Mattiello J, Starkman S, Vinuela F, Duckwiler G, et al. (2000) Thrombolytic reversal of acute human cerebral ischemic injury shown by diffusion/perfusion magnetic resonance imaging. *Annals of Neurology*, **47**, 462–9.

50 Uno M, Harada M, Okada T & Nagahiro S (2000) Diffusion-weighted and perfusion-weighted magnetic resonance imaging to monitor acute intra-arterial thrombolysis. *Journal of Stroke and Cerebrovascular Diseases*, **9**, 113–20.

51 Lutsep HL, Nesbit GM, Berger RM, Coshow WR & Clark WM (2000) Does reversal of ischemia on diffusion-weighted imaging reflect higher ADC values? *Neurology*, **54** Suppl 3, A95.

52 Marks MP, de Crespigny A, Lentz D, Enzmann DR, Albers GW & Moseley ME (1996) Acute and chronic stroke: navigated spin-echo diffusion-weighted MR imaging. *Radiology*, **199**, 403–8.

53 Marks MP, Tong DC, Beaulieu C, Albers GW, de Crespigny A & Moseley ME (1999) Evaluation of early reperfusion and i.v. tPA therapy using diffusion- and perfusion-weighted MRI. *Neurology*, **52**, 1792–8.

54 Schellinger PD, Jansen O, Fiebach JB, Heiland S, Steiner T, Schwab S, et al. (2000) Monitoring intravenous recombinant tissue plasminogen activator thrombolysis for acute ischemic stroke with diffusion and perfusion MRI. *Stroke*, **31**, 1311–17.

55 Li F, Han SS, Tatlisumak T, Liu K, Garcia JH, Sotak CH, et al. (1999) Reversal of acute apparent diffusion coefficient abnormalities and delayed neuronal death following transient focal cerebral ischemia in rats. *Annals of Neurology*, **46**, 333–42.

56 Li F, Silva MD, Sotak CH & Fisher M (2000) Temporal evolution of ischemic injury evaluated with diffusion-, perfusion-, and T2-weighted MRI. *Neurology*, **54**, 689–96.

57 Dijkhuizen RM, Knollema S, van der Worp HB, Ter Horst GJ, De Wildt DJ, Berkelbach van der Sprenkel JW, et al. (1998) Dynamics of cerebral tissue injury and perfusion after temporary hypoxia–ischemia in the rat: evidence for region-specific sensitivity and delayed damage. *Stroke*, **29**, 695–704.

58 van Lookeren Campagne M, Thomas GR, Thibodeaux H, Palmer JT, Williams SP, Lowe DG, et al. (1999) Secondary reduction in the apparent diffusion coefficient of water, increase in cerebral blood volume, and delayed neuronal death after middle cerebral artery occlusion and early reperfusion in the rat. *Journal of Cerebral Blood Flow & Metabolism*, **19**, 1354–64.

59 Busch E, Krüger K, Allegrini PR, Kerskens CM, Gyngell ML, Hoehn-Berlage M, et al. (1998) Reperfusion after thrombolytic therapy of embolic stroke in the rat: magnetic resonance and biochemical imaging. *Journal of Cerebral Blood Flow & Metabolism*, **18**, 407–18.

60 Hallenbeck JM & Dutka AJ (1990) Background review and current concepts of reperfusion injury. *Archives of Neurology*, **47**, 1245–54.

61 Rordorf G, Koroshetz WJ, Copen WA, Cramer SC, Schaefer PW, Budzik RF Jr, et al. (1998) Regional ischemia and ischemic injury in patients with acute middle cerebral artery stroke as defined by early diffusion-weighted and perfusion-weighted MRI. *Stroke*, **29**, 939–43.

62 Kidwell CS, Alger JR, Saver JL, Mattiello JH, Woods RP, Starkman SS, et al. (2000) MR signatures of infarction vs. salvageable penumbra in acute human stroke: a preliminary model. *Stroke*, **31**, 285 (Abstract).

30

Diffusion and perfusion magnetic resonance imaging in the evaluation of acute ischemic stroke

Michael P. Marks

Stanford Stroke Center and Departments of Radiology and Neurosurgery,
Stanford University Medical Center, Stanford, CA

Introduction

Diffusion and perfusion imaging are playing a greater role in the clinical setting of acute ischemic stroke. These newer imaging techniques are already utilized in stroke diagnosis, and in the future may be used for prognosis and treatment triage. Diffusion-weighted imaging (DWI) has already been proven to sensitively show tissue injured by ischemic stroke early in the postictal state [1–6]. Lesion volumes have been observed with DWI to enlarge over time after an acute stroke. Baird et al. [7], Barber et al. [8] and van Everdingen et al. [9] reported that 43%, 44% and 41% of their respective patients showed increases in lesion volume after the first imaging time point. Recently there has been an emphasis on the combined use of perfusion-weighted imaging (PWI) and DWI in the acute stroke setting in the hope that they will help to define tissue at risk for injury. Several studies have shown that the perfusion deficit (measured as a prolonged mean transit time or time-to-peak delay) is initially larger in this acute setting [3,5,7,10,11]. It appears that, in 70% to 80% of patients imaged within the first 6 hours of stroke, measured PWI deficits are greater than DWI deficits [5,8,10,11]. In addition, this pattern where PWI> DWI is larger on the initial image has been shown to predict DWI expansion into the surrounding lesion [8,12–15]. Many of these studies of DWI and PWI have, however, included patients imaged rather late in the time course of acute stroke (24 to 60 hours postictus) and included outcome measurements made early in the sub-acute period after stroke (within the first 7 days postictus).

Recombinant tissue-type plasminogen activator (rtPA) is currently the only known effective agent for the acute treatment of ischemic stroke. rtPA administered intravenously within 3 hours of symptom onset has been shown to improve long-term functional outcome in patients undergoing acute ischemic stroke [16]. No difference in rtPA benefit could be found based upon classification by stroke subtype (large vessel occlusive, lacunar, cardioembolic), although this stroke subtype classification was based solely on clinical prerandomization information. Indeed, it has been argued that patients with small infarcts such as lacunar infarcts and patients who have undergone spontaneous recanalization may have no benefit from thrombolytic therapy [17]. In addition, patients who have already sustained injury in all of the territory at risk for injury and those who have spontaneously recanalized may not benefit from rtPA. This may prove important as there is an increased risk of symptomatic hemorrhage with rtPA treatment [16].

This study sought to evaluate DWI and PWI changes seen earlier within the hyperacute time period after stroke (within the first 7 hours postictus) and systematically to follow the imaging changes seen over approximately 30 days. The study was designed to follow the evolution of PWI and DWI findings as well as the relationship between early findings and final outcome. In addition, we have sought to evaluate the effect of rtPA therapy on early imaging and to study the role of early reperfusion in serial imaging changes and the final outcome. Many of these results have recently been reported in two publications [12,13].

Methods

Twenty-one patients were studied within 7 hours of symptom onset. Eleven patients were treated with intravenous rtPA prior to the first magnetic resonance imaging (MRI) examination as part of accepted medical practice. Fourteen were randomized to possible treatment with putative neuroprotective agents (7 nalmafene, 4 lubeluzole, 2 basic fibroblast growth factor, 1 aptiganel hydrochloride). Thrombolytic infusion was initiated a mean ($\pm$ standard deviation) of 100 ± 40 minutes after symptom onset for those who received it. There was no significant difference in the time to imaging between the rtPA-treated (mean 4.3 ± 0.8 hours) and non-rtPA-treated (mean 5.3 ± 1.1 hours) groups. Patients were studied at five time points: less than 7 hours postictus (t1), 3 to 6 hours later (t2), at 24 to 36 hours (t3), 5 to 7 days (t4) and at approximately 30 days (t5). Six patients were not imaged at 30 days because one refused, two had died, two were bedridden and one left the state. Three patients did not have a successful PWI examination at the first time point. Neurological examinations were done by a certified neurologist and reported on a clinical scale using the National Institutes of Health Stroke Scale (NIHSS) score.

DWI utilized single-shot spin-echo, echo-planar imaging to obtain 16 oblique slices, each with a 5 mm thickness and a 2.5 mm gap. Images with ($b = 829 \, \text{s/mm}^2$) and without ($b = 0 \, \text{s/mm}^2$) diffusion-weighting were obtained. DWIs were acquired with the diffusion-sensitizing gradients applied along the X, Y and Z directions,

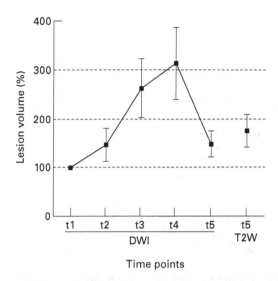

Figure 30.1   The temporal evolution of ischemic lesion volume averaged at five time points: <7 hours after stroke onset (t1) and then 3 to 6 hours (t2), 24 to 36 hours (t3), 5 to 7 days (t4) and ~30 days (t5) later. The lesion volumes are normalized relative to the lesion volume on DWI at the first time point. The mean volume ± SEM is shown. T2W, T_2-weighted. (Reprinted from ref. 13, with permission. Beaulieu C, de Crespigny A, Tong DC, Moseley ME, Albers GW & Marks MP (1999) Longitudinal magnetic resonance imaging study of perfusion and diffusion in stroke: evolution of lesion volume and correlation with clinical outcome. *Annals of Neurology,* **46,** 568–78.)

sequentially and were averaged to obtain trace images. Two images without diffusion weighting and two images with diffusion weighting were obtained in each direction to improve the apparent diffusion coefficient (ADC) calculation.

PWI was done as a single-shot gradient-echo, echo-planar imaging after an intravenous gadolinium bolus (0.2 mmol Gd-DTPA/kg). PWI utilized the same matrix size, slice thickness, interslice gap and field-of-view as DWI, but used a relaxation time (TR) of 2000 ms and an excitation time (TE) of 60 ms. Twelve slices were acquired every 2 seconds for 35 time points. Images were processed to yield maps of time-to-peak, which provided a high contrast between normally and abnormally perfused tissue.

Results

All patients demonstrated DWI abnormalities at the first imaging time (t1). The mean DWI lesion volume at t1 was $45 \pm 44 \, cm^3$ (range: 0.7 to 153.2 cm^3). Figure 30.1 shows the evolution in lesion volume (t2 to t5) expressed as a percentage of t1. The mean lesion volume reached a maximum of $320 \pm 80\%$ (mean ± standard

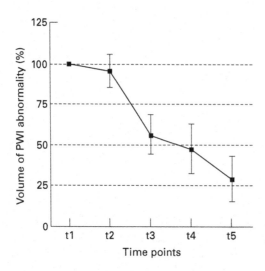

Figure 30.2 The temporal evolution of the volume of perfusion abnormality averaged over 21 patients for five time points: <7 hours after stroke onset (t1) and then 3 to 6 hours (t2), 24 to 36 hours (t3), 5 to 7 days (t4) and ~30 days (t5) later. The volumes are normalized relative to the first time point for each patient. The volume of perfusion abnormality drops markedly by the third time point and then continues to decrease over the subsequent month. The mean ± SEM is presented. (Reprinted from ref. 13 with permission. Beaulieu C, de Crespigny A, Tong DC, Moseley ME, Albers GW & Marks MP (1999) Longitudinal magnetic resonance imaging study of perfusion and diffusion in stroke: evolution of lesion volume and correlation with clinical outcome. *Annals of Neurology*, **46,** 568–78.)

error) at 5 to 7 days (t4) after stroke onset. This volume then decreased to 180 ± 30% at ~30 days (t5). The change in DWI lesion volume described for the entire group also held true for the individual patient. Increases in lesion volume from t1 to t4 were observed in 95% (18/19) of patients (two patients died prior to t4).

PWI time-to-peak maps showed a delay in contrast arrival in 16 patients (89%), while two patients (11%) had no perfusion abnormalities at t1. Three patients had suboptimal PWIs at t1. The mean time-to-peak delay within the ischemic territory was 9.9 ± 5.6 seconds at t1 when compared with a similar region of interest (ROI) in the normal contralateral hemisphere. The evolution after infarction of the PWI lesion was quite different from the DWI lesion volume (Figure 30.2). The abnormal perfusion volume remained relatively constant over the first two time points, and then showed a steady decrease through to t5. This decrease was most marked from t2 to t3 (24 to 36 hours). Eleven patients did demonstrate persistent perfusion abnormalities through t4, while eight showed resolution by t4.

In order to evaluate the DWI and PWI volume changes seen in patients who received rtPA versus non-rtPA-treated patients, the first six patients in the study (who received rtPA) were formally compared with the first six who did not receive rtPA [12]. rtPA was given in the standard intravenous dose prior to MRI. Patients were evaluated on the basis of the time to resolution of perfusion abnormalities. "Early reperfusers" were defined as patients experiencing a complete or near complete resolution of PWI abnormalities by t3 (24 to 36 hours). Patients without early reperfusion who had persistent PWI abnormalities at t3 constituted the other group. Differences in evolution of the ADC within the ischemic lesion delineated on DWI were assessed for the two groups.

The rtPA-treated patients did not differ significantly from the non-rtPA-treated patients in the initial NIHSS score, age or time to initial MRI. The average NIHSS score for all subjects was 11 ± 9. PWI was successfully performed at t1 in 11/12 patients. At this initial time point, the volume of the PWI abnormality was less than the volume of the DWI abnormality (PWI$<$DWI) in 5/6 (83%) rtPA-treated patients. In contrast, PWI$<$DWI was present in only 1/5 (20%) of the non-rtPA-treated patients ($P=0.08$, Fisher's exact test). In addition, early reperfusion (by t2 or t3) was seen in 5/6 (83%) rtPA-treated patients compared with 1/5 (20%) of the non-rtPA-treated patients ($P=0.08$, Fisher's exact test). Moreover 5/6 (83%) rtPA-treated patients showed a $>$50% decrease in PWI volume by t2 when compared with the t1 PWI volume, whereas 0/5 (0%) of the non-rtPA-treated patients showed a $>$50% decrease in PWI by t2. PWI was successfully performed at t3 in 11/12 patients and PWI normalization by this time (i.e., early reperfusion) was observed in 6/11 patients. Five of these patients received rtPA and one did not.

The aggregate ADC value determined from the ROI of the DWI abnormality in the early reperfusion group was significantly greater than in the non-reperfusion group by t2 at ~10 hours after symptom onset (unpaired t test, $P=0.04$) (Figure 30.3). The difference remained significant at t3 and t4 ($P=0.002$ and $P=0.0005$, respectively). A relative difference in ADC values between the two groups (early reperfusion versus no early reperfusion) increased from t2 to t4, but did converge at t5. Elevated signal regions were seen within the abnormal area of the ADC maps (rADC = ipsilateral ADC/contralateral ADC = 1.46 ± 0.19) by t3 in 5/6 (83%) early reperfusers vs. 0/5 (0%) non-early reperfusers ($P=0.015$, Fisher's exact test). The signal intensities on T_2-weighted (fluid-attenuated inversion recovery (FLAIR)) images for the infarct regions were also compared for the early reperfusion group vs. the non-early reperfusion group (Figure 30.4).

In order to investigate how the initial perfusion–diffusion mismatch and reperfusion affected the lesion volume evolution a comparison was made between those where PWI$>$DWI with no early reperfusion and those where PWI$\leq$DWI with early reperfusion. As shown in Figure 30.5, the presence of a perfusion–diffusion mismatch appears to influence the evolution of the DWI and the final infarct volume. Both groups did show a DWI volume increase. Volume peaked at t4 in

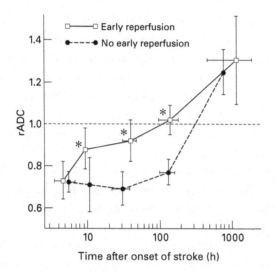

Figure 30.3 Comparison of the temporal evolution of the mean relative ADC values (rADC=ADC in lesion/ADC in contralateral ROI) in early reperfusers ($n=6$) vs. non-early reperfusers ($n=5$). Early reperfusion is defined as regaining normal perfusion by 24 to 36 hours. The rADC values are reduced in both groups immediately after stroke onset (~5 hours postictus), but become significantly different by the second time point (~10 hours). The rADC is higher in the early reperfusers throughout the first week and then it converges to elevated values at the chronic time point that are similar to the non-early reperfusers. The rADC values given are mean±SD throughout the entire lesion identified on DWI. * $P<0.05$. (Reprinted from ref. 12 with permission. Marks MP, Tong DC, Beaulieu C, Albers GW, de Crespigny A & Moseley ME (1999) Evaluation of early reperfusion and i.v. tPA therapy using diffusion- and perfusion-weighted MRI. *Neurology*, **52**, 1792–8.)

those where PWI ≥ DWI without early reperfusion and at t3 in those with PWI≤ DWI and early reperfusion. The final lesion volume as measured by the T_2-weighted images at t5 grew to 200±80% of the DWI volume at t1 in the PWI> DWI group. The final volume did not increase in the PWI≤DWI group. Here, the final lesion volume was 100%±20% at time t5.

Conclusion

The longitudinal evolution of DWI and PWI after ischemic stroke has allowed us to make several observations. The volume of tissue that is abnormal in the DWIs is quite dynamic in the several weeks after stroke. It appears to peak at approximately 5 to 7 days after the infarct and then decline at chronic time points. Overall for the entire group, however, the final infarct volume as measured by T_2-weighted imaging increased to 180% of the initial DWI volume seen in the first 7 hours. This

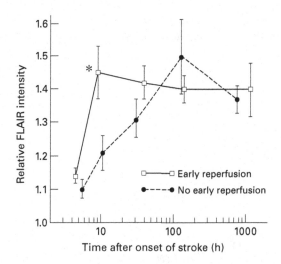

Figure 30.4 Comparison of the temporal evolution of the mean relative FLAIR (fluid-attenuated inversion recovery) signal intensity (intensity in lesion / intensity in contralateral ROI) in early reperfusers ($n=6$) vs. non-early reperfusers ($n=5$). The relative FLAIR intensities are near normal (i.e., value close to 1) in both groups immediately after stroke onset (~5 hours postictus), but there is a much more rapid increase in signal intensity in the group of early reperfusers. The later time points demonstrate similar hyperintensities on FLAIR for both groups. The relative signal intensity values given are mean $\pm$ SEM throughout the entire lesion identified on DWI. * $P<0.05$. (Reprinted from ref. 12, with permission. Marks MP, Tong DC, Beaulieu C, Albers GW, de Crespigny A & Moseley ME (1999) Evaluation of early reperfusion and i.v. tPA therapy using diffusion- and perfusion-weighted MRI. *Neurology*, **52**, 1792–8.)

observed growth, when compared with the initial DWI volume, suggests that there may indeed be salvageable tissue, i.e., tissue that is not injured on the basis of the DWI seen in the first several hours after onset of ischemia.

The observation that PWI volumes were less than DWI volumes in 5/6 (83%) of the thrombolytic-treated patients compared with only 1/5 (20%) of the patients not receiving thrombolytic therapy 3 to 7 hours postictus (t1), suggests that rapid imaging with PWI shows early changes in perfusion brought about by rtPA treatment. It has been postulated that the mismatch between PWI and DWI where PWI > DWI identifies tissue at risk for injury in the ischemic penumbra. Our observation that lesion growth between the first 7 hours and the final lesion volume (at 30 days) was seen in those patients where the PWI > DWI and there was no early reperfusion, but not seen in those patients where PWI ≤ DWI with early reperfusion, supports this hypothesis. Indeed, the fact that the final lesion volume did not grow in the group where PWI ≤ DWI with early reperfusion suggests that this group of patients may already be maximally injured at the time of imaging. If lesion

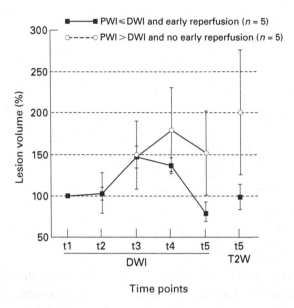

Figure 30.5 The dependence of the temporal evolution of ischemic lesion volume (defined on DWI and then T_2 for final time point) on the initial mismatch between the volume of perfusion abnormality and the diffusion lesion volume, as well as the occurrence of early reperfusion for five time points: <7 hours after stroke onset (t1) and then 3 to 6 hours (t2), 24 to 36 hours (t3), 5 to 7 days (t4) and ~30 days (t5) later. Two groups that had all five DWIs are presented: PWI>DWI at t1 and no early reperfusion (n=5) and PWI ≤ DWI at t1 and early reperfusion (n=5). The lesion volumes are normalized relative to the lesion volume on DWI at the first time point for each patient. The final lesion volume at t5 days increases to 200±80% (P=0.14 cf t1) in the PWI>DWI/no early reperfusion group, whereas it remains relatively stable (100±20%; P=0.54 cf t1) in the PWI ≤ DWI/early reperfusion group. The mean±SEM is presented. T2W, T_2 weighted.

volume change data such as these prove to hold true and be significant in larger groups of patients, this may have profound implications for the use of MRI as a triage tool for thrombolytic therapy.

Acknowledgments

I wish to acknowledge my colleagues from the Stanford University School of Medicine who made this work possible: Gregory Albers, M.D., and David Tong, M.D., of the Department of Neurology; and Christian Beaulieu, Ph.D., Alexander deCrespigny, Ph.D., and Michael Moseley, Ph.D., of the Department of Radiology.

REFERENCES

1 Marks MP, de Crespigny A, Lentz D, Enzmann DR, Albers GW & Moseley ME (1996) Acute and chronic stroke: navigated spin-echo diffusion-weighted MR imaging. [erratum: *Radiology*, **200**, 289, 1996] *Radiology*, **199**, 403–8.

2 Lutsep HL, Albers GW, DeCrespigny A, Kamat GN, Marks MP & Moseley ME (1997) Clinical utility of diffusion-weighted magnetic resonance imaging in the assessment of ischemic stroke. *Annals of Neurology*, **41**, 574–80.

3 Sorensen AG, Buonanno FS, Gonzalez RG, Schwamm LH, Lev MH, Huang-Hellinger FR, Reese TG, Weisskoff RM, Davis TL, Suwanwela N, Can U, Moreira JA & Copen WA (1996) Hyperacute stroke: evaluation with combined multisection diffusion-weighted and hemodynamically weighted echo-planar MR imaging. *Radiology*, **199**, 391–401.

4 Warach S, Chien D, Li W, Ronthal M & Edelman RR (1992) Fast magnetic resonance diffusion-weighted imaging of acute human stroke. [erratum: *Neurology*, **42**, 2192, 1992] *Neurology*, **42**, 1717–23.

5 Warach S, Dashe JF & Edelman RR (1996) Clinical outcome in ischemic stroke predicted by early diffusion-weighted and perfusion magnetic resonance imaging: a preliminary analysis. *Journal of Cerebral Blood Flow & Metabolism*, **16**, 53–9.

6 Schlaug G, Siewert B, Benfield A, Edelman RR & Warach S (1997) Time course of the apparent diffusion coefficient (ADC) abnormality in human stroke. *Neurology*, **49**, 113–19.

7 Baird AE, Benfield A, Schlaug G, Siewert B, Lovblad KO, Edelman RR & Warach S (1997) Enlargement of human cerebral ischemic lesion volumes measured by diffusion-weighted magnetic resonance imaging. *Annals of Neurology*, **41**, 581–9.

8 Barber PA, Darby DG, Desmond PM, Yang Q, Gerraty RP, Jolley D, Donnan GA, Tress BM & Davis SM (1998) Prediction of stroke outcome with echoplanar perfusion- and diffusion-weighted MRI. *Neurology*, **51**, 418–26.

9 van Everdingen KJ, van der Grond J, Kappelle LJ, Ramos LM & Mali WP (1998) Diffusion-weighted magnetic resonance imaging in acute stroke. *Stroke*, **29**, 1783–90.

10 Rordorf G, Koroshetz WJ, Copen WA, Cramer SC, Schaefer PW, Budzik RF Jr, Schwamm LH, Buonanno F, Sorensen AG & Gonzalez G (1998) Regional ischemia and ischemic injury in patients with acute middle cerebral artery stroke as defined by early diffusion-weighted and perfusion-weighted MRI. *Stroke*, **29**, 939–43.

11 Darby DG, Barber PA, Desmond PM, Yang Q, Gerraty RP, Tress TM & Davis SM (1999) Patterns and frequency of acute ischemic stroke topography as depicted by combined perfusion- and diffusion-weighted magnetic resonance imaging. *Stroke*, **30**, 235.

12 Marks MP, Tong DC, Beaulieu C, Albers GW, de Crespigny A & Moseley ME (1999) Evaluation of early reperfusion and i.v. tPA therapy using diffusion- and perfusion-weighted MRI. *Neurology*, **52**, 1792–8.

13 Beaulieu C, de Crespigny A, Tong DC, Moseley ME, Albers GW & Marks MP (1999) Longitudinal magnetic resonance imaging study of perfusion and diffusion in stroke: evolution of lesion volume and correlation with clinical outcome. *Annals of Neurology*, **46**, 568–78.

14 Jansen O, Schellinger P, Fiebach J, Hacke W & Sartor K (1999) Early recanalisation in acute ischaemic stroke saves tissue at risk defined by MRI. *Lancet,* **353,** 2036–7.

15 Kidwell CS, Saver JL, Mattiello J, Starkman S, Vinuela F, Duckwiler G, Gobin YP, Jahan R, Vespa P, Kalafut M & Alger JR (2000) Thrombolytic reversal of acute human cerebral ischemic injury shown by diffusion/perfusion magnetic resonance imaging. *Annals of Neurology,* **47,** 462–9.

16 The National Institute of Neurological Disorders; Stroke rtPA Stroke Study Group (1995) Tissue plasminogen activator for acute ischemic stroke. *New England Journal of Medicine,* **333,** 1581–7.

17 Caplan LR, Mohr JP, Kistler JP & Koroshetz W (1997) Should thrombolytic therapy be the first-line treatment for acute ischemic stroke? Thrombolysis – not a panacea for ischemic stroke. *New England Journal of Medicine,* **337,** 1309–10.

31

Early recanalization in acute ischemic stroke saves tissue at risk defined by stroke magnetic resonance imaging

Olav Jansen[1] & Peter D. Schellinger[2]

[1] Department of Neuroradiology, University of Heidelberg Medical School, Heidelberg, Germany
[2] Department of Neurology, University of Heidelberg Medical School, Heidelberg, Germany

Introduction

The target for most therapeutic interventions for focal ischemia should be ischemic tissue that can respond to treatment and is not irreversibly injured. Such tissue will be defined as potentially salvageable ischemic tissue and must be distinguished from non-salvageable ischemic tissue that has evolved to a status at which recovery is no longer possible. Characterization of potentially reversible vs. irreversible ischemic tissue is based on the ischemic penumbra hypothesis [1]. Ideally, before any aggressive therapeutic approach (i.e., thrombolysis) is undertaken, four important questions concerning the individual stroke situation should be addressed using only one optimal diagnostic imaging procedure:

1 Does the patient have acute cerebral ischemia or is another underlying pathology responsible for the stroke symptoms (e.g., intracerebral hemorrhage, tumor)?
2 Is there already an area of irreversibly damaged ischemic tissue and what is the size of this infarct core?
3 Is there a tissue of risk ("penumbra") that can be preserved from damage by therapeutic intervention, and what is the size of this area?
4 Is the vessel that is responsible for the ischemia still occluded or has there been a spontaneous recanalization?

The ideal imaging modality will be able to address all of these questions within an acceptable amount of time before a specific treatment is begun.

Magnetic resonance imaging in early ischemic stroke

Diffusion-weighted imaging

Since the description of early findings in acute experimental ischemic stroke with diffusion-weighted imaging (DWI), it has been predicted that this technique might become an important tool for the identification of very early ischemic injury in patients [2]. In the last 5 years several clinical works have been published showing the feasibility of this motion-sensitive technique, even in patients with acute stroke. Since the availability of echo-planar imaging (EPI) on clinical scanner systems, DWI can be performed more often in the clinical routine. DWI is sensitive to the microscopic motion of water protons (molecular brownian movement). With DWI, structures with fast diffusion are dark, structures with slower diffusion are bright. By acquiring images with different diffusion values, the apparent diffusion coefficient (ADC) and ADC maps can be calculated.

A hyperacute infarction becomes hyperintense in early DWI and dark in ADC maps [3], and can be detected with this technique within minutes after vessel occlusion, whereas standard magnetic resonance imaging (MRI) (i.e., T_2-weighted) does not have the capability of detecting an acute infarction within the first 6 hours [4].

Perfusion-weighted imaging

Perfusion-weighted imaging (PWI) makes use of the signal loss that occurs during the dynamic tracking of the first pass of an intravenous paramagnetic contrast agent. A concentration time course is consequently derived voxel by voxel. Different hemodynamic parameters such as relative mean transit time (rMTT) and relative cerebral blood volume and flow can then be calculated and displayed as perfusion maps from the entire brain [5]. Although PWI is not able to measure absolute cerebral blood volume or flow values, relative maps demonstrate areas of minor perfusion in comparison with the unaffected brain.

Perfusion images are usually obtained with an EPI spin-echo sequence. The contrast bolus is administered with an injector via a large-bore cannula in the antecubital fossa (i.e., 0.1 mmol/kg). The total imaging time is approximately between 1 and 2 minutes with an additional time needed for postprocessing the hemodynamic maps. The rMTT maps usually show perfusion deficits of a greater volume and with a clearer distinction to the unaffected tissue than other hemodynamic measurements. In the daily routine many centers use the rMTT maps only as a basis for describing the hemodynamic situation in a patient with acute stroke.

The Heidelberg multimodal MRI approach in patients with acute ischemic stroke

At the beginning of rapid and functional MRI use, several groups tried to address the most relevant questions regarding the patient with acute stroke, using one of the described techniques, alone. DWI, especially, seemed to have enough potential to differentiate between the irreversibly damaged infarct core and the still salvage-able penumbra or another kind of tissue at risk. However, these attempts were not successful and the concept of a multimodal MRI approach with a standardized stroke protocol was created [6]. The protocol consists of a regular, fast T_2-weighted image, a magnetic resonance angiography (MRA), DWI and PWI. This combina-tion of different imaging techniques is the most practicable and promising stroke imaging protocol.

The standardized Heidelberg stroke MRI protocol uses a three-dimensional time-of-flight (TOF) angiography (aquisition time (AT): 2 minutes), a T_2-weighted fast spin-echo sequence with an echo-train length of 32 (AT: 1 minute), an isotropic diffusion-weighted spin-echo EPI sequence with four different b values (AT: 3 minutes) and a perfusion-weighted gradient-echo EPI sequence during bolus administration of contrast media (AT: 2 minutes). The whole protocol, including positioning of the patient, tuning and shimming of the MR machine, requires 15 to 20 minutes.

The regular T_2-image is obtained to rule out severe non-ischemic lesions and to show older vascular lesions either of micro- or macroangiopathic etiology. MRA has been well accepted as a reliable method to demonstrate vessel occlusion in the arteries of the circle of Willis. To save time, a very short sequence with reduced res-olution is used. However, the quality of the MRA should be good enough to com-pletely evaluate the major brain vessels and the proximal parts of the M2 segments of the middle cerebral artery (MCA). Instead of a TOF-MRA with reduced resolu-tion, a percutaneous angiography with only a few sections in the coronal plane can be obtained. The slab thickness must be large enough to demonstrate the patency or occlusion of the major brain vessels.

Our approach with PWI and DWI in acute stroke patients presumes a simplifi-cation in the interpretation of the data from these techniques. In this concept it is speculated that DWI lesions present irreversibly damaged tissue, the infarct core. PWI and especially the rMTT maps demonstrate the area of reduced perfusion in patients with acute vessel occlusion. The correlation of DWI lesions with PWI lesions results either in a match (PWI = DWI) or in a mismatch (PWI > DWI; PWI < DWI) (Figure 31.1). We speculate that the mismatch area (with PWI > DWI) represents an area of brain tissue that is at risk for infarction. In these patients, the area of abnormal and reduced perfusion is larger than the already damaged area. With an increase in edema or a slight decrease in systemic blood pressure, patients with a mismatch have a high risk of larger infarctions at follow-up due to secon-dary failure of leptomeningeal collaterals. However, in mismatch patients with a successful recanalization or maintaining of patency of sufficient collaterals, the tissue at risk can be saved from infarction. Patients with a match between PWI and DWI do not show tissue at risk. In these patients the whole infarct has already

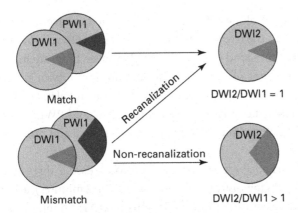

Figure 31.1   Concept of match and mismatch based on the correlation between PWI and DWI in patients with acute stroke. Match patients do not have tissue at risk or an increase in infarct size. The DWI lesion on day 2 after stroke is approximately the same size as on day 1. Mismatch patients do have tissue at risk, which can be preserved from infarction by early recanalization. In the case of non-recanalization, the tissue at risk can be damaged and the infarct size can increase from day 1 to day 2.

developed and in those cases with no additional vascular event the infarct size should not grow significantly during the follow-up in comparison with the initial DWI lesion. The third group of patients show a mismatch with the PWI smaller than the DWI. This kind of inverse mismatch is not very often observed in hyperacute and acute patients [7,8] and occurs in cases with a spontaneous recanalization. The perfusion in the already damaged tissue (DWI lesions) has improved or normalized and there is no risk of an increase in the infarct size.

Detection of hyperacute hemorrhage with stroke MRI

Fifteen to 20% of all patients suffering from acute stroke show not cerebral ischemia but acute intracerebral hemorrhage. An imaging method, which should be used to select ideal candidates for acute ischemic stroke therapy (i.e., thrombolysis), must also be able to show or rule out acute cerebral hemorrhage. For a long time it has been formulated that MRI is not able to detect or differentiate hyperacute hemorrhage. Therefore, we started a small series of patients with hyperacute intracerebral hemorrhage, where computed tomography (CT) and stroke MRI were performed immediately one after another with a mean time interval of 2 hours [9]. All nine patients suffered from hyperacute intracerebral hemorrhage, which was easily identified on all stroke MRIs. Volumetry showed the highest sensitivity for very fresh intracerebral blood for the T_2-weighted images, which are already included in the stroke MRI protocol with the source PWIs. In comparison to CT these T_2-weighted images overestimated hematoma size, which means that they were more sensitive for hyperacute hematoma. We are in agreement with other groups in supposing that additional CT is no longer necessary to rule out intracerebral hemorrhage in hyperacute stroke when stroke MRI is performed [10,11].

The Heidelberg stroke MRI study

On the basis of the described concept of stroke MRI, we performed an open, prospective clinical trial from September 1997 to July 1999. The purpose of this study was to evaluate whether stroke MRI is able to identify a subgroup of patients who show a significant morphological and clinical benefit from early recanalization of their initially occluded cerebral arteries. We included patients who had had an ischemic stroke within the last 12 hours and a baseline National Institutes of Health Stroke Scale (NIHSS) score of at least 3, but preferred a time window of 6 hours after symptom onset. All patients were examined with 1.5 T whole body MRI (EDGE, Picker International, Cleveland, OH) equipped with enhanced gradient hardware for EPI. We performed stroke MRI on days 1 (initial scan), 2 and 5 (day 5 without PWI). Lesion volumes on DWI and PWI were measured in a semiautomatic fashion.

We examined 64 patients (36 men, 28 women) with stroke MRI. The mean age was 60.9 years (range 29 to 83 years). The median NIHSS score at baseline was 12 (range 3 to 25), only one patient having an NIHSS score of less than 5. With the exception of one patient, the quality of all MR images/sequences obtained was satisfactory for interpretation, without disturbing motion artifacts. One patient did not tolerate the examination despite mild sedation, so that only the DWI sequences were interpretable (feasibility of stroke MRI = 98.4%). On the second day, follow-up stroke MRI could not be performed in 11 patients who were intubated and ventilated due to either hemicraniectomy or therapeutic hypothermia. In another seven patients the examination could not be completed because of a lack of patient tolerance, so that PWI was not performed on 17 patients on day 2.

In the initial MRI study a DWI abnormality was seen in all patients, 62 patients had lesions in the MCA territory or MCA and anterior cerebral artery territory, one patient each had lesions in the posterior or anterior territory only. Comparison of lesion size by PWI and DWI showed a PWI > DWI mismatch in 44 patients (68.75%). Forty-three of these 44 mismatch patients showed a cerebral artery occlusion in the MRA. Twenty of 64 patients showed a match between PWI and DWI, of these only seven demonstrated an occlusion in the MRA.

A day-2 MRA demonstrated a recanalization in 15 of the 50 patients who had an artery occlusion on day-1 MRA. Twenty of 50 patients with artery occlusion on MRA received intravenous recombinant tissue plasminogen activator (rtPA). On day 2, in 11 of these 20 patients recanalization of the occlusion could be shown by MRA, which resulted in a recanalization rate of 55% with intravenous rtPA.

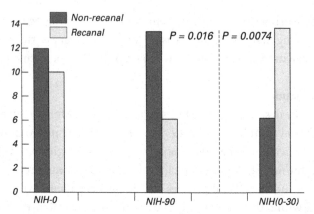

Figure 31.2 In patients with a mismatch comparison of NIHSS at day 90 between recanalization (Recanal) and non-recanalization (Non-recanal), a significantly better outcome was seen after recanalization.

Follow-up on day 2 of the 43 patients with a mismatch and MRA-proven occlusion of the artery showed recanalization in 15 patients and non-recanalization in 28 patients. Plate 31.1 demonstrates two examples of mismatch patients, one patient with recanalization and one without.

Last year we reported the midterm clinical and morphological results of a cohort of 35 mismatch patients (16 men, 19 women) aged 29 to 83 years (mean 62 years) [8]. Twenty-one of these 35 patients were identified by the initial MRI to have a considerable mismatch between the abnormal area on DWI and the abnormal area on PWI (PWI/DWI > 1.2). In all of these patients MRA at day 1 showed occlusion of a main cerebral artery (intracranial internal carotid artery or MCA). Fourteen of 35 patients did not have a PWI/DWI mismatch. In these patients MRA did not show major vessel occlusion. Eleven of 21 patients of the mismatch group received rtPA, five of them received the drug after 3 hours from symptom onset. MRA at day 2 showed recanalization in eight of 21 patients with a mismatch, six of whom had received rtPA intravenously within 5 hours after symptom onset. Two had spontaneous recanalization; in the other 13 patients, the vessel remained occluded. Of the six patients who received rtPA and had early recanalization, three were treated within the first 3 hours of stroke onset and three were treated between 3 and 5 hours.

Clinical follow-up examination showed a significantly better outcome on day 30 for the recanalization group (NIHSS score, $P=0.0016$; Standardized Stroke Scale (SSS), $P=0.003$; Barthel Index (BI), $P=0.0013$; Rankin Scale (RS) $P=0.0011$) and on day 90 (NIHSS score, $P=0.017$; SSS, $P=0.011$; BI, $P=0.005$; RS, $P=0.006$). There was also significantly greater improvement from day 1 to day 30 (NIHSS score $P=0.0074$). The significance regarding improvement disappeared though, at day 90 (NIHSS score: $P=0.49$), as there was one late death in this group due to cardiopulmonary embolism (Figure 31.2). Follow-up MRI showed significantly

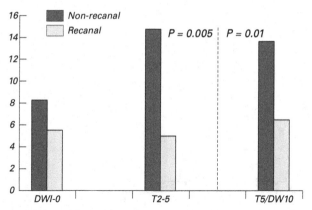

Figure 31.3 In patients with a mismatch comparison of infarct size at day 5 between recanalization (Recanal) and non-recanalization (Non-recanal), significantly smaller infarcts were seen after recanalization.

smaller infarcts in the recanalization group than in the non-recanalization group at day 2, as evident on DWI ($P=0.0016$), and at day 5, as evident on T_2-weighted imaging ($P=0.0005$). Furthermore, the increase of infarct size from day 1 to day 2 on DWI ($P=0.0055$) and from day 1 to day 5 on T_2-weighted imaging ($P=0.0011$) was significantly smaller in the recanalization group than in the non-recanalization group (Figure 31.3). A recently published follow-up analysis of patients who received stroke MRI and were treated with thrombolytic therapy showed this finding to be consistent [12].

Demonstration of "time is brain" with stroke MRI

The quotient of PWI/DWI measures the size of the tissue at risk in acute stroke patients. The concept of "time is brain", i.e., a reduction of salvageable brain tissue with progressing time, is shown by comparing this quotient with the time window between stroke onset and MRI investigation in an acute stroke population. In our population this comparison showed a continuous decrease of the quotient over time and demonstrated that stroke MRI is able to show that "time is brain" (Figure 31.4). However, the same figure shows that there are patients far beyond the 6 hour window, who had significant tissue at risk. These data challenge the concept of a rigid and universal time window for the treatment of acute ischemic stroke [13].

The progressive reduction of the therapeutic target (tissue at risk) is also ruled out by comparing patients with a relevant PWI/DWI mismatch ($>20\%$) over time. While in the 3 hour cohort, 80% of the patients show a mismatch, this is reduced to 40% in the 12 hour cohort (Figure 31.5). The mean PWI/DWI quotient in the 3 hour cohort was 20.2, in the 6 hour cohort 8.9, in the 9 hour cohort 1.7 and in the 12 hour cohort 0.5. This means that in the 9 hour cohort the mean PWI/DWI quotient still showed a relevant mismatch.

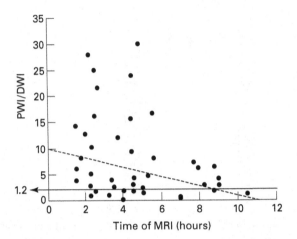

Figure 31.4   Correlation between PWI/DWI and time of the MRI (hours) after onset of symptoms in an acute stroke population of 64 patients. 1.2 defines the cutoff value of a 20% mismatch between PWI and DWI.

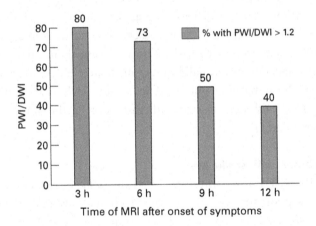

Figure 31.5   Decrease in the portion of patients with a relevant PWI/DWI quotient (>1.2) in an acute ischemic stroke population of 64 patients.

Conclusion

With the advent of sufficient therapies for acute ischemic stroke, the availability of accurate brain imaging information assumes an increasingly important role in patient management. Currently, CT is still the most widely used brain imaging technique for patients with acute stroke. However, stroke MRI has the potential to supply stroke physicians with all necessary information to select patients who may show a benefit from more aggressive therapies. Stroke MRI with DWI and PWI in combination with MRA and T_2-weighted imaging can: (i) demonstrate location and extent of the ischemic area; (ii) show the region of disturbed microvascular perfusion; (iii) demonstrate major vessel occlusions; and (iv) rule out hemorrhage or tumor, which may be responsible for stroke-like symptoms.

The Heidelberg trial on stroke MRI showed that acute stroke patients can be examined with a standardized stroke MRI protocol with a very high feasibility rate (98%). Stroke MRI with its major elements, PWI and DWI, is able to demonstrate the therapeutic target for any aggressive stroke therapy. This target is the mismatch between PWI and DWI (PWI > DWI), which demonstrates the individual size of the tissue at risk. Stroke MRI shows that this tissue at risk continuously decreases with time. However, it can be shown that, even after a quite long time window of more than 9 hours after stroke onset, the ischemic stroke patient can show a relevant mismatch and therefore relevant tissue at risk. Our follow-up study clearly shows that successful recanalization saves tissue at risk as defined by stroke MRI. This results in significantly smaller infarcts and significantly better clinical outcome. Therefore, stroke MRI is an ideal tool for identifying patients for recanalization therapy.

REFERENCES

1 Astrup J, Siesjö B & Symon L (1981) Thresholds in cerebral ischemia – the ischemic penumbra. *Stroke*, 12, 723–5.

2 Moseley ME, Kucharczyk J, Mintorovitch J, Cohen Y, Kurhanewicz J, Derugin N, Asgari H & Norman D (1990) Diffusion-weighted MR imaging of acute stroke: correlation with T2-weighted and magnetic susceptibility-enhanced MR imaging in cats. *AJNR: American Journal of Neuroradiology*, 11, 423–9.

3 Warach S, Gaa J, Siewert B, Wielopolski P & Edelman RR (1995) Acute human stroke studied by whole brain echo planar diffusion-weighted magnetic resonance imaging. *Annals of Neurology*, 37, 231–41.

4 Mohr JP, Biller J, Hilal SK, Yuh WTC, Tatemichi TK, Hedges S, Tali E, Nguyen H, Mun I, Adams HP Jr, Grimsman K & Marler JR (1995) Magnetic resonance vs. computed tomographic imaging in acute stroke. *Stroke*, 26, 807–12.

5 Belliveau JW, Rosen BR, Kantor HL, Rzedzian RR, Kennedy DN, McKinstry RC, Vevea JM, Cohen MS, Pykett IL & Brady TJ (1990) Functional cerebral imaging by susceptibility-contrast NMR. *Magnetic Resonance in Medicine*, 14, 538–46.

6 Moseley ME, Wendland MF & Kucharczyk J (1991) Magnetic resonance imaging of diffusion and perfusion. *Topics in Magnetic Resonance Imaging*, 3, 50–67.

7 Tong DC, Yenari MA, Albers GW, O'Brien M, Marks MP & Moseley ME (1998) Correlation of perfusion- and diffusion-weighted MRI with NIHSS score in acute (< 6.5 hour) ischemic stroke. *Neurology*, 50, 864–70.

8 Jansen O, Schellinger P, Fiebach J, Hacke W & Sartor K (1999) Early recanalisation in acute ischaemic stroke saves tissue at risk defined by MRI. *Lancet*, **353**, 2036–7.

9 Schellinger PD, Jansen O, Fiebach JB, Hacke W & Sartor K (1999) A standardized MRI stroke protocol: comparison with CT in hyperacute intracerebral hemorrhage. *Stroke*, **30**, 765–8.

10 Linfante I, Llinas RH, Caplan LR & Warach S (1999) MRI features of intracerebral hemorrhage within 2 hours from symptom onset. *Stroke*, **30**, 2263–7.

11 Patel MR, Edelman RR & Warach S (1996) Detection of hyperacute primary intraparenchymal hemorrhage by magnetic resonance imaging. *Stroke*, **27**, 2321–4.

12 Schellinger PD, Jansen O, Fiebach JB, Heiland S, Steiner T, Schwab S, Pohlers O, Ryssel H, Sartor K & Hacke W (2000) Monitoring intravenous recombinant tissue plasminogen activator thrombolysis for acute ischemic stroke with diffusion and perfusion MRI. *Stroke*, **31**, 1318–28.

13 Baron JC, von Kummer R & del Zoppo GJ (1995) Treatment of acute ischemic stroke: challenging the concept of a rigid and universal time window. *Stroke*, **26**, 2219–21.

Part X

Risk factors, clinical trials, and new therapeutic horizons

Co-Chairs: Vladimir Hachinski, John R. Marler,
Gregory W. Albers & Marc Fisher

32

Vascular factors in Alzheimer's disease

José G. Merino[1] & Vladimir Hachinski[2]

Department of Clinical Neurological Sciences, University of Western Ontario, Ontario, Canada

Introduction

The presence of cerebrovascular disease and vascular risk factors are generally considered to be exclusion criteria for the clinical diagnosis of Alzheimer's disease (AD). The high prevalence of cerebrovascular disease and AD in the elderly population means that the category of patients with dementia, stroke and vascular dementia, includes patients with AD [1]. The criteria used to diagnose AD were established by consensus, with vascular abnormalities becoming an artificial border between vascular dementia and AD. However, growing evidence suggests that the distinction is not clear cut [2]. Half of all patients with vascular disease who become demented also have AD [3] and a third of patients with pathologically confirmed AD have evidence of vascular lesions [4]. Brain infarcts may play an important role in determining the presence and severity of clinical symptoms of AD [5]. Data from large population studies give validity to the construct of mixed AD/vascular dementia [6]. It is not known whether the cerebral vascular pathology found in the brains of patients with AD is coincident or causal. Is there a direct interaction between the two pathological processes? Alternatively, does cerebrovascular disease unmask subclinical AD? Data supporting both arguments exist. The puzzle remains. Understanding the interaction between cerebrovascular and neurodegenerative disorders demands a radical shift in framework and thought process.

Coexistence of AD and vascular pathology

Several longitudinal studies [5,7,8] have demonstrated that the changes of cerebrovascular disease and neurodegeneration with Alzheimer-type pathology have synergistic effects on cognition [9]. The Nun Study evaluated cognitive functions and the prevalence of dementia in a group of elderly women [5]. Mixed dementia was common; at autopsy 47% (of 102 brains studied) had neuropathological changes of AD and at least one infarct. Among the nuns with a pathological diagnosis of AD, 57% had clinical dementia. Among those having the pathological diagnosis of AD plus cortical infarcts, 75% were demented. When the infarcts were subcortical, 93% were demented. Participants with lacunar infarcts in the basal ganglia, thalamus or deep white matter had a specially high prevalence of dementia as compared with those without infarcts (odds ratio for dementia with large lobe infarcts, 6.7, 95% confidence interval (CI) 0.9 to 48.3; odds ratio for dementia with lacunar infarcts, 20.7, 95% CI 1.5 to 288) [5]. Fewer neuropathological lesions of AD resulted in dementia in those with lacunar infarcts compared with those without infarcts [5]. A few small infarcts in strategic regions of the brain may be sufficient to produce dementia in those made vulnerable by abundant neuropathological AD lesions in the cortex. In this study infarcts were not associated with increased AD pathology in the entire group (i.e., those without dementia), suggesting that both processes are independent but that cerebrovascular disease can precipitate clinical AD at pathological stages that would not otherwise be clinically apparent [5].

Similar results were found in subjects with autopsy-proven AD studied by the Consortium to Establish a Registry for Alzheimer's Disease (CERAD) [8]. Patients with concomitant cerebral infarcts or lacunar lesions had a more severe dementia at the time of the last follow-up visit than patients with changes of AD alone [8]. Both groups had similar cognitive profiles on entry into the CERAD study. Subsequently, patients with AD and vascular lesions performed worse on verbal fluency, the Boston Naming Test and the Mini-Mental State Examination [8]. The presence of cerebral infarcts did not affect performance on constructional praxis, word list learning and delayed word recall tasks; these deficits had been detected in patients with mixed dementia in the Nun Study [5].

Coexistent cerebrovascular pathology means that a lower load of Alzheimer-type lesions is needed to produce clinical dementia. In the Nun Study, the degree of Alzheimer-type pathology required to produce a detectable clinical deficit was lower in patients with concomitant strokes than in patients with AD alone [5]. Similar results were found by the Oxford Project to Investigate Memory and Ageing, a longitudinal prospective study of dementia [7]. In addition, the major determinant of cognitive deficit in patients with AD alone was the density of neurofibrillary tangles, and in the presence of vascular disease it was the amount of amyloid laid down as plaques [7]. The CERAD investigators did not find this correlation between cerebrovascular pathology and the amount of neurofibrillary tangles and senile plaques needed to produce a clinical deficit [8]. However, CERAD used semiquantitative ratings; the others used quantitative measurements [8].

Cognitive impairment after stroke

Cognitive impairment after stroke is very common. It varies along a wide spectrum from isolated cognitive deficits to incapacitating, full-blown dementia. Between one quarter and one third of patients with an acute stroke meet standardized criteria for dementia at 3 months [10–13], and a proportion of these patients have mixed dementia. An even higher percentage (26.8% to 61%) does not meet these criteria but shows evidence of cognitive impairment (defined as impaired performance on one or more domains of cognitive testing) [12–14]. The incidence of poststroke dementia or cognitive impairment remains high after taking into account the existence of prestroke cognitive decline [12,15]. The effects of stroke on cognitive function persist for a long time after the vascular event. A risk factor for dementia in the Kungsholmen Project was a stroke that had occurred up to 3 years prior to a patient's entry into the study [16]. A study done at the Mayo Clinic [17] found that the incidence of dementia in the first year after a stroke was nine time greater than expected. In individuals who did not develop dementia by the first year, the subsequent risk of dementia was about twice the risk in the general population. After the first year, a 50% increase was observed in AD in the cohort compared with that in the community. Some of these cases may represent subclinical AD.

Strokes may precipitate, aggravate or accelerate a pre-existing process or predisposition [18]. A proposed explanation for this interaction is that ischemic events induce the amyloid precursor protein and other Alzheimer pathology-associated factors that may interact with glial cells to generate lesions in hypoperfused areas of the brain [19]. This could be a result of early microglial cyclooxygenase-2 induction by ischemia [20]. This is particularly intriguing given evidence from large epidemiological studies showing that chronic use of aspirin and other non-steroidal anti-inflammatory agents is associated with a decreased risk of AD [21] through suppression of microglial activity [22].

Risk factors in common

AD and vascular disease share some risk factors. These may be causally related or they may share common environmental and genetic determinants. Cerebrovascular disease, hypertension, hyperlipidemia, smoking and male gender accelerate cerebral degenerative changes, cognitive decline and dementia [23].

Epidemiological studies show a link between hypertension and AD. In a cross-sectional study in Kuopio, high systolic blood pressure correlated with increased risk of AD (1.01, 95% CI 1.0 to 1.03) [24]. In the Göteborg Longitudinal Study [25] patients who developed Alzheimer-type dementia at ages 79 to 85 years had higher systolic and diastolic blood pressure at age 70 than those who did not develop dementia. Patients with white matter lesions on computed tomography at age 85 had a higher blood pressure at age 70 than those without such lesions [25]. The authors of the study conclude that hypertension possibly increased the risk of dementia by inducing small vessel disease and white matter lesions [25]. Blood pressure declined in the years preceding the dementia [25]. A similar finding was also noted in the cross-sectional Kungsholmen Project. Both systolic and diastolic blood pressure were related inversely to the prevalence of dementia [26]. Patients with isolated systolic hypertension who were treated with antihypertensives in the Systolic Hypertension in Europe trial had a lower incidence of dementia than those who were not treated [27]. Most patients who became demented, in the placebo and the treatment groups, fulfilled the criteria for AD or mixed dementia [27].

Pathological evidence also links AD and hypertension. Hypertensive patients without dementia had an increased prevalence of senile plaques and neurofibrillary tangles than did patients with normal blood pressure [28].

Heart disease is associated with AD [29]. Significant associations between dementia and cardiovascular risk factors (electrocardiographic evidence of ischemia, systolic hypertension, smoking) were found in the UK Medical Research Council Elderly Hypertension Trial [30]. A significant positive association among atrial fibrillation and dementia and impaired cognitive function was found in the Rotterdam Study [31]. Interestingly, the strongest association was found with AD, not with vascular dementia [31].

Necropsy studies have shown that the brains of patients without dementia who died from coronary artery disease had more senile plaques than brains from patients without heart disease [32]. The distribution of plaques in patients with heart disease is similar to that in AD patients, albeit less numerous [33]. No difference exists in the number of neurofibrillary tangles between patients with and without heart disease [33].

High serum cholesterol during middle age confers an increased risk of AD in old age [34]. In the Rotterdam Study [35], all indicators of atherosclerosis that were examined (vessel wall thickness, carotid plaque, ankle to brachial systolic blood pressure ratio) were associated with dementia, with AD, and with vascular dementia. The frequency of all dementia, AD and vascular dementia, increased with the degree of atherosclerosis. The odds ratio of AD in those with severe atherosclerosis compared with those without atherosclerosis was 3.0 (95% CI 1.5 to 6.0) [35].

Diabetes mellitus is a risk factor for AD. In a population-based study [36] patients with adult onset diabetes had an increased risk of developing dementia (relative risk [RR] 1.66, 95% CI 1.34 to 2.05) and AD (RR for men 2.27, 95% CI 1.55 to 3.31; RR for women 1.37, 95% CI 0.94 to 2.01). Diabetes almost doubled the risk of dementia (RR 1.9, 95% CI 1.3 to 2.8) and AD (RR 1.9, 95% CI 1.2 to 3.1) in the Rotterdam Study [37]. Those patients who required treatment with insulin were at the highest risk of developing dementia (RR 4.3, 95% CI 1.7 to 10.5) [37]. The risk attributable to diabetes was 8.8% [37]. In a cross-sectional population study of 980 people aged 69 to 78 years in Kuopio, 4.7% of the patients were classified as having possible or probable AD. Features of the insulin resistance syndrome were found to be associated with AD independently of the apolipoprotein E (ApoE) ε4 phenotype [24].

The role of smoking is not clear. A meta-analysis of 11 case-controlled studies showed a statistically significant inverse association between AD and smoking [38]. The Rotterdam Study found that smoking was associated with a doubling of the risk of dementia and AD [39].

Genetic links

Genetic susceptibility factors for AD have been identified. Significantly, these may provide a link between this condition and heart disease.

APOE is the product of the APOE gene on chromosome 19. It plays a role in triglyceride-rich lipoprotein metabolism and cholesterol homeostasis [40]. The presence of the APOE ε4 isoform has been associated with coronary heart disease in middle-aged men [41] and with the development of atherosclerosis [42].

APOE has an important role in central nervous system repair. It influences recovery after a variety of neurological insults [43] such as head trauma and stroke, and it may have neurotrophic, immunomodulatory and antioxidant effects [43]. The presence of the ε4 isoform has been associated with poor repair after neuronal damage that results from amyloid-β peptide deposition, oxidative stress and excitotoxic amino acids [44]. The increased density of senile plaques seen in hypertensive patients seems to correlate with the APOE ε4 allele dose frequency [45].

APOE ε4 is a susceptibility gene that accelerates the rate of an ongoing, universal, metabolic process [46]. It is a genetic risk factor for dementia with stroke, including AD and vascular dementia [24, 35, 47]. The presence of APOE ε4 was associated with poor performance on cognitive testing in the Cardiovascular Health Study [48]. In the Zutphen Elderly Study cohort [49], cerebrovascular disease and the presence of APOE ε4 had a synergistic effect on cognitive decline. This finding was corroborated by a study that pooled data from two population-based studies (Rotterdam and New York City). Patients with dementia and stroke had a higher frequency of APOE ε4 allele than controls [47].

Atherosclerosis was a risk factor for dementia and its major subtypes, AD and vascular dementia, in patients enrolled in the Rotterdam Study [35], particularly in APOE carriers. Elevated cholesterol concentrations in middle age may be an intermediate factor through which the APOE ε4 allele is associated with the risk of AD

[34]. However, the risk of AD and vascular dementia in the presence of the APOE ε4 allele is independent of the presence of atherosclerosis [1].

Patients older than 85 years with white matter lesions have an increased risk of dementia only if they also have the APOE ε4 allele. Possession of APOE ε4 is associated with an increased risk of dementia only in subjects who have white matter lesions [50]. APOE may neither be sufficient nor necessary to produce dementia in old age. Dementia in the very old results from the interaction of several pathological processes [50].

Other candidate links between AD and vascular risk are the components of the renin–angiotensin system [51]. The angiotensin-converting enzyme (ACE) D allele has been associated with cardiovascular diseases (a higher risk of myocardial infarction) [52,53]. Some [54], but not all [55–57], epidemiological studies have found the presence of the ACE D allele as a risk factor for the development of AD. Physiopathological studies have shown that learning in animals can be influenced by the manipulation of the renin–angiotensin system [58], and the use of ACE inhibitors for blood pressure control has been associated with improved work performance and cognitive function [59].

Cerebrovascular pathology in AD

A variety of cerebrovascular lesions are found in the brains of patients with AD: cerebral amyloid angiopathy, endothelial and vascular smooth muscle degeneration, macroscopic infarction, microinfarction, hemorrhage and white matter lesions related to small vessel disease [60]. Cerebral amyloid angiopathy is found in the leptomeningeal and cortical arteries of 62% to 97% of patients with AD [61, 62]. In the CERAD study, 83% of patients had at least a mild degree of amyloid angiopathy [63]. It has been hypothesized that cerebral amyloid angiopathy may compromise vascular function and lead to a state of chronic hypoperfusion, although the proof remains elusive [18]. It is also a cause of intracerebral hemorrhage; up to 10% of patients with AD have evidence of intracerebral hemorrhage [62].

Patients with AD have microvascular pathology independent of amyloid deposition [60,64]. These abnormalities relate to blood–brain barrier function and imply abnormalities in the patency of brain microvasculature [60]. The abnormalities include degeneration of vascular smooth muscle cells, focal constrictions and degenerative changes in smooth muscle cells, degeneration and focal necrotic changes in the endothelium, vascular basement membrane alterations accompanied by accumulation of collagen, loss of perivascular nerve plexus, decreased mitochondrial content, increased pinocytic vesicles and loss of tight junctions [60]. Accumulating knowledge of the vasoactive properties of amyloid and of the role of the endothelium in health and disease will lead to a new understanding of the relationship between blood vessels and AD [18]. White matter lesions have been described in AD [65]. Long-standing hypertension leads to lipohyalinosis and possibly to white matter lesions. This may be an explanation for the link between hypertension and AD.

Conclusion

The use of vascular risk factors and cerebrovascular disease as exclusion criteria in traditional definitions of AD has hindered progress in the discovery of the relationship between AD and vascular disease. The situation is changing. Longitudinal epidemiological studies show that cardiovascular risk factors are associated with AD. It has also become evident that cerebrovascular disease can precipitate or potentiate neurodegenerative dementia. This new knowledge may lead to preventive and therapeutic interventions. These potential opportunities will become real when the new knowledge becomes true understanding.

REFERENCES

1 Slooter AJC, Cruts M, Ott A, Bots ML, Witteman JCM, Hofman A, Van Broeckhoven C, Breteler MMB & van Duijn CM (1999) The effect of APOE on dementia is not through atherosclerosis: the Rotterdam Study. *Neurology*, **53**, 1593–5.

2 Gold G, Giannakopoulos P & Bouras C (1998) Reevaluating the role of vascular changes in the differential diagnosis of Alzheimer's disease and vascular dementia. *European Neurology*, **40**, 121–9.

3 O'Brien MD (1994) How does cerebrovascular disease cause dementia? *Dementia*, **5**, 133–6.

4 Gearing M, Mirra SS, Sumi SM, Hansen L, Hedreen J & Heyman A (1995) The Consortium to Establish a Registry for Alzheimer's Disease (CERAD) part X: neuropathology confirmation of the clinical diagnosis of Alzheimer's disease. *Neurology*, **45**, 461–6.

5 Snowdon DA, Greiner LH, Mortimer JA, Riley KP, Greiner PA & Markersbery WR (1997) Brain infarction and the clinical expression of Alzheimer disease. The Nun Study. *Journal of the American Medical Association*, **277**, 813–17.

6 Rockwood K, Macknight C, Wentzel C, Black S, Bouchard R, Gauthier S, Feldman H, Hogan D, Kertesz A & Montgomery P (2000) The diagnosis of "mixed" dementia in the Consortium for the Investigation of Vascular Impairment of Cognition (CIVIC). *Annals of the New York Academy of Sciences*, **903**, 522–8.

7 Nagy Z, Esiri MM, Jobst KA, Morris JH, King EM, McDonald B, Joachim C, Litchfield S, Barnetson L & Smith AD (1997) The effects of additional pathology on the cognitive deficit in Alzheimer disease. *Journal of Neuropathology & Experimental Neurology*, **56**, 165–70.

8 Heyman A, Fillenbaum GG, Welsh-Bohmer KA, Gearing M, Mirra SS, Mohs RC, Peterson BL & Pieper CF (1998) Cerebral infarcts in patients with autopsy-proven Alzheimer's disease: CERAD, part XVIII. *Neurology*, **51**, 159–62.

9 Hachinski V (1983) Multi-infarct dementia (Symposium on Cerebrovascular Disease). *Neurologic Clinics*, **1**, 27–36.

10 Tatemichi TK, Desmond DW, Mayeux R, Paik M, Stern Y, Sano M, et al. (1992) Dementia after stroke: baseline frequency, risks, and clinical features in a hospitalized cohort. *Neurology*, **42**, 1185–93.

11 Tatemichi TK, Paik M, Bagiella E, Desmond DW, Stern Y, Sano M, Hauser WA & Mayeux R (1994) Risk of dementia after stroke in a hospitalized cohort: results of a longitudinal study. *Neurology*, **44**, 1885–91.

12 Pohjasvaara T, Erkinjuntti T, Vataja R & Kaste M (1997) Dementia three months after stroke. Baseline frequency and effect of different definitions of dementia in the Helsinki Stroke Aging Memory Study (SAM) cohort. *Stroke*, **28**, 785–92.

13 Desmond DW, Moroney JT, Paik MC, Sano M, Mohr JP, Aboumatar S, Tseng C-L, Chan S, Williams JBW, Remien RH, Hauser WA & Stern Y (2000) Frequency and clinical determinants of dementia after ischemic stroke. *Neurology*, **54**, 1124–31.

14 Tatemichi TK, Desmond DW, Stern Y, Paik M, Sano M & Bagiella E (1994) Cognitive impairment after stroke: frequency, patterns, and relationship to functional abilities. *Journal of Neurology, Neurosurgery & Psychiatry*, **57**, 202–7.

15 Hénon H, Pasquier F, Durieu I, Godefroy O, Lucas C, Lebert F & Leys D (1997) Preexisting dementia in stroke patients. Baseline frequency, associated factors, and outcome. *Stroke*, **28**, 2429–36.

16 Zhu L, Fratiglioni L, Guo Z, Winblad B & Viitanen M (2000) Incidence of stroke in - relation to cognitive function and dementia in the Kungsholmen project. *Neurology*, **54**, 2103–7.

17 Kokmen E, Whisnant JP, O'Fallon WM, Chu CP & Beard CM (1996) Dementia after ischemic stroke: a population-based study in Rochester, Minnesota (1960–1984). *Neurology*, **46**, 154–9.

18 Hachinski V & Munoz D (2000) Vascular factors in cognitive impairment – where are we now? *Annals of the New York Academy of Sciences*, **903**, 1–5.

19 Kalaria RN, Bhatti SU, Palatinsky EA, Pennington DH, Shelton ER, Chan HW, Perry G & Lust WD (1993) Accumulation of the β amyloid precursor protein at sites of ischemic injury in rat brain. *Neuroreport*, **4**, 211–14.

20 Sairanen T, Ristimaki A, Karjalainen-Lindsberg ML, Paetau A, Kaste M & Lindsberg PJ (1998) Cyclooxygenase-2 is induced globally in infarcted human brain. *Annals of Neurology*, **43**, 738–47.

21 Stewart WF, Kawas C, Corrada M & Metter EJ (1997) Risk of Alzheimer's disease and duration of NSAID use. *Neurology*, **48**, 626–32.

22 Mackensie IRA & Munoz DG (1998) Nonsteroidal anti-inflammatory drug use and Alzheimer-type pathology in aging. *Neurology*, **50**, 986–90.

23 Meyer JS, Rauch GM, Rauch RA, Haque A & Crawford K (2000) Cardiovascular and other risk factors for Alzheimer's disease and vascular dementia. *Annals of the New York Academy of Sciences*, **903**, 411–23.

24 Kuusisto J, Koivisto K, Mykkanen L, Helkala EL, Vanhanen M, Hanninen T, Kervinen K, Kesaniemi YA, Riekkinen PJ & Laakso M (1997) Association between features of the insulin resistance syndrome and Alzheimer's disease independently of apolipoprotein E4 phenotype: cross sectional population based study. *BMJ*, **315**, 1045–9.

25 Skoog I, Lernfelt B, Landahl S, Palmertz B, Andreasson L-A, Nilsson L, Persson G, Oden A & Svanborg A (1996) 15-year longitudinal study of blood pressure and dementia. *Lancet*, **347**, 1141–5.

26 Guo Z, Viitanen M, Fratiglioni L & Winblad B (1996) Low blood pressure and dementia in elderly people: the Kungsholmen project. *BMJ*, **312**, 805–8.

27 Forette F, Seux M-L, Staessen JA, Thijs L, Birkenhager WH, Babarskiene M-R, Babeanu S, Bossini A, Gil-Extremera B, Girerd X, Laks T, Lilov E, Moisseyev V, Tuomilehto J, Vanhanen H, Webster J, Yodfat Y & Fagard R (1998) Prevention of dementia in randomised double-blind placebo-controlled Systolic Hypertension in Europe (Syst-Eur) trial. *Lancet*, **352**, 1347–51.

28 Sparks DL, Scheff SW, Liu H, Landers TM, Coyne CM & Hunsaker JC III (1995) Increased incidence of neurofibrillary tangles (NFT) in non-demented individuals with hypertension. *Journal of the Neurological Sciences*, **131**, 162–9.

29 Stewart R (1998) Cardiovascular factors in Alzheimer's disease. *Journal of Neurology, Neurosurgery & Psychiatry*, **65**, 143–7.

30 Prince M, Cullen M & Mann A (1994) Risk factors for Alzheimer's disease and dementia: a case-control study based on the MRC elderly hypertension trial. *Neurology*, **44**, 97–104.

31 Ott A, Breteler MMB, de Bruyne MC, van Harskamp F, Grobbee DE & Hofman A (1997) Atrial fibrillation and dementia in a population-based study. The Rotterdam Study. *Stroke*, **28**, 316–21.

32 Sparks DL, Hunsacker JC III, Scheff SW, Kryscio RJ, Henson JL & Markesbery WR (1990) Cortical senile plaques in coronary artery disease, aging and Alzheimer's disease. *Neurobiology of Aging*, **11**, 601–7.

33 Soneira CF & Scott TM (1996) Severe cardiovascular disease and Alzheimer's disease: senile plaque formation in cortical areas. *Clinical Anatomy*, **9**, 118–27.

34 Notkola IL, Sulkava R, Pekkanen J, Erkinjuntti T, Ehnholm C, Kivinen P, Tuomilehto J & Nissinen A (1998) Serum total cholesterol, apolipoprotein E ε4 allele, and Alzheimer's disease. *Neuroepidemiology*, **17**, 14–20.

35 Hofman A, Ott A, Breteler MMB, Bots ML, Slooter AJC, van Harskamp F, van Duijn CN, Van Broeckhoven C & Grobbee DE (1997) Atherosclerosis, apolipoprotein E, and prevalence of dementia and Alzheimer's disease in the Rotterdam Study. *Lancet*, **349**, 151–4.

36 Leibson CL, Rocca WA, Hanson VA, Cha R, Kokmen E, O'Brien PC & Palumbo PJ (1997) Risk of dementia among persons with diabetes mellitus: a population-based cohort study. *American Journal of Epidemiology*, **145**, 301–8.

37 Ott A, Stolk RP, van Harskamp F, Pols HAP, Hofman A & Breteler MMB (1999) Diabetes mellitus and the risk of dementia: the Rotterdam Study. *Neurology*, **53**, 1937–42.

38 Graves AB, van Duijn CM, Chandra V, Fratiglioni L, Heyman A, Jorm AF, et al. (1991) Alcohol and tobacco consumption as risk factors for Alzheimer's disease: a collaborative re-analysis of case-control studies. EURODEM Risk Factors Research Group. *International Journal of Epidemiology*, **20** Suppl 2, S48–S57.

39 Ott A, Slooter AJC, Hofman A, van Harskamp F, Witteman JCM, Van Broeckhoven C, van Duijn CM & Breteler MMB (1998) Smoking and risk of dementia and Alzheimer's disease in a population-based cohort study: the Rotterdam Study. *Lancet*, 351, 1840–3.

40 Curtiss LK & Boisvert WA (2000) Apolipoprotein E and atherosclerosis. *Current Opinion in Lipidology*, 11, 243–51.

41 Wilson PWF, Myers RH, Larson MG, Ordovas JM, Wolf PA & Schaefer EJ (1994) Apolipoprotein E alleles, dyslipidemia, and coronary heart disease: the Framingham offspring study. *Journal of the American Medical Association*, 272, 1666–71.

42 Davignon J, Gregg RE & Sing CF (1988) Apolipoprotein E polymorphism and atherosclerosis. *Arteriosclerosis*, 8, 1–21.

43 Laskowitz DT, Horsburgh K & Roses AD (1998) Apolipoprotein E and the CNS response to injury. *Journal of Cerebral Blood Flow & Metabolism*, 18, 465–71.

44 Mahley RW & Huang Y (1997) Apolipoprotein E: from atherosclerosis to Alzheimer's disease and beyond. *Current Opinion in Lipidology*, 10, 207–17.

45 Sparks DL, Scheff SW, Liu H, Landers T, Danner F, Coyne CM & Hunsaker JC III (1996) Increased density of senile plaques (SP), but not neurofibrillary tangles (NFT), in non-demented individuals with the apolipoprotein E4 allele: comparison to confirmed Alzheimer's disease patients. *Journal of the Neurological Sciences*, 138, 97–104.

46 Goedert M, Strittmatter WJ & Roses AD (1994) Alzheimer's disease. Risky apolipoprotein in the brain. *Nature*, 372, 45–6.

47 Slooter AJ, Tang MX, van Duijn CM, Stern Y, Ott A, Bell K, Breteler MM, Van Broeckhoven C, Tatemichi TK, Tycko B, Hofman A & Mayeux R (1997) Apolipoprotein E ε4 and the risk of dementia with stroke. A population-based investigation. *Journal of the American Medical Association*, 277, 818–21.

48 Kuller LH, Shemanski L, Manolio T, Haan M, Fried L, Bryan N, Burke GL, Tracy R & Bhadelia R (1998) Relationship between APOE, MRI findings, and cognitive function in the Cardiovascular Health Study. *Stroke*, 29, 388–98.

49 Kalmijn S, Feskens EJM, Launer LJ & Kromhout D (1996) Cerebrovascular disease, the apolipoprotein ε4 allele, and cognitive decline in a community-based study of elderly men. *Stroke*, 27, 2230–5.

50 Skoog I, Hesse C, Aevarsson O, Landahl S, Wahlström J, Fredman P & Blennow K (1998) A population study of apoE genotype at the age of 85: relation to dementia, cerebrovascular disease, and mortality. *Journal of Neurology, Neurosurgery & Psychiatry*, 64, 37–43.

51 Amouyel P, Richard F, Berr C, David-Fromentin I & Helbecque N (2000) The renin angiotensin system and Alzheimer's disease. *Annals of the New York Academy of Sciences*, 903, 437–41.

52 Cambien F, Poirier O, Lecerf L, Evans A, Cambou JP, Arveiler D, Luc G, Bard JM, Bara L, Ricard S, Tiret L, Amouyel P, Alhencgelas F & Soubrier F (1992) Deletion polymorphism in the gene for angiotensin-converting enzyme is a potent risk factor for myocardial infarction. *Nature*, 359, 641–4.

53 Hamon M, Amant C, Bauters C, Lablanche J-M, Bertrand M & Amouyel P (1996) ACE polymorphism, a genetic predictor of occlusion after coronary angioplasty. *American Journal of Cardiology*, 78, 679–81.

54 Amouyel P, Richard F, Cottel D, Amant C, Codron V & Helbecque N (1996) The deletion allele of the angiotensin I converting enzyme gene as a genetic susceptibility factor for cognitive impairment. *Neuroscience Letters*, **217**, 203–5.

55 Tysoe C, Galinsky D, Robinson D, Brayne CE, Easton DF, Huppert FA, Dening T, Paykel ES & Rubinsztein DC (1997) Analysis of alpha-1 antichymotrypsin, presenilin-1, angiotensin-converting enzyme, and methylenetetrahydrofolate reductase loci as candidates for dementia. *American Journal of Medical Genetics*, **74**, 207–12.

56 Scacchi R, De Bernardini L, Mantuano E, Vilardo T, Donini LM, Ruggeri M, Gemma AT, Pascone R & Corbo RM (1998) DNA polymorphisms of apolipoprotein B and angiotensin I-converting enzyme genes and relationships with lipid levels in Italian patients with vascular dementia or Alzheimer's disease. *Dementia & Geriatric Cognitive Disorders*, **9**, 186–90.

57 Chapman J, Wang N, Treves TA, Korczyn AD & Bornstein NM (1998) ACE, MTHFR, factor V Leiden, and APOE polymorphisms in patients with vascular and Alzheimer's dementia. *Stroke*, **29**, 1401–4.

58 Wright JW & Harding JW (1994) Brain angiotensin receptor subtypes in the control of physiologic and behavioral responses. *Neuroscience and Biobehavioral Reviews*, **18**, 21–53.

59 Croog SH, Levine S, Testa MA, Brown B, Bulpitt CJ, Jenkins CD, Klerman GL & Williams GH (1986) The effects of antihypertensive therapy on the quality of life. *New England Journal of Medicine*, **314**, 1657–64.

60 Kalaria RN & Ballard C (1999) Overlap between pathology of Alzheimer disease and vascular dementia. *Alzheimer Disease and Associated Disorders*, **13** Suppl 3, S115–S123.

61 Vinters HV (1987) Cerebral amyloid angiopathy: a critical review. *Stroke*, **18**, 311–24.

62 Premkumar DRD, Cohen DL, Hedera P, Friedland RP & Kalaria RN (1996) Apolipoprotein E ε4 alleles in cerebral amyloid angiopathy and cerebrovascular pathology in Alzheimer's disease. *American Journal of Pathology*, **148**, 2083–95.

63 Ellis RJ, Olichney JM, Thal LJ, Morris JC, Beekly D & Heyman A (1996) Cerebral amyloid angiopathy in the brains of patients with Alzheimer's disease. The CERAD experience, part XV. *Neurology*, **46**, 1592–6.

64 Kalaria RN (1996) Cerebral vessels in ageing and Alzheimer's disease. *Pharmacology and Therapeutics*, **72**, 193–214.

65 Díaz JF, Merskey H, Hachinski VC, Lee DH, Boniferro M, Wong CJ, Mirsen TR & Fox H (1991) Improved recognition of leukoaraiosis and cognitive impairment in Alzheimer's disease. *Archives of Neurology*, **48**, 1022–5.

33

Beyond neuroprotection: the protection of axons and oligodendrocytes in cerebral ischemia

James McCulloch[1], Katalin Komajti[2], Valerio Valeriani[3] &
Deborah Dewar[4]

[1,3,4] Wellcome Surgical Institute and Hugh Fraser Neuroscience Laboratories, University of Glasgow, Glasgow, Scotland

[2] Experimental Research Department, 2nd Institute of Physiology, Budapest, Hungary

Neuroprotection and anti-ischemic drug development

A decade ago, there was little compelling evidence that pharmacological intervention could radically alter outcome after cerebral ischemia, even in experimental animals. By 1996, the pace of advance was such that a large number of drugs targeted at neurotransmitter receptors, and related mechanisms involved in ischemic damage, had advanced to clinical trials in stroke and head injury [1]. The transformation of the pharmacology of cerebral ischemia had been achieved for two major reasons: first, the elucidation of neurochemical cascades initiated by ischemia, which revealed potential targets for intervention; and, second, the systematic assessment of drug efficacy using robust end-points (quantitative histopathology) in the most pertinent animal models. Since the elucidation of the excitotoxic cascade, numerous other pathological mechanisms have been identified by which neuroprotection can be achieved in ischemia. However, excitotoxicity remains central to current concepts of neuronal cell death and provides the prototype for anti-ischemic drug development for new pharmacological targets, i.e., reduction of the volume of neuronal perikaryal damage in models of focal cerebral ischemia.

Animal models of focal cerebral ischemia are generally recognized as the most pertinent in relation to human stroke. The most widely used models of focal cerebral ischemia involve occlusion of the middle cerebral artery (MCA) either by surgical division [2,3] or intraluminal suture placement [4]. Occlusion of the MCA produces necrosis in the territory supplied by the artery, with the final lesion size being established after approximately 3 hours of ischemia [5], although enlargement of the lesion, as distinct from edema development, may occur at later times, particularly with mild ischemia [6,7]. The pattern of ischemia produced after MCA occlusion (MCAO) results in a sharp boundary between viable and damaged tissue on histological examination and this lends itself to volumetric assessment of the lesion in gray matter [8]. While the volume of the ischemic lesion is generally well defined when putative anti-ischemic drugs are evaluated, the histological definition of the lesion is often rudimentary. At best, it involves mapping the distribution of eosinophilic neuronal perikarya; at worst, it means simply mapping the area of tissue pallor using triphenyltetrazolium staining. This limited histological definition of ischemic pathology in many pharmacological investigations has contributed to a neglect of ischemic white matter pathology where the definition of ischemic damage is difficult.

Based on their proven ability to reduce gray matter damage in animal models, a large number of drugs targeted at neurotransmitter receptors and related mechanisms involved in ischemic damage have advanced to clinical trials in stroke and head injury [1,9]. At the time of writing, the outcome of the clinical trials of neuroprotective drugs has been disappointing. The notable exception in clinical trials for stroke is the benefit demonstrated with tissue plasminogen activator [10], where the putative mechanism of action is restoration of blood flow, not neuroprotection. Although the failure to translate insight gained in animal models into therapy is multifactorial, we have suggested that the inability of the first generation of neuroprotective drugs to improve function after human stroke is their inability to protect white matter [11]. Many drugs (e.g., N-methyl-D-aspartate (NMDA) receptor antagonists) are targeted at receptors that are not present to any extent in axons or oligodendrocytes. The protection of myelinated fiber tracts by drugs has hitherto been largely neglected in preclinical investigations of drug action. However, in humans, it is obvious that improved *functional* outcome after drug treatment depends not only on the protection of cortical gray matter but also the simultaneous protection of associated white matter.

Assessment of ischemic pathology in white matter

The neuronal axon and its associated oligodendrocytes exhibit rapid structural damage in response to an anoxic or ischemic challenge. Structural damage to axons occurs in the form of cytoskeletal breakdown and consequent disruption of fast axonal transport. In the isolated optic nerve, 60 minutes of anoxia was sufficient to induce loss of both microtubule and neurofilament components of the axonal cytoskeleton [12]. Short periods (2 to 4 hours) of focal cerebral ischemia in vivo were also associated with cytoskeletal breakdown and disturbances in fast axonal transport in myelinated fiber tracts. Structural damage to the cytoskeleton was indicated by marked disruption in the patterns of immunostaining for a variety of microtubule proteins, including tau and microtubule-associated proteins 1 and 5, as well as the neurofilament protein 68kDa subunit [13–15]. The functional consequences of cytoskeletal disruption were indicated by the accumulation in ischemic axons of proteins that are normally transported by fast axonal transport [16–18]. The time course of the cytoskeletal dysfunction in these studies was consistent with axonal damage per se and not as a consequence of secondary degenerative processes in perikarya.

Acute structural changes in oligodendrocytes also occurred after short periods of focal cerebral ischemia. Swelling of oligodendroglia occurred within 30 minutes to 3 hours after induction of ischemia in the rat [19], while abnormalities of microtubules were also detected within the affected cells [20]. Cytoskeletal pathology in ischemic oligodendrocytes was also indicated by alterations in the immunostaining of the microtubule-associated protein, tau [13,21]. Increased tau immunostaining in oligodendrocytes in subcortical white matter after permanent MCAO in rats occurred rapidly after induction of ischemia [21] and highlights the particular sensitivity of oligodendrocytes to experimental ischemia in vivo.

Quantitative techniques have been developed to assess the extent of both axonal and oligodendrocyte pathology in experimental models of focal cerebral ischemia, using immunohistochemistry. Axonal pathology can be detected by accumulation of amyloid precursor protein (APP) staining within damaged axons (Figure 33.1). Assessment of the extent of axonal damage can then be achieved by semiquantitative scoring or by plotting the distribution of staining and using a grid counting system. Oligodendrocyte pathology can be detected by increased immunostaining of the microtubule-associated protein tau (Figure 33.1). Assessment of the extent of oligodendrocyte pathology can then be achieved by cell counting or by plotting the distribution of labeled cells and determining the volume of tissue in which they are present [17,21–23].

NMDA receptor blockade fails to protect axons or oligodendrocytes

The ability of the NMDA receptor antagonist MK-801 to protect myelinated axons after focal cerebral ischemia has been examined in the cat [23]. In contrast to the compelling evidence that MK-801 reduces the volume of ischemic damage to neuronal perikarya in this species [24–27], MK-801 failed to alter the extent of axonal damage as reflected by the APP accumulation score (Figure 33.2). In consequence, the relationship between axonal and perikaryal pathology was significantly altered in the MK-801-treated cats compared with the vehicle-treated cats. That is, there was disproportionately greater axonal pathology after MK-801 treatment because of reduced perikaryal damage [23]. In the rat, MK-801 failed to modify the extent of oligodendrocyte pathology induced by focal cerebral ischemia [21].

Tau in oligodendrocytes

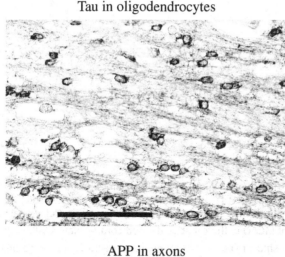

APP in axons

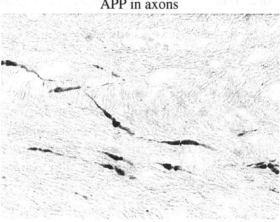

Figure 33.1   Axons and oligodendrocytes comprise the functional unit of the myelinated fiber. Oligodendrocytes are highly vulnerable to ischemia in vivo and exhibit abnormalities of the cytoskeletal protein tau. The top photograph shows numerous tau-positive oligodendrocytes in the subcortical white matter 1 hour after induction of focal cerebral ischemia in the rat. In non-ischemic white matter oligodendrocytes are not immunostained with tau antibodies. Quantification of tau-positive glia in white matter can be used to assess the effects of potential anti-ischemic intervention strategies on oligodendrocyte pathology (see Figures 33.3 and 33.4). The sensitivity of oligodendrocytes to ischemia and the numerical relationship that exists between one oligodendrocyte and the internodal segments of its associated axons could mean that damage to one oligodendrocyte may affect multiple axons and thus have a marked functional effect within a given myelinated fiber tract. Axons themselves are also vulnerable to ischemic damage in vivo. The bottom photograph shows axonal damage detected with APP immunostaining 6 hours after middle cerebral artery occlusion in the cat. Damaged axons exhibit a characteristic "string of sausages" or bulb-like appearance indicative of cytoskeletal breakdown and obstruction of fast axonal transport. Quantification of APP accumulation in white matter can be used to determine the effects of anti-ischemic agents on axonal pathology (see Figures 33.2, 33.3 and 33.4). Bar = 10 μm.

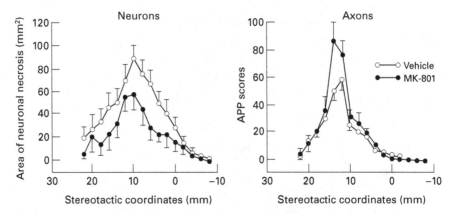

Figure 33.2 The effect of MK-801 on the amount of cortical neuronal necrosis and axonal injury 6 hours after permanent MCAO in the cat at 16 defined coronal planes. Although MK-801-treated animals had a smaller area of cortical neuronal necrosis at each coronal plane, there was no reduction in the APP score compared with the vehicle-treated animals. Data points are the mean at each coronal plane (stereotactic coordinates); bars represent SEM. Vehicle, $n = 10$; MK-801, $n = 6$. (Redrawn from ref. 23.)

Oligodendrocytes are known to be insensitive to NMDA [28,29] but vulnerable to free radicals [30,31]. After MCAO in the rat, the spin trap agent α-phenyl-tert-butyl-nitrone prevented the rapid alteration of tau immunostaining in oligodendrocytes [21]. The failure of NMDA antagonists to improve functional outcome after human stroke [1,32] may be a reflection of their inability to protect axons and oligodendrocytes from ischemic pathology.

Early reperfusion protects all cellular elements

To validate the quantitative methods that have been developed for assessing axonal and oligodendrocyte pathology in focal ischemia, the impact of restoration of blood flow 2 hours after the onset of intraluminal thread occlusion of the MCA was assessed and contrasted with permanent occlusion of the vessel. Reperfusion after 2 hours of ischemia resulted not only in smaller volumes of neuronal perikaryal damage than observed with permanent occlusion, but also in significantly less axonal and oligodendrocyte pathology (Figure 33.3). In animals with transient MCAO, the reduction in axonal pathology was most marked in the more caudal planes examined, whereas the reductions in oligodendrocyte and neuronal perikaryal damage were most marked in rostral brain areas (Figure 33.4). These data provide compelling evidence that the methodology that we have developed can demonstrate salvage of white matter. Power calculation indicates that the techniques are as equally potent in detecting alterations in white matter as the established

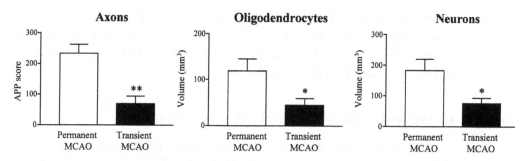

Figure 33.3 Transient occlusion of the middle cerebral artery is associated with significantly less damage to axons, oligodendrocytes and neuronal perikarya than permanent occlusion. Data are the total hemispheric APP scores and volumes of oligodendrocyte pathology and neuronal necrosis derived from area measurements at eight predetermined coronal planes. Data are expressed as mean ± SEM, $n=6$ per group. ** $P<0.002$; * $P<0.05$. (Redrawn from ref. 22.)

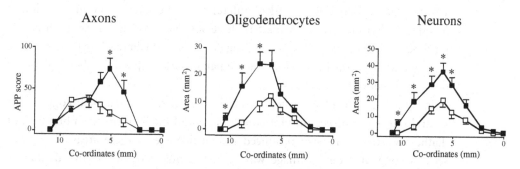

Figure 33.4 Rostrocaudal extents of axon, oligodendrocyte and neuronal perikarya damage in the transient and permanent occlusion groups. APP scores, areas of tau-positive oligodendrocytes and areas of neuronal necrosis are shown at each of the eight coronal planes analyzed. Coordinates (millimeters) are from the interaural line. The APP score in the transient occlusion group was significantly lower than in the permanent occlusion group at two of the more caudal coronal planes, whereas the areas of oligodendrocyte and neuronal pathology were significantly lower at more rostral coronal planes. Data are mean ± SEM, $n=6$ per group. ** $P<0.01$; * $P<0.05$. (Redrawn from ref. 22.).

technique for assessing volume of neuronal perikaryal damage. The technology can now be used to examine in vivo the ability of drugs targeted at mechanisms that have been implicated in axonal or oligodendrocyte pathology in vitro, with Na$^+$ channel blockade, α-amino-3-hydroxy-5-methyl-4-isoxazole propionic acid (AMPA) blockade and free radicals among the most interesting possibilities [11]. The ability of reperfusion to protect all cell types from pathology not only validates the methodological approach but also offers an explanation as to why functional outcome after stroke can be improved by tissue plasminogen activator but not by NMDA receptor blockade. Namely, early restoration of blood flow will protect all cellular elements upon which function depends, whereas NMDA blockade can salvage only those elements (neuronal cell bodies) on which the receptors are located.

Blood flow to white matter and ischemia model selection

A range of therapeutic interventions produce similar effects in the rat irrespective of the approach used to occlude the MCA (i.e., intraluminal thread or diathermy occlusion) provided the experimental end-point is the extent of neuronal damage. For example, NMDA and AMPA receptor blockade, calcium entry blockade and hypothermia, *inter alia* reduce the volume of neuronal perikaryal damage after diathermy MCAO or intraluminal thread occlusion [33–38]. However, we have identified fundamental differences in the topography of axonal damage in these two most widely utilized rat models of focal ischemia. Moreover, differences in axonal pathology are due to marked differences in the severity and distribution of blood flow alterations in white matter. These observations have major implications for model selection in anti-ischemic drug development where white matter as well as gray matter is considered and may be particularly important when functional outcome is being assessed after ischemia.

Intraluminal thread occlusion invariably produced axonal pathology in the ventral internal capsule, anterior commissure and median forebrain bundle, but diathermy occlusion never produced axonal damage in these areas. A circumscribed zone of axonal damage was found in only two of the five diathermy occluded rats in the most dorsal aspect of the internal capsule, where it penetrates the caudate nucleus. By contrast, damage in this area was frequently observed (five of six rats) after intraluminal thread occlusion. Axonal pathology in the external capsule was an almost invariable observation with both modes of occlusion (five of six animals with intraluminal thread occlusion, five of five animals with diathermy occlusion). The different distribution of axonal pathology in the two models was not a reflection of differences in the size of the neuronal perikarya pathology, which was similar in the two groups, but rather is a consequence of occlusion of additional vessels, notably the anterior choroidal artery, with the intraluminal thread approach.

MCAO produced widespread reductions in cerebral blood flow (CBF) in myelinated fiber tracts in the ipsilateral hemisphere irrespective of the mode of occlusion. However, the anatomical distribution of the changes in CBF differed markedly between the two models of MCAO (Figure 33.5). In the ventral internal capsule, median forebrain bundle and anterior commissure, blood flow was reduced only after occlusion with an intraluminal thread, but was minimally altered by diathermy

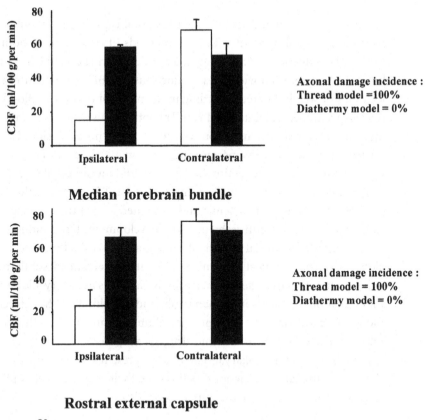

Ventral internal capsule

Median forebrain bundle

Rostral external capsule

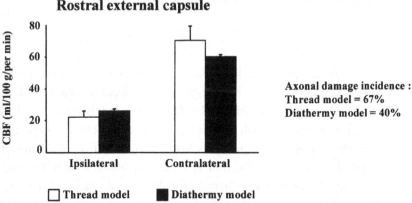

Axonal damage incidence :
Thread model =100%
Diathermy model = 0%

Axonal damage incidence :
Thread model = 100%
Diathermy model = 0%

Axonal damage incidence :
Thread model = 67%
Diathermy model = 40%

☐ Thread model   ■ Diathermy model

Figure 33.5 Cerebral blood flow (CBF) was assessed using [^{14}C]iodoantipyrine autoradiography 1 hour after MCAO by either intraluminal thread or diathermy. The autoradiographic technique was modified in order to optimize measurement of low CBF in white matter. Autoradiographic measurements were made in a number of white matter tracts ipsilateral and contralateral to the occluded MCA. There were marked differences between the two models in the distribution and severity of white matter tract ischemia. This corresponds to differences in the distribution of axonal pathology, assessed by APP immunostaining in separate groups of animals 24 hours after MCAO by either method. Data are mean ± SEM CBF study: thread model $n = 6$; diathermy model $n = 5$. APP study: thread model $n = 6$; diathermy model $n = 6$.

occlusion. In subcortical white matter (external capsule and cingulum) CBF was reduced to a similar extent with both methods of occlusion. In both models of MCAO the reduction in CBF was greater in the external capsule than in the cingulum. MCAO produced widespread reductions in CBF in gray matter regions, the locations of which differed according to the mode of occlusion. Blood flow in the nucleus accumbens, globus pallidus and hypothalamus was significantly reduced by intraluminal thread occlusion but not with diathermy occlusion. In the caudate nucleus (with its extensive permeating white matter tracts), diathermy occlusion produced more severe reductions in CBF than did intraluminal thread occlusion.

The difference between the two models of focal ischemia in the location and severity of white matter ischemia and associated axonal tract damage has significant implications for anti-ischemic drug development. Drug-induced reductions in the volume of neuronal perikaryal damage are increasingly viewed as insufficient alone to warrant clinical assessment [39]. Improvement in subtle behaviors in animals after drug treatment is increasingly viewed as necessary additional support for evaluations of agents in human stroke and head injury. While the choice of rat models of focal cerebral ischemia (intraluminal thread or diathermy) has only rarely impacted on anti-ischemic drug development when the end-point was volume of neuronal perikaryal damage, the present data suggest that, after focal ischemia in the rat, the functional deficits and their modification by pharmacological intervention may be highly model dependent.

Conclusion

From the perspective of functional recovery (the end-point of most clinical trials in stroke and head injury) it is axiomatic that all cell types and cellular components, not solely neuronal perikarya, should be protected. Irrespective of the outcome of the neuroprotective trials that will report over the next few years, the refocusing of the pharmacology of cerebral ischemia from selective protection of gray matter toward total brain protection is timely. Pharmacological approaches that also protect white matter in ischemia provide therapies that would be both *additional,* were current clinical trials of neuroprotection to succeed, and *alternative,* were current trials to fail, to existing therapeutic approaches.

REFERENCES

1 Dyker AG & Lees KR (1998) Duration of neuroprotection treatment for ischemic stroke. *Stroke,* **29,** 535–42.

2 Tamura A, Graham DI, McCulloch J & Teasdale GM (1981) Focal cerebral ischaemia in the rat: 1. Description of technique and early neuropathological consequences following middle cerebral artery occlusion. *Journal of Cerebral Blood Flow & Metabolism*, 1, 53–60.

3 Tamura A, Graham DI, McCulloch J & Teasdale GM (1981) Focal cerebral ischaemia in the rat: 2. Regional cerebral blood flow determined by [^{14}C]iodoantipyrine autoradiography following middle cerebral artery occlusion. *Journal of Cerebral Blood Flow & Metabolism*, 1, 61–9.

4 Zea Longa E, Weinstein PR, Carlson S & Cummins R (1989) Reversible middle cerebral artery occlusion without craniectomy in rats. *Stroke*, 20, 84–91.

5 Jones TJ, Morawetz RB, Crowell RM, Marcoux FW, FitzGibbon SJ, DeGirolami U & Ojemann RG (1981) Thresholds of focal cerebral ischemia in awake monkeys. *Journal of Neurosurgery*, 54, 773–82.

6 Du C, Hu R, Csernansky CA, Hsu CY & Choi DW (1996) Very delayed infarction after mild focal cerebral ischaemia: a role for apoptosis? *Journal of Cerebral Blood Flow & Metabolism*, 16, 195–201.

7 Touzani O, Young AR, Derlon J-M, Beaudouin V, Marchal G, Rioux P, Mézenge F, Baron J-C & MacKenzie ET (1995) Sequential studies of severely hypometabolic tissue volumes after permanent middle cerebral artery occlusion: a positron emission tomographic investigation in anesthetized baboons. *Stroke*, 26, 2112–19.

8 Osborne KA, Shigeno T, Balarsky AM, Ford I, McCulloch J, Teasdale GM & Graham DI (1987) Quantitative assessment of early brain damage in a rat model of focal cerebral ischaemia. *Journal of Neurology, Neurosurgery and Psychiatry*, 50, 402–10.

9 McCulloch J (1992) Excitatory amino acid antagonists and their potential for the treatment of ischemic brain damage in man. *British Journal of Clinical Pharmacology*, 34, 106–14.

10 The National Institute of Neurological Disorders and Stroke rtPA Stroke Study Group (1995) Tissue plasminogen activator for acute ischemic stroke. *New England Journal of Medicine*, 333, 1581–7.

11 Dewar D, Yam P & McCulloch J (1999) Drug development for stroke: importance of protecting cerebral white matter. *European Journal of Pharmacology*, 375, 41–50.

12 Waxmann SG, Black JA, Stys PK & Ransom BR (1992) Ultrastructural concomitants of anoxic injury and early post-anoxic recovery in rat optic nerve. *Brain Research*, 574, 105–19.

13 Dewar D & Dawson D (1995) Tau protein is altered by focal cerebral ischaemia in the rat: an immunohistochemical and immunoblotting study. *Brain Research*, 684, 70–8.

14 Dewar D & Dawson D (1996) Changes of cytoskeletal protein immunostaining in myelinated fibre tracts after focal cerebral ischaemia in the rat. *Acta Neuropathologica*, 93, 71–7.

15 Yam PS, Dewar D & McCulloch J (1998) Axonal injury caused by focal cerebral ischemia in the rat. *Journal of Neurotrauma*, 15, 441–50.

16 Stephenson DT, Rash K & Clemens JA (1992) Amyloid precursor protein accumulates in regions of neurodegeneration following focal cerebral ischemia in the rat. *Brain Research*, 393, 128–35.

17 Yam PS, Takasago T, Dewar D, Graham DI & McCulloch J (1997) Amyloid precursor protein in white matter at the margin of a focal ischaemic lesion. *Brain Research*, 760, 150–7.

18 Dietrich WD, Kraydieh S, Prado R & Stagliano NE (1998) White matter alterations following thromboembolic stroke: a β-amyloid precursor protein immunocytochemical study in rats. *Acta Neuropathologica*, **95**, 524–31.

19 Patoni L, Garcia JH & Gutierrez JA (1996) Cerebral white matter is highly vulnerable to ischemia. *Stroke*, **27**, 1641–7.

20 Petito CK (1986) Transformation of postischemic perineuronal glial cells. I. Electron microscopic studies. *Journal of Cerebral Blood Flow & Metabolism*, **6**, 616–24.

21 Irving EA, Yatsuhiro K, McCulloch J & Dewar D (1997) Rapid alteration of tau in oligodendrocytes after focal ischemic injury in the rat: involvement of free radicals. *Journal of Cerebral Blood Flow & Metabolism*, **17**, 612–22.

22 Valeriani V, Dewar D & McCulloch J (2000) Quantitative assessment of ischemic pathology in axons, oligodendrocytes, and neurons: attenuation of damage after transient ischemia. *Journal of Cerebral Blood Flow & Metabolism*, **20**, 765–71.

23 Yam PS, Dunn LT, Graham DI, Dewar D & McCulloch J (2000) NMDA receptor blockade fails to alter axonal injury in focal cerebral ischemia. *Journal of Cerebral Blood Flow & Metabolism*, **20**, 772–9.

24 Ozyurt E, Graham DI, Woodruff GN & McCulloch J (1988) Protective effect of the glutamate antagonist, MK-801 in focal cerebral ischemia in the cat. *Journal of Cerebral Blood Flow & Metabolism*, **8**, 138–43.

25 Park CK, Nehls DG, Graham DI, Teasdale GM & McCulloch J (1988) Focal cerebral ischaemia in the cat: treatment with the glutamate antagonist MK-801 after induction of ischaemia. *Journal of Cerebral Blood Flow & Metabolism*, **8**, 757–62.

26 Uematsu D, Araki N, Greenberg JH, Sladky J & Reivich M (1991) Combined therapy with MK-801 and nimodipine for protection of ischemic brain damage. *Neurology*, **41**, 88–94.

27 Dezsi L, Greenberg JH, Hamar J, Sladky J, Karp A & Reivich M (1992) Acute improvement in histological outcome by MK-801 following focal cerebral ischemia and reperfusion in the cat independent of blood flow changes. *Journal of Cerebral Blood Flow & Metabolism*, **12**, 390–9.

28 Yoshioka A, Hardy M, Younkin DP, Grinspan JB, Stern JL & Pleasure D (1995) α-Amino-3-hydroxy-5-methyl-4-isoxazolepropionate (AMPA) receptors mediate excitotoxicity in the oligodendroglial lineage. *Journal of Neurochemistry*, **64**, 2442–8.

29 Sánchez-Gómez MV & Matute C (1999) AMPA and kainate receptors each mediate excitotoxicity in oligodendroglial cultures. *Neurobiology of Disease*, **6**, 475–85.

30 Kim YS & Kim SU (1981) Oligodendroglial cell death induced by oxygen radicals and its protection by catalase. *Journal of Neuroscience Research*, **29**, 100–6.

31 Oka A, Belliveau MJ, Rosenberg PA & Volpe JJ (1993) Vulnerability of oligodendroglia to glutamate: pharmacology, mechanisms, and prevention. *Journal of Neuroscience*, **13**, 1441–53.

32 Lees KR, Asplund K, Carolei A, Davis SM, Diener H-C, Kaste M, Orgogozo J-M, Whitehead J and the GAIN International Investigators (2000) Glycine antagonist (gavestinel) in neuroprotection (GAIN International) in patients with acute stroke: a randomised controlled trial. *Lancet*, **355**, 1949–56.

33 Simon RP, Swan JH, Griffiths T & Meldrum BS (1984) Blockade of N-methyl-D-aspartate receptors may protect against ischemic damage in the brain. *Science*, **226**, 850–2.

34 Albers GW, Goldberg MP & Choi DW (1992) Do NMDA antagonists prevent neuronal injury? Yes. *Archives of Neurology*, **49**, 418–20.

35 Ma J, Endres M & Moskowitz MA (1998) Synergistic effects of caspase inhibitors and MK 801 in brain injury after transient focal cerebral ischaemia in mice. *British Journal of Pharmacology*, **124**, 756–62.

36 DeGraba TJ, Ostrow P, Hanson S & Grotta JC (1994) Motor performance, histologic damage, and calcium influx in rats treated with NBQX after focal ischemia. *Journal of Cerebral Blood Flow & Metabolism*, **14**, 262–8.

37 Wood NI, Barone FC, Benham CD, Brown TH, Campbell CA, Cooper DG, Evans ML, Feuerstein GZ, Hamilton TC, Harries MH, King PD, Meakin JE, Murkitt KL, Patel SR, Price WJ, Roberts JC, Rothaul AL, Samson NA, Smith SJ & Hunter AJ (1997) The effects of SB 206284A, a novel neuronal calcium-channel antagonist, in models of cerebral ischemia. *Journal of Cerebral Blood Flow & Metabolism*, **17**, 421–9.

38 Ginsberg MD, Sternau LL, Globus MY, Dietrich WD & Busto R (1992) Therapeutic modulation of brain temperature: relevance to ischemic brain injury. *Cerebrovascular & Brain Metabolism Reviews*, **4**, 189–225.

39 Stroke Therapy Academic Industry Roundtable (STAIR) (1999) Recommendations for standards regarding preclinical neuroprotective and restorative drug development. *Stroke*, **30**, 2752–8.

34

Combining neuroprotection with thrombolysis: how to translate laboratory success to our clinical trials

James Grotta

Department of Neurology, University of Texas-Houston Medical School, Houston, TX

Introduction

My assignment in this book highlighting the cutting edge in the battle against stroke in the experimental laboratory is to describe how the results of this research might be translated into positive results in a clinical experiment. I want to emphasize that what we need to carry out in the laboratory *and* at the bedside are both experiments. To date, many such experiments have been positive in the laboratory, but most have been negative at the bedside. What have we learned from these experiences? It is logical to me that at the bedside we need to emulate the conditions under which the laboratory experiment turns out positive; in other words, we need to do the "rat experiment" in humans. Those clinical studies that have adhered to this dictum, such as tests of recombinant tissue plasminogen activator (rtPA) [1] and ancrod [2] given within 3 hours of stroke onset, and of prourokinase given only to patients with documented middle cerebral artery occlusion (MCAO) [3], have been the only positive clinical trials to date.

Figure 34.1 depicts the general design of the rat transient MCAO model that is most often used to test neuroprotective drugs, which are the focus of this chapter. It also depicts the general design of the sort of clinical trial that I postulate must be done to get positive results with such a drug in stroke patients. There are four main areas where clinical trials have departed most from this model. In rats, we take pains to produce lesions of standardized severity and location with small variability in order to better detect a treatment effect, we start our evaluations giving the drug soon after the onset of stroke and then determine how long we can wait and still see the effect, we use models of temporary rather than permanent middle cerebral artery occlusion, and we increase the dose of the drug until we see a therapeutic effect.

Table 34.1. Issues in study design

1. Comparable stroke severity
2. Time
3. With thrombolysis
4. Dose
5. Potency combinations

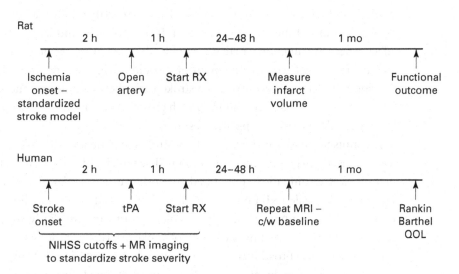

Figure 34.1   Proposed algorithm for studying neuroprotective drugs in laboratory animals and human stroke patients. RX, drug; tPA, tissue plasminogen activator; MRI, magnetic resonance imaging; c/w, compare with.

These factors, all of which must be addressed in the design of future clinical trials, are listed in Table 34.1 along with one other important point. We need to find drugs or drug combinations in the laboratory that are substantially more potent than those that have failed in clinical trials. I will discuss each of these points in more detail.

Standardize stroke severity

Logically, the outcome after stroke is closely related to its initial severity. In animal models, the deeper the degree of ischemia, and the longer it lasts, the worse the outcome measured either histologically or functionally [4]. In animal models, the depth of ischemia can be adjusted according to the number of vessels occluded and the location of the occlusion, and the duration of ischemia can be adjusted by reversing the arterial occlusion after a prespecified interval. Stroke severity also varies according to the location of the infarct, i.e., cortex or striatum, and rat strain, age and gender. Therefore, when designing an experimental evaluation of a drug in the laboratory, researchers will carefully standardize the severity of the stroke by subjecting both the treatment and vehicle groups to the same duration of ischemia and by using the same model in the same strain, age and gender of rat.

There are two reasons why standardizing stroke severity is important in these experiments. Both relate to optimizing the ability to see a treatment effect between the drug and vehicle groups if one exists. If stroke severity is too great, then animals die whether or not they receive treatment. If severity is too mild, there is a "floor" effect, where the functional deficit cannot be detected or the lesion is so small that any differences between treatment groups would be tiny. Second, if by chance the distribution of initial severity of the stroke varies between the treatment groups, the effect of this imbalance could be much greater than any effect of the treatment, leading to false negative or positive results.

Attempts to standardize the severity of strokes in patients randomized into clinical trials is important for the same reasons. The severity of stroke is reflected in the neurological examination, quantified for instance in the National Institutes of Health Stroke Scale (NIHSS) [5]. In most clinical studies, the baseline NIHSS is clearly the most important variable predicting outcome [6]. Early studies made little attempt to achieve standardization of stroke severity, using long time windows for treatment, and broad inclusion and few exclusion criteria [7]. Many trials that included very severely affected patients were stopped, perhaps prematurely, because of high mortality in one or both groups [8]. Others arrived at equivocal or misleading results because of imbalances in the distribution of stroke severity between the groups [9]. This led to attempts to find differences in subgroups based on a segment of patients with NIHSS scores matched along the severity continuum. But since these were always post hoc analyses based on small numbers of patients, they were usually misleading. Recent studies have made more of an attempt to achieve standardization of stroke severity by using low and high NIHSS cutoffs [10], by trying to select patients with signs of cortical damage on the NIHSS [11], and by ensuring that treatment groups are matched in distribution of NIHSS scores. However, the NIHSS is not a precise reflection of what is going on at the tissue level.

Might our stroke standardization be better accomplished by assessing tissue viability? This notion creates a dilemma. Just as in animal models, stroke severity should optimally be standardized by standardizing the depth of ischemia and its effect on the viability of the brain tissue at risk, *and* by including patients only within a very narrow time window (duration of arterial occlusion). The dilemma is that our ability to determine the state of tissue viability is still inexact, not available in many centers, and, most importantly, takes time. The most successful clinical strategy so far, as will be described later, is to include patients with only a brief (<3 hours) duration of ischemia. Keeping the time-to-treatment (TTT) brief may itself help to standardize the severity of stroke, since all patients would have ischemia of relatively brief duration and consequently most would probably still have some reversibly damaged tissue. But adhering to a very narrow time window does not allow for ancillary tests to determine the depth of ischemia or tissue viability.

Emerging technology may provide an imaging tool to enable us to identify salvageable tissue. Such a test has, up to now, been the elusive "Holy Grail" of diagnostic studies for stroke. Initially, clinicians used measurements of cerebral blood flow to establish the profundity of ischemia, but these methods had many disadvantages. Either they lacked regional or quantitative information, or they were invasive [12]. The only method of measuring cerebral blood flow in the acute setting that is still in use is xenon-enhanced computed tomography (CT) [13]. The consensus of most investigators is that the future of stroke standardization rests with magnetic resonance imaging (MRI) technology [14]. The details of how to determine tissue viability by MRI in the acute stroke setting are still uncertain, but probably rest in some correlation between diffusion and perfusion imaging [15]. Furthermore, just as in rats, we measure the ability of a therapy to reduce infarct volume, and MRI may help us to compare the effect of drugs on the volume of tissue at risk that goes on to infarction. These studies are now being embodied into clinical trials. Attempts will be made to see whether a certain MRI profile can help to identify those patients with the severity of damage that is best targeted by neuroprotective therapy, and can help to measure the effect of such therapy on eventual infarction size.

Another variable affecting severity of stroke in rats that has not been controlled in most human studies is the number of occluded vessels, which obviously affects the depth and location of ischemia. Only one study, the PROACT trial of an intraarterially administered thrombolytic [3], was designed to limit the patients enrolled to only those who had one type of vascular lesion. The study was limited only to patients with documented MCAO of less than 6 hours' duration. The results were positive, again reflecting the wisdom of designing clinical studies to closely emulate what we do in animals. Non-invasive techniques such as transcranial ultrasound, magnetic resonance angiography or contrast-enhanced CT angiography may help us to standardize patients enrolled into future trials by quantifying and localizing the offending arterial occlusion [16].

Finally, depending on the proposed mechanism of action of the drug, we place our laboratory stroke lesions either in the cortex, striatum, or both. Although there is proportionately much less white matter in rodents than in humans, striatal lesions involve more white matter damage than do cortical strokes (Figure 34.2).

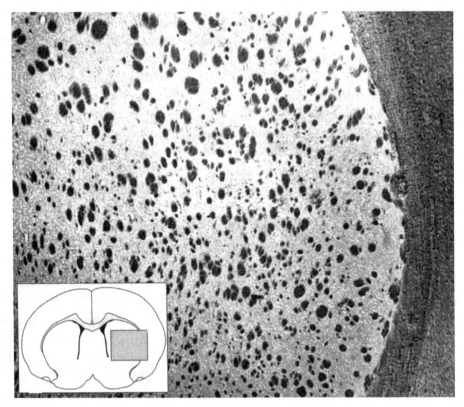

Figure 34.2 Histological section from designated area in rat caudate demonstrating white matter tracts stained with trypan blue.

Many drugs work less well in the striatum [17], not only because the depth of blood flow reduction may be greater in the striatum, but also because the drug may have an effect on neurotransmitters or receptors that are present only on neuronal cell bodies. In testing such drugs in humans, we need to enrich the proportion of cortical strokes. This can be done to some extent by including only patients with cortical abnormalities on their NIHSS [11], but would be far more exact if MRI could be incorporated into the screening process.

In summary, for now we need to standardize the types of stroke we try to treat in clinical trials by controlling the TTT, range and distribution of the NIHSS score, and exclusion of very aged patients. In the future, we need to learn how to utilize MRI to detect those patients with viable tissue at risk (and to help to measure outcome). Finally, we might want to limit our trials to those with certain patterns of arterial occlusion likely to produce cortical lesions amenable to our neuroprotective therapies.

Time to treatment

In assessing the effect of a drug in the laboratory, two variables are adjusted, the TTT and the drug dose. As mentioned in the previous section, other variables are held constant. Seeing a gradual decrease in effect on outcome as TTT increases and an enhancing effect as the dose increases, are basic findings that confirm a pharmacological effect on the mechanism causing the stroke. I will discuss dose later. In the laboratory, the investigator always starts with a brief TTT and then gradually prolongs it until an effect is no longer seen [18]. This is just the opposite of what has been done in almost all clinical studies.

Researchers in the field of neuroprotection might learn important lessons by comparing results in the laboratory with clinical studies that use thrombolysis to achieve tissue reperfusion in stroke patients. In the laboratory, brain tissue must be reperfused within 2 to 4 hours, depending on the model, to see a reduction of infarct size as compared with animals with permanent occlusion [19]. Clinical studies using intravenous rtPA begun within 3 hours showed a positive effect [1], with more benefit associated with earlier treatment within that window. If begun after 3 hours, rtPA had little or no benefit [20], though many investigators believe there may be some benefit in selected patients. Considering that it takes 30 to 90 minutes for a clot to dissolve after beginning intravenous rtPA therapy, the TTT for reperfusion in clinical studies correlates very nicely with what has been found in laboratory models (Figure 34.3). Similar laboratory results have been seen with neuroprotective drugs.

Preclinical studies have shown that all neuroprotective drugs are less effective the later they are given, and most are ineffective if started more than 2 to 4 hours after the onset of ischemia. Yet no clinical trial has yet included enough patients within that 4 hour time window to reach any conclusions about efficacy. The rtPA investigators have shown that it is possible to treat patients and conduct a randomized placebo-controlled trial within this narrow TTT. Obviously, however, such a brief time window will limit the number of patients that can be treated. Seduced by imaging studies reporting "penumbral" tissue more than 6 hours after stroke onset [21], pharmaceutical companies, naturally interested in establishing the largest market for their drug, have abandoned the laboratory data and extended the TTT in most studies to 6 hours or more.

In summary, further clinical testing of neuroprotective agents should follow the example of preclinical laboratory studies and positive clinical trials of thrombolysis. Design the first efficacy experiments with very early treatment, and then work outward in prolonging the TTT. This might be a second arm of the initial study, or a separate trial, and positive results with delayed therapy might be more likely if

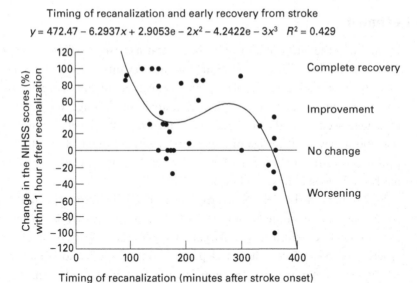

Figure 34.3 Outcome measured by change in NIHSS score (*y*-axis) related to time to reperfusion after stroke onset as determined by transcranial Doppler (*x*-axis).

selection of patients is based on imaging evidence of continued reversibly injured tissue. Finally, there are fewer risks associated with most neuroprotective drugs than with thrombolytics, and they might be useful in a wider spectrum of patients. Therefore, the market may be considerably larger than that of rtPA even if the drug is only effective if given in the first few hours.

Combine neuroprotection with reperfusion

Another lesson from laboratory stroke models is that neuroprotective therapy is generally more effective if given to animals with reversible rather than permanent arterial occlusion [22]. One reason for this is obvious. For a neuroprotective drug to work, it must reach the injured tissue. The fastest, safest and most convenient way to get a drug to the brain in a stroke patient is by iv infusion. An occluded artery would not allow as much blood flow into the injured region as would one that is opened. Consequently, drug delivery to the target would be greater if reperfusion of the injured tissue occurred either before or at the same time as the drug is given.

An occluded artery that is opened within a certain time frame is likely to produce quantitatively less severe injury than one that is left blocked. As mentioned in the first two sections, the depth of ischemia and its duration largely determine the fate of the tissue. By lessening both of these variables, reperfusion models therefore probably produce a proportionately larger area of sublethal and reversible tissue damage.

In fact, it is possible that the type of tissue injury associated with reperfusion may be qualitatively different from what occurs with permanent occlusion. Reperfusion is associated with tissue reoxygenation producing free radicals that attack a variety of cellular components. It is also associated with excitotoxicity after a second wave of glutamate release. Early reperfusion may allow protein synthesis to continue or restart, leading to the manufacture of proteins necessary to initiate an inflammatory response and apoptosis. These mechanisms might be quite amenable to reversal by neuroprotective drugs.

Laboratory studies support the existence of such "reperfusion injury" [23], a mechanism also seen with cardiac ischemia and organ transplantation. In rats, we are able to show in several models that if the artery is opened, it actually produces *more* damage than if it were left occluded. This is seen in models of moderate severity; it is not seen after deep ischemia as occurs with arterial occlusion in spontaneously hypertensive rats. We have also found that neuroprotective drugs, especially those that attack free radicals, inhibit protein synthesis, reduce inflammation, or prevent apoptosis, are particularly effective, reducing the final infarct size by up to 80%.

Is it possible to design a study combining reperfusion and neuroprotection? Thrombolytic therapy with iv rtPA, according to established guidelines, is associated with at least partial recanalization in up to 70% of cases, and has been shown to increase tissue reperfusion. Even better, intra-arterial administration of a lytic drug is associated with at least partial recanalization in 80% of occluded MCAs, and provides the advantage of possible direct administration of the neuroprotectant through the arterial catheter into the arterial blood perfusing the injured tissue. Therefore combining the neuroprotective drug with thrombolytic therapy can recreate the setting of reperfusion in which neuroprotection is most effective in the laboratory.

It might be difficult to randomize patients to an investigational neuroprotective drug while at the same time determining eligibility for thrombolysis and administering both within 3 hours of symptom onset. However, this can be done. In a recent safety study of lubeluzole combined with rtPA [24], all patients received iv rtPA within 3 hours of stroke onset and were begun on the study drug within 1 hour of starting rtPA, on average 3.3 hours after stroke onset (Figure 34.4). Furthermore, patients were enrolled at a rate of more than 0.5 patients per month.

In summary, reperfusion is the best setting to see the beneficial effect of neuroprotection in the laboratory. Concomitant administration of a neuroprotective drug with a thrombolytic agent can reproduce this paradigm in the clinical arena.

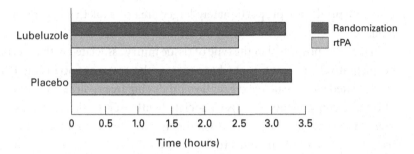

Figure 34.4 Time to starting intravenous treatment with rtPA and lubeluzole or placebo in a recently completed multicenter randomized trial of lubeluzole vs. placebo in stroke patients receiving rtPA. According to the protocol, rtPA was given to all patients within 3 hours of stroke onset and lubeluzole or placebo had to be started before the end of the 1 hour rtPA infusion.

Dose

Whether the artery is open or not, a sufficient amount of drug must reach the injured region to have the desired biological effect. Unfortunately, this has not been achieved in many clinical trials.

Side effects have been the Achilles' heel limiting the doses of neuroprotective drugs given to stroke patients. Many side effects seen in humans, such as mild hypotension, sedation and other behavioral effects can be hard to detect or do not occur in a rat. Consequently, with many drugs it is possible to dose rats until a "ceiling" is reached where no larger amount produces benefit. This is not the case with humans. Recent stroke victims seem particularly vulnerable to cardiovascular or sedative effects of a drug [7,25]. Perhaps because of a disrupted blood–brain barrier and consequently more tissue bioavailability of the drug in the stroke patient than with the same dose in normal volunteers, stroke patients often have drug reactions not predicted by phase I studies in normal volunteers. Also, for any given drug there may be different rates of absorption, metabolic pathways or rates, tissue uptake mechanisms, receptor availability and other biological differences between species. These considerations make it difficult to translate the blood levels we can achieve in rats, and even in normal human volunteers, to those we can expect to reach safely in our acute stroke patients.

Even with drugs where side effects do not limit the dose, many trials have used the minimal effective dose or blood level from preclinical studies when choosing the dose or target blood level for stroke patients [26]. Then, when the pivotal efficacy trial is carried out, it is determined that lower blood levels were achieved than expected and most patients were therefore not exposed to a potentially therapeutic amount of drug.

In designing a clinical neuroprotective trial, it would seem logical to always begin with a dose escalation study (with blood level correlation) in stroke patients similar to those you intend to include in the pivotal trial. The highest tolerable dose should then be chosen for the pivotal trial. Ideally, the next step would be to demonstrate that the dose chosen is able to achieve a measurably beneficial effect on the target biological process. An example would be to demonstrate that the dose of thombolytic drug to be used in a study is able to lyse the clot in a sample of patients studied angiographically. Unfortunately, such tests in living stroke patients are not available for most neuroprotective drugs that have their effect on cellular mechanisms. In that case, one is forced to rely on the ability to achieve blood levels that are on the high side of the range that is effective in preclinical animal studies.

In summary, it is likely that effective drugs have been discarded because insufficient blood levels were achieved in their therapeutic testing in humans. It is also likely that futile studies, with doses that had little hope of successfully reaching therapeutic brain levels, have wasted time, money, energy and the cooperation of our stroke patients. More time should be devoted to pilot studies aimed at determining the maximal tolerated dose, and detecting whether this has the desired biological effect and the ability to achieve blood levels clearly in the therapeutic range determined by preclinical studies.

Finding a more effective drug

Most of the neuroprotective drugs subjected to clinical evaluation have been able to reduce relative infarct volume and improve behavioral outcome by about 50% as compared with controls in well-standardized preclinical stroke models. It is possible that even if we adhere to the principles described in the preceding pages, this effect is not enough for detection in our stroke patients. Perhaps the biology of ischemic damage in the rat is so different from that of humans that positive results in the former cannot be extrapolated to the latter.

I think that a better explanation for our clinical failures, in addition to our failure to design trials to mimic what has been successful in the laboratory, is that the drugs we have chosen are too weak. A firm conclusion cannot be made because of weaknesses in clinical study design to date. However, based on our inability to translate preclinical results to the bedside, we probably should no longer move forward with clinical evaluation of a monotherapy that reduces damage by only 50% in a rat. We need to find drugs that reduce damage by 80% in these models. This is possible with some drugs we are now studying in our laboratory [27] (Figure 34.5). Surprisingly, the most effective agents, particularly in our reperfusion model, are drugs that affect downstream biological consequences of ischemia such as inflammatory mechanisms and apoptosis.

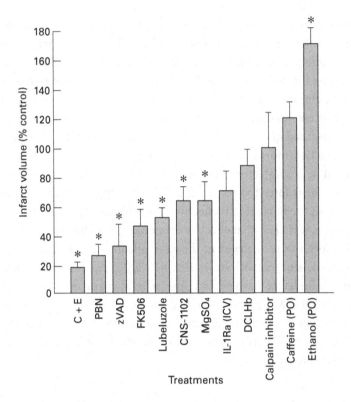

All animals: LE rats with 180 min MCA/CCA occlusion
All drugs: Started 15 min postischemia

Figure 34.5 Comparison of the effect of various neuroprotective drugs in a reperfusion injury model in rat. Long–Evans rats were subjected to 180 minutes of reversible MCA/common carotid artery (CCA) occlusion followed by 24 hours of reperfusion, which leads to larger infarction than if the MCA is left permanently occluded [23]. All treatments were given intravenously unless otherwise noted, and begun 15 minutes after the onset of MCAO. y-axis is infarct volume measured as percentage of control group. * Statistically significantly different from control. C + E, caffeine and ethanol; PBN, N-tert-butyl-alpha-phenylnitrone; IL-1Ra, interleukin-1 receptor antagonist; ICV, intracerebroventricular; DCLHb, diaspirin cross-linked hemoglobin; PO, orally.

Selecting a drug that affects a single pathway in the process of brain injury after stroke has scientific and regulatory purity. However, this strategy has proven ineffective clinically. It is time to look for combinations of drugs that have a stronger effect. We need to work on the regulatory and financial impediments for conducting such trials. Regulatory agencies will accept combination trials if the combination provides more effect than merely a summation of the effect of each drug alone. An example of such is our interesting finding that while caffeine has

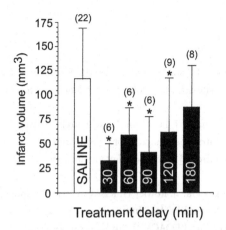

Figure 34.6 Infarct volume ± SD (mm³) following 180 minutes of unilateral MCAO/common carotid artery occlusion in Long–Evans rats after an iv bolus plus infusion that delivered a total of 0.65 g ethanol/kg (10% solution) plus 10 mg caffeine/kg initiated 30, 60, 90, 120, and 180 minutes after induction of ischemia vs. saline control. Caffeine and ethanol were dissolved in 3 ml of saline; 0.5 ml was injected as a bolus and then the remaining 2.5 ml as a continuous infusion over 2.5 hours. *Statistically different ($P<0.05$) from saline-treated (control) group. Numbers in parentheses represent numbers of animals per group.

little effect on stroke outcome, and ethanol makes it worse, a combination of low doses given acutely to naïve rats is more effective than any monotherapy we have yet evaluated in our reperfusion model [18] (Figures 34.5 and 34.6). The stroke research community will need to be even more creative in designing and finding funding for such a combination trial. However, stroke is a huge public health problem. If finding a potent and safe combination therapy is the only way that neuroprotection will work, I am optimistic that eventually funding agencies and industry will support this approach.

Conclusion

In summary, current approaches to neuroprotection have succeeded in the laboratory but not at the bedside. To succeed, clinicians need better trial designs to reflect the conditions under which drugs work in the laboratory, and basic researchers need to discover more potent and safe therapies than those that have already been tried at the bedside.

REFERENCES

1 The National Institute of Neurological Disorders and Stroke rtPA Stroke Study Group (1995) Tissue plasminogen activator for acute ischemic stroke. *New England Journal of Medicine*, 333, 1581–7.

2 Sherman DG, Atkinson RP, Chippendale T, Levin KA, Ng K, Futrell N, Hsu CY & Levy DE, for the STAT Participants (2000) Intravenous ancrod for treatment of acute ischemic stroke: the STAT Study: a randomized controlled trial. *Journal of the American Medical Association*, 283, 2395–403.

3 Furlan A, Higashida R, Wechsler L, Gent M, Rowley H, Kase C, Pessin M, Ahuja A, Callahan F, Clark WM, Silver F & Rivera F, for the PROACT Investigators (1999) Intra-arterial prourokinase for acute ischemic stroke. The PROACT II Study: a randomized controlled trial. *Journal of the American Medical Association*, 282, 2003–11.

4 Jones TH, Morawetz RB, Crowell RM, Marcoux FW, FitzGibbon SJ, DeGirolami U & Ojemann RG (1981) Thresholds of focal cerebral ischemia in awake monkeys. *Journal of Neurosurgery*, 54, 773–82.

5 Lyden P, Brott T, Tilley B, Welch KMA, Mascha EJ, Levine S, Haley EC, Grotta J, Marler J & the NINDS TPA Stroke Study Group (1994) Improved reliability of the NIH Stroke Scale using video training. *Stroke*, 25, 2220–6.

6 The NINDS t-PA Stroke Study Group (1997) Generalized efficacy of t-PA for acute stroke: subgroup analysis of the NINDS t-PA stroke trial. *Stroke*, 28, 2119–25.

7 The American Nimodipine Study Group (1992) Clinical trial of nimodipine in acute ischemic stroke. *Stroke*, 23, 3–8.

8 Hemodilution in Stroke Study Group (1989) Hypervolemic hemodilution treatment of acute stroke. Results of a randomized multicenter trial using pentastarch. *Stroke*, 20, 317–23.

9 Albers GW, Alberts MJ, Broderick JP, Lyden PD & Sacco RL (2000) Recent advances in stroke management. *Stroke and Cerebrovascular Disease*, 9, 95–105.

10 Davis SM, Lees KR, Albers GW, Diener HC, Markabi S, Karlsson G & Norris J, for the ASSIST Investigators (2000) Selfotel in acute ischemic stroke: possible neurotoxic effects of an NMDA antagonist. *Stroke*, 31, 347–54.

11 Gribkoff VK, Starrett JE, Hewawasam P, Dworetzy SK, Ortiz AA, Kinney GG, Boissard CG, Post-Munson DJ, Trojnacki JT, Huston KM, Signor LJ, Lombardo LA, Reid SA, Hibbard JR, Myers RA, Moon SL, Yeleswaram S, Pajor LM, Johnson G & Molinoff PB (2000) A novel maxi-K potassium channel opener, BMS-204352, reduced cortical infarct size in stringent rodent models of acute focal stroke. *Neurology*, 54 Suppl 3, A68.

12 Lassen NA (1990) Pathophysiology of brain ischemia as it relates to the therapy of acute ischemic stroke. *Clinical Neuropharmacology*, 13, S1.

13 Kaufmann AM, Firlik AD, Fukui MB, Wechsler LR, Jungries CA & Yonas H (1999) Ischemic core and penumbra in human stroke. *Stroke*, 30, 93–9.

14 Moseley ME, Kucharczyk J, Mintorovitch J, Cohen Y, Kurhanewicz J, Derugin N, Asgari H & Norman D (1990) Diffusion-weighted MR imaging of acute stroke: correlation with T2-

weighted and magnetic susceptibility-enhanced MR imaging in cats. *American Journal of Neuroradiology*, **1**, 423–9.

15 Beaulieu C, de Crespigny A, Tong DC, Moseley ME, Albers GW & Marks MP (1999) Longitudinal magnetic resonance imaging study of perfusion and diffusion in stroke: Evolution of lesion volume and correlation with clinical outcome. *Annals of Neurology*, **46**, 568–78.

16 Alexandrov AV, Demchuk AM, Wein TH & Grotta JC (1999) Yield of transcranial Doppler in acute cerebral ischemia. *Stroke*, **30**, 1604–9.

17 Roussel S, Pinard E & Seylaz J (1992) Effect of MK-801 on focal brain infarction in normotensive and hypertensive rats. *Hypertension*, **19**, 40–6.

18 Strong R, Grotta JC & Aronowski AJ (2000) Combination of low dose ethanol and caffeine protects brain from damage produced by focal ischemia in rats. *Neuropharmacology*, **39**, 515–22.

19 Kaplan B, Brint S, Tanabe J, Jacewicz M, Wang XJ & Pulsinelli W (1991) Temporal thresholds for neocortical infarction in rats subjected to reversible focal cerebral ischemia. *Stroke*, **22**, 1032–9.

20 Hacke W, Kaste M, Fieschi C, Toni D, Lesaffre E, von Kummer R, Boysen G, Bluhmki E, Höxter G, Mahagne M-H & Hennerici M, for the ECASS Study Group (1995) Intravenous thrombolysis with recombinant tissue plasminogen activator for acute hemispheric stroke. The European Cooperative Acute Stroke Study (ECASS). *Journal of the American Medical Association*, **274**, 1017–25.

21 Baron JC, von Kummer R & del Zoppo GJ (1995) Treatment of acute ischemic stroke. Challenging the concept of a rigid and universal time window. *Stroke*, **26**, 2219–21.

22 Zang RL, Chopp M, Jiang N, Tang WX, Prostak J, Manning AM & Anderson DC (1995) Anti-intercellular adhesion molecule-1 antibody reduces ischemic cell damage after transient but not permanent middle cerebral artery occlusion in the Wistar rat. *Stroke*, **26**, 1438–42.

23 Aronowski J, Strong R & Grotta J (1997) Reperfusion injury: demonstration of brain damage produced by reperfusion after transient focal ischemia in rats. *Journal of Cerebral Blood Flow & Metabolism*, **17**, 1048–56.

24 Grotta JC (2000) Combination therapy stroke trial: rtPA +/− lubeluzole. *Stroke*, **31**, 278.

25 Davis SM, Albers, GW, Diener HC, Lees KR & Norris J (1997) Termination of acute stroke studies involving selfotel treatment. *Lancet*, **349**, 32.

26 Grotta J, for the US and Canadian Lubeluzole Ischemic Stroke Study Group (1997) Lubeluzole treatment of acute ischemic stroke. *Stroke*, **28**, 2338–46.

27 Grotta J (1999) Acute stroke therapy at the millennium: consummating the marriage between the laboratory and bedside. The Feinberg Lecture. *Stroke*, **30**, 1722–8.

35

Prospects for improved neuroprotection trials in stroke

Kennedy R. Lees

University Department of Medicine & Therapeutics, Western Infirmary, Glasgow, Scotland

Introduction

The experimental basis for neuroprotection is well founded. In a range of animal models of ischemic stroke, drugs acting by a variety of mechanisms can be administered up to several hours after the ischemic insult and reductions in infarct volume can be demonstrated. Whilst individual models have their proponents and their disadvantages, numerous strategies have been sufficiently convincing to encourage clinical development. Examples of drugs reaching large clinical trials range from free radical scavengers, γ-aminobutyric acid (GABA) agonists and calcium antagonists, through a range of drugs acting on the glutamate cascade to precursors of membrane constituents such as citicoline [1–8]. Unfortunately, the range of drugs and mechanisms that has been tested in the clinic and has so far failed, exactly parallels the former list (Table 35.1). In most cases, the result has been neutral but a few drugs had adverse effects that were not anticipated from the preclinical studies [7,9].

In the face of these disappointments, some pessimism amongst the clinical researchers would be understandable, but instead a cautious optimism remains. This is based on sound scientific analysis of the progress that has been made and the prospects for adjusting the development strategy for future compounds.

Potential reasons for the failure of previous clinical trials have been widely reviewed [8,10–12]. Most are speculative, but the principles that underlie them can readily be tested and bear repetition. First, the translation from animal models to human stroke demands certain assumptions. Rodent brains, in which most compounds are initially tested, are extremely small and have very little white matter. Effects that occur at the margin of an infarct in a rodent brain are capable of reducing infarct volume by large percentages; in contrast, a similar reduction in infarct diameter in the human brain has a disproportionately smaller effect on volume. Coupled with this, protection of cortical cells in the human brain without

Table 35.1. Recent large neuroprotection trials

Drug class	Drug	Status [ref.]
Aminosteroid (free radical scavenger)	Tirilazad	Abandoned, neutral [1,62]
NMDA glutamate recognition site antagonist	Selfotel	Abandoned, adverse [5,7]
NMDA ion channel blocker	Aptiganel	Abandoned, unpublished data [19]
NMDA polyamine site antagonist	Eliprodil	Abandoned, unpublished
NMDA glycine site antagonist	Gavestinel	Completed, neutral [8]
Sodium channel blocker/NOS inhibitor	Lubeluzole	Completed, neutral [3,4,49]
GABA agonist	Clomethiazole	Completed, neutral [6]
Anti-ICAM-1 antibody	Enlimomab	Abandoned, adverse [9]
Membrane precursor	Citicoline	Completed, neutral
Maxi-K potassium channel opener	BMS-204352	Completed, neutral
Nitrone (free radical scavenger)	NXY-059	Planned [63]
Physiological Ca^{2+}/NMDA antagonist	Magnesium	In progress (30,31 and Y. Yang et al., unpublished data)
Anti-inflammatory (anti-CD11b)	Neutrophil inhibitory factor	Planned [64]

Notes:
NMDA, *N*-methyl-D-aspartate; NOS, nitric oxide synthase; GABA, γ-aminobutyric acid; ICAM, intercellular adhesion molecule.

preservation of their axonal connections through white matter is unlikely to be translated into functional benefit [13]. There is increasing evidence that classes of compounds such as *N*-methyl-D-aspartate (NMDA) antagonists, which were exciting candidate neuroprotective compounds a few years ago, are incapable of rescuing white matter from ischemic damage [14]. Unfortunately, good animal models of white matter ischemia have not until recently become available [13]. Recommendations such as those produced by the STAIR group do not presently include specific testing for brain protection rather than neuroprotection, but the need to replicate studies in several laboratories in several animal species and to employ both functional and histological end-points may partially achieve this aim [15]. It is crucial to realize that reperfusion strategies such as thrombolysis with alteplase lead to preservation of white matter as well as cortical tissue [13]. Thus the first conclusion to be drawn is that clinical trials with the many compounds studied so far have been consistent with the pre-clinical evidence.

A second major criticism of the clinical trials concerns selection of dose. In animal studies, safety and side effects take second place to efficacy, whereas in clinical trials adequate dosing is often limited by side effects, whether real or perceived.

For example, the competitive glutamate receptor antagonist selfotel was neuroprotective in rats at plasma concentrations of approximately 40 µg/ml. In stroke patients, plasma concentrations of 21 µg/ml were achieved at the doses used for efficacy trials [7,16,17]. Higher doses were associated with intolerable psychotomimetic and sedative effects [17]. Likewise, plasma concentrations of aptiganel that could be achieved in humans were on the threshold of adequate neuroprotection based on extrapolation from animal models [18,19]. A relatively small phase II trial with lubeluzole showed possible increases in mortality as compared with placebo with a 20 mg dose in stroke patients and an apparent reduction in mortality with 10 mg [4]. The lower dose was taken forward into phase III trials [3,4]. On the basis of plasma concentration data, the lower of these doses attains approximately half of the concentration that was associated with neuroprotection when the drug was given very early after permanent middle cerebral artery occlusion in the rat. A retrospective concentration–response analysis supports the hypothesis that the dose used in the phase III trials may have been insufficient [20].

Preferable approaches to dose selection involve selection of a target plasma, or preferably brain, concentration based on preclinical studies, which can be used as a decision point for clinical development. If that target concentration cannot be achieved or exceeded without intolerable side effects, then development of the compound should cease. Where concentration data are not available to guide dosing, a surrogate marker of pharmacological effect may be considered.

This approach places considerable reliance on extrapolation from the animal models and assumes that protein binding in plasma, penetration into the brain and the time course of the brain pharmacokinetics are similar in animals and humans. These assumptions do not always hold. For example, gavestinel exhibits extensive plasma protein binding in both rats and humans, but the free fraction is so small at under 1% in the rat and under 0.1% in humans that at least a 10-fold difference in free drug concentrations will exist between the species [21]. The target concentration approach also has disadvantages if the dose–response relationship for the drug is not monotonic, i.e., if high doses of the drug are associated with some loss of efficacy as compared with moderate doses. This may conceivably occur when the drug has hemodynamic effects at higher doses, which may offset potential neuroprotective benefits: this may be why elderly females receiving lifarizine appeared to fare poorly compared with a trend toward benefit in other groups [22]. An attempt to achieve a maximum tolerated dose that exceeds a target concentration may unnecessarily lead to failure. Clearly, what is required is an approach that selects the dose based on therapeutic response in humans, provided that there is *prima facie* evidence that potentially neuroprotective concentrations are being achieved.

The traditional approach to dose finding involves dose escalation studies in small groups of patients until the maximum tolerated dose has been identified and then an arbitrary selection of doses for further study. The subsequent trial is often underpowered to detect a drug effect, let alone differences between doses, and the resultant choice of dose for phase III efficacy studies is better suited to the casino than the clinic. Fortunately, this may now be a relic of the past.

One of the most exciting recent developments in stroke trial design has been the attempt to select doses based on an adaptive randomization design. With this approach, modern technology, established principles of clinical pharmacology and a statistical technique developed by the Reverend Bayes in the 18th century are combined [23]. In summary, a small number of patients is studied at each of a wide range of potentially interesting doses. The patients' therapeutic responses are assessed and are compared with the expected response based on previous experience and on the outcome of patients receiving placebo. Trends toward benefit at particular doses are then explored further by allowing the outcome information to interact with the randomization procedure in a way favoring allocation of doses that appear to be producing therapeutic benefit. In this manner, the number of patients treated at ineffective doses is minimized. The ultimate aims are to identify the dose that is associated with 95% of maximal therapeutic benefit and to recognize the earliest stage in the trial at which that dose becomes apparent. Whilst this approach will not necessarily reach a conclusion with a smaller number of patients than traditional trials, it optimizes the choice of dose, and the decision on progression to phase III is based on hard facts rather than soft impressions. It also maximizes the information that can be obtained from individual patients participating in phase II trials and is thus ethically attractive.

A third criticism of existing trial methodology continues the theme of maximizing contributions. Unfortunately, many patients who are entered into clinical trials have a small chance of contributing useful information to the result. This may be because the outcome measure is one that can only realistically be achieved by patients with moderate severity of initial stroke. Severely affected patients are unlikely to improve sufficiently to attain the target outcome measure, for example a Barthel Index score of 95 or 100. In contrast, mildly affected patients will almost inevitably recover to this degree whether or not they receive a neuroprotective treatment. Other patients will fail to contribute because they are treated too late for the drug to have realistic benefit or because the stroke type, location or etiology is one that is not appropriate for the mechanism of action of the drug. Some hints that this may have clinical relevance derive from the CLASS Study of clomethiazole [6]. Within the phase III trial, there was an overall neutral effect of clomethiazole but, within the subgroup of patients with large middle cerebral artery infarcts, a trend toward benefit with clomethiazole was seen. Clearly, this may be purely a chance result from subgroup analysis but, in the light of experimental data that suggest that the penumbra is primarily present in large cortical infarcts and that some neuroprotectants operate primarily in the cortical region, there is a reasonable case to test the hypothesis further. Accordingly, a further CLASS trial is nearing completion, in which patients with large cortical infarcts are specifically targeted.

This move toward enrichment of the population under study reverses a trend that had been led by the marketing departments of pharmaceutical companies. A major disadvantage of thrombolysis relates to the small target population of patients with proven ischemic stroke who seek medical assistance less than 3 hours from onset [24]. It was assumed that to be commercially viable a neuroprotectant should be suitable for widespread use, i.e., without the need for cerebral imaging and at later times from stroke onset. Whilst this certainly is an attractive scenario, it is first necessary to prove that the drug has therapeutic benefit. The difficulties in establishing this fact must take priority over marketing considerations. Thus every practical strategy that can be used to select patients in whom a favorable drug effect may be demonstrated should be employed. Strategies include: selection according to time from stroke onset on the premise that benefit decays as the time elapsed increases [25]; selection of patients with ischemic stroke on the grounds that, whilst the penumbra may be present around a primary cerebral hemorrhage, this is not the primary determinant of outcome; and for most neuroprotectants, selection of patients who have involvement of the cortex may be justified. In addition, depending on the end-points selected it may be sensible to restrict recruitment to patients within a certain range of stroke severity though the interaction of stroke severity with age must not be ignored. There has also been considerable interest in imaging studies to aid patient selection [26,27].

The presence of a large perfusion deficit on magnetic resonance (MR) perfusion imaging that is not matched by a large deficit on a diffusion-weighted scan, taken to represent tissue already infarcting, is a theoretically attractive means of selecting patients. It does, however, suffer from practical hurdles in arranging complex scans around the clock in acutely ill patients. These difficulties can be overcome, as illustrated by the GAIN trials [8,28,29]. Between the two phase III clinical studies with gavestinel, GAIN International and GAIN Americas, there were over 300 centers recruiting approximately 3400 patients, with 2700 being eligible for the primary efficacy analysis. A subset of 20% of these centers participated in GAIN MR imaging (MRI) and were able to consider 5% of the total patients, with 3% completing the MRI trial. This final number is approximately half of that currently considered appropriate for a reasonably powered MRI trial, where the end-point is based on comparison of final infarct volume with initial imaging features. The cost of this trial was probably approximately 5% of the cost of the large clinical studies and thus a potential financial saving is possible at the expense of slower recruitment. The number of centers capable of undertaking acute MRI studies is steadily increasing and this approach is becoming more realistic for each subsequent trial.

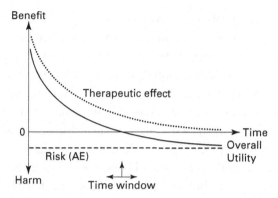

Figure 35.1   Utility of acute stroke treatment is a function of therapeutic benefit less harm, vs. time from stroke onset; and the therapeutic window for a drug thus depends on the extent of benefit, the potential for harmful effects and the time at which utility function crosses the abscissa. AE, adverse effect.

Another possible approach that combines clinical and imaging criteria has not yet been fully evaluated. Diffusion-weighted imaging is relatively simple to perform on most clinically available MRI scanners. By contrast, perfusion-weighted imaging requires more complex software, higher field strengths and careful attention to injection technique. There are reasonable grounds for supposing that the clinical presentation of the patient will parallel the perfusion deficit that is still present and thus reasonable cause to assume that a mismatch between the clinical deficit and the diffusion-weighted image may be a suitable substitute for perfusion/diffusion mismatch.

Whilst time from stroke onset is a critical factor that will determine neuroprotective efficacy, the useful time window calculated from thrombolysis studies is not necessarily applicable to neuroprotection. The utility of a drug depends on its therapeutic benefit and the degree to which this is offset by adverse effects, i.e., harm (Figure 35.1). Whilst therapeutic benefit is probably greatest when the drug is administered early after onset of ischemia and then decays exponentially, harm may be a constant negative factor or may even increase as time from stroke onset elapses. For example, a drug that carries a small risk of an idiosyncratic allergic response is likely to produce this effect regardless of the time at which the drug is administered relative to stroke onset. In contrast, a drug that promotes intracerebral bleeding may be relatively safe at times when spontaneous hemorrhagic transformation is unlikely, e.g., within the first hour or two of stroke onset, but may be much more dangerous later when spontaneous transformation is occurring with a higher frequency. It is therefore conceivable that thrombolytic therapy will have utility only in the early hours after stroke onset, whereas a neuroprotectant drug with an excellent safety profile may continue to have a diminishing but still useful benefit several hours later. This is one of the reasons that the international IMAGES trial is testing magnesium not only within the first 6 hours but also within a group of patients treated between 6 and 12 hours after stroke onset [30,31]. Magnesium is neuroprotective in a range of animal models of cerebral ischemia, including models of white matter injury, it rapidly penetrates the brain in humans and has an excellent safety profile in elderly patients with cardiovascular disease, as evidenced by the ISIS-4 trial [32–48] (Y. Yang, Q. Li, F. Ahmad, A. Shuaib, unpublished data). Its low price and simplicity mean that even a small benefit would be highly cost effective and its safety profile suggests that it could readily be administered by less experienced health care workers including paramedical staff.

Selection criteria for trials are inevitably closely linked with the intended primary end-point. The strategy of excluding patients with mild or severe stroke could be taken to extreme, if the optimal population for a traditional end-point were to be chosen. Thus, if the measure of success within a trial is defined as the proportion of patients reaching a Barthel Index score of 95 to 100, or a Rankin Scale score of 0 to 1, then patients with moderate or severe stroke should all be excluded, along with very mildly affected patients. This dichotomization of functional scores is robust but relatively insensitive to change. Alternative choices of end-point are now being explored. These include stratified responses, where improvements are measured on a neurological score such as the National Institutes of Health Stroke Scale, and "success" requires a greater improvement for severely affected rather than mildly affected patients. Other trials have used dual measures of success: the GAIN trials employed a trichotomy analysis, with Barthel split 95 to 100, 60 to 90 and 0 to 55 [8].

A fifth criticism of existing clinical trials relates to confounding issues. There are numerous examples of phase II trials involving small numbers of patients, in which randomization has left important imbalances in prognostic variables between the treatment groups [17,48,49]. Such differences are likely to account for the apparent adverse effects of the higher dose and beneficial effects of the lower dose in the phase II study with lubeluzole [49]. They are also likely to account for the almost statistically significant trend in favor of placebo treatment within the overview of gavestinel phase II studies [50]. The neutral effect of gavestinel in most of the phase II studies [50] that was confirmed by both GAIN International [8] and GAIN Americas [29] was in striking contrast to the poorer outcome with gavestinel in the GAIN European phase II trial [48]. In this trial, death and disability occurred in 60 out of 86 patients treated with gavestinel vs. 14 out of 42 treated with the control. There were substantial imbalances in the baseline stroke severity and in the proportion of patients with primary intracerebral hemorrhage in the gavestinel vs. the control groups. The lesson was learned from these phase II trials, and GAIN

International used stratified randomization based on age and stroke severity, with the result that a near-perfect balance in prognostic variables was achieved. This led to a result of the trial that was considered unequivocal, though disappointingly neutral [8].

Stratification is suitable for controlling a limited number of variables, but block sizes become too small if multiple variables are involved, and treatment packaging and supply issues become a problem. Adaptive randomization can be used instead. This is a form of minimization in which a computer algorithm allocates patients to receive placebo or active treatment in a random manner, with adjustment according to the available prognostic information [51]. The algorithm may adjust on 12 or more factors simultaneously, ensuring that not only are individual factors balanced but that interactions between factors may also be considered. This approach improves study power as compared with simple stratification on only four factors, equivalent to a sample size increase of 8%, but more importantly assures that the result will not be confounded by a predictable flaw [52].

Other features that have not yet been adequately controlled within clinical trials include issues such as the approach to management of hypertension or hypotension [53–57], the management of blood sugar (which is strongly associated with outcome) [58,59] and pyrexia/infection, which again is profoundly associated with infarct volume in preclinical studies [60,61]. The likely effect of these variables, which in some cases may double mortality, would easily outweigh the therapeutic benefit that we are seeking with neuroprotective drugs. Perhaps it is salutary that the one trial that controlled blood pressure, albeit on an empirical basis, was the only trial to demonstrate significant improvement in functional outcome [24,55].

Certainly, protocols for clinical trials should stipulate that complications potentially caused by the drug under study must be actively managed. There are examples of adverse events occurring in patients participating in trials that have led to withdrawal of the patient from the trial and a Do Not Resuscitate order, at a stage when side effects of the drug may still be responsible (K.R.L., unpublished observation). Since some neuroprotectants have proven sedative or have psychotomimetic effects that can mimic stroke progression, this clearly is inappropriate. The glutamate receptor antagonist selfotel was associated with an increase in early brain deaths and development was abandoned [5,7]. Had this early mortality not been noted, an improvement in final death and disability may have occurred [7]. A known side effect of selfotel was early sedation with a time course that mimics stroke progression [17].

In summary, compounds selected for study in future stroke trials will have their efficacy tested in a range of preclinical models that will include effects on functional outcome and on white matter ischemia. Target concentrations will be defined on the basis of animal studies and only compounds that can be dosed to this level will

Table 35.2. Recent large neuroprotection programs assessed according to empirical criteria likely to contribute to success or failure

	pMCAO	External validation	Target concentration	Short time window	Brain PK	Stratified randomization	Confounding factors	Adequate power	Appropriate end-point	Result
Tirilazad	✗	✓	✓	✓?	✓	✗	✗	✓	✓	✗
Selfotel	✓	✓	✗	✓?	✗	✗	✗	✓	✓	✗
Aptiganel	✓	✓	✓	✓?	✓	✗	✗	✗	✓	✗
Lubeluzole	✓	✗	✗	✗?	✓	✗	✗	✓	?	✗
Clomethiazole	?	?	?	✗	✓	?	✗	✓	✓	?
GV150526	✓	✗?	✓	✓?	✗	✓	✗	✓	✓	✗

Notes:

✓, satisfies criteria; ✗, fails criteria; ?, uncertain/equivocal; PK, phosphokinase. Factors considered are preclinical testing in a permanent middle cerebral artery occlusion ischemia model (pMCAO); external validation of preclinical efficacy data, i.e., in an independent laboratory and different model; attainment in acute stroke of a target plasma or brain concentration expected from animal models to be neuroprotective; treatment within a short time window (maximum 6 hours); reasonable prospect of rapid penetration of brain by neuroprotectant or other reason to expect that it reaches the site of action; stratified randomization or other measure to assure balance in baseline prognostic variables between treatment groups; control of confounding factors such as concomitant medication, treatment of hemodynamic, metabolic and temperature regulation disturbances; study powered to detect an effect size of 5% or less; choice of functional end-point, with appropriate analysis; a positive trial result on the primary end-point.

reach later stage clinical trials. Modern statistical and modeling techniques will be used to identify the optimal clinical dose. Clinical trials, at least at the proof of concept stage, will use enrichment procedures to maximize the proportion of patients who can contribute to the scientific experiment testing therapeutic efficacy. Selection features will include time, presence of cortical symptoms and mismatch of either perfusion/diffusion imaging or between clinical symptoms and diffusion imaging. Outcome assessment will be based on more than one possible end-point. These will include growth of lesion assessed by MRI; patient-specific end-points adjusted according to the initial stroke severity or type; and, where scales such as the Barthel Index or Rankin Scale are categorized, use of a trichotomy rather than dichotomy analysis. Finally, greater degrees of control will be used within trials, involving stratified or adaptive randomization and measures to improve the consistency of management of concomitant medical conditions or complications. So far, whilst there is increasing evidence that NMDA antagonists may be ineffective in human stroke, no clinical development program has yet definitively tested its hypothesis as evidenced by Table 35.2. With these numerous potential improvements in clinical trial design and the improved attention to selection of candidate molecules, the prospects for identifying a useful neuroprotective drug remain good.

REFERENCES

1 Peters GR, Hwang L-J, Musch B, Brosse DM & Orgogozo JM (1996) Safety and efficacy of 6 mg/kg/day tirilazad mesylate in patients with acute ischemic stroke (TESS Study). *Stroke*, **27**, 195 (Abstract).

2 Diener H-C (1999) Lubeluzole in acute ischemic stroke treatment: lack of efficacy in a large phase III study with an 8-hour window. *Stroke*, **30**, 234 (Abstract).

3 Diener HC, for the European and Australian Lubeluzole Ischemic Stroke Study Group (1998) Multinational randomised controlled trial of lubeluzole in acute ischaemic stroke. *Cerebrovascular Diseases*, **8**, 172–81.

4 Grotta J, for the US and Canadian Lubeluzole Ischemic Stroke Study Group (1997) Lubeluzole treatment of acute ischemic stroke. *Stroke*, **28**, 2338–46.

5 Davis SM, Albers GW, Diener HC, Lees KR & Norris J (1997) Termination of acute stroke studies involving selfotel treatment: ASSIST Steering Committee. *Lancet*, **349**, 32.

6 Wahlgren NG, Ranasinha KW, Rosolacci T, Franke CL, van Erven PMM, Ashwood T & Claesson L, for the CLASS Study Group (1999) Clomethiazole Acute Stroke Study (CLASS). Results of a randomized, controlled trial of clomethiazole vs. placebo in 1360 acute stroke patients. *Stroke*, **30**, 21–8.

7 Davis SM, Lees KR, Albers GW, Diener HC, Markabi S, Karlsson G & Norris J, for the ASSIST Investigators (2000) Selfotel in acute ischemic stroke. Possible neurotoxic effects of an NMDA antagonist. *Stroke*, **31**, 347–54.

8 Lees KR, Asplund K, Carolei A, Davis SM, Diener H-C, Kaste M, Orgogozo J-M & Whitehead J, for the GAIN International Investigators (2000) Glycine antagonist (gavestinel) in neuroprotection (GAIN International) in patients with acute stroke: a randomised controlled trial. *Lancet*, **355**, 1949–54.

9 Schneider D, Berrouschot J, Brandt T, Hacke W, Ferbert A, Norris SH, Polmar SH & Schafer E (1998) Safety, pharmacokinetics and biological activity of enlimomab (anti-ICAM-1 antibody): an open-label, dose escalation study in patients hospitalized for acute stroke. *European Neurology*, **40**, 78–83.

10 Grotta JC (1994) The current status of neuronal protective therapy: why have all neuronal protective drugs worked in animals but none so far in stroke patients? *Cerebrovascular Diseases*, **4**, 115–20.

11 Muir KW & Grosset DG (1999) Neuroprotection for acute stroke. Making clinical trials work. *Stroke*, **30**, 180–2.

12 De Keyser J, Sulter G & Luiten PG (1999) Clinical trials with neuroprotective drugs in acute ischaemic stroke: are we doing the right thing? *Trends in Neurosciences*, **22**, 535–40.

13 Valeriani V, Dewar D & McCulloch J (2000) Quantitative assessment of ischemic pathology in axons, oligodendrocytes, and neurons: attenuation of damage after transient ischemia. *Journal of Cerebral Blood Flow & Metabolism*, **20**, 765–71.

14 Yam PS, Dunn LT, Graham DI, Dewar D & McCulloch J (2000) NMDA receptor blockade fails to alter axonal injury in focal cerebral ischemia. *Journal of Cerebral Blood Flow & Metabolism*, **20**, 772–9.

15 Stroke Therapy Academic Industry Roundtable (STAIR) (1999) Recommendations for standards regarding preclinical neuroprotective and restorative drug development. *Stroke*, **30**, 2752–8.

16 Steinberg GK, Pérez-Pinzón MA, Maier CM, Sun GH, Yoon E, Kunis DM, Bell TE, Powell M, Kotake A & Giffard R (1995) CGS-19755: correlation of in vitro neuroprotection, protection against experimental ischemia and CSF levels in cerebrovascular surgery patients. *Proceedings, 5th International Symposium on Pharmacology of Cerebral Ischemia*, Marburg, 20–22 July 1994, 28 (Abstract).

17 Grotta J, Clark W, Coull B, Pettigrew LC, Mackay B, Goldstein LB, Meissner I, Murphy D & LaRue L (1995) Safety and tolerability of the glutamate antagonist CGS 19755 (selfotel) in patients with acute ischemic stroke. Results of a phase IIa randomized trial. *Stroke*, **26**, 602–5.

18 Muir KW, Grosset DG, Gamzu E & Lees KR (1994) Pharmacological effects of the non-competitive NMDA antagonist CNS1102 in normal volunteers. *British Journal of Clinical Pharmacology*, **38**, 33–8.

19 Dyker AG, Edwards KR, Fayad PB, Hormes JT & Lees KR (1999) Safety and tolerability study of aptiganel hydrochloride in patients with an acute ischemic stroke. *Stroke*, **30**, 2038–42.

20 Ford GA & Freemantle N, on behalf of LUB-INT-13 Investigators (2000) Lubeluzole plasma concentrations and outcome in acute ischaemic stroke. *Cerebrovascular Diseases*, **10**, 78 (Abstract).

21 Hoke JF, Dyker AG, Barnaby R & Lees KR (2000) Pharmacokinetics of a glycine antagonist (gavestinel) following multiple dosing in patients with acute stroke. *European Journal of Clinical Pharmacology*, **55**, 867–72.

22 Squire IB, Lees KR, Pryse-Phillips W, Kertesz A & Bamford J (1996) The effects of lifarizine in acute cerebral infarction: a pilot safety study. *Cerebrovascular Diseases*, **6**, 156–60.

23 Malakoff D (1999) Bayes offers a 'new' way to make sense of numbers. *Science*, **286**, 1460–4.

24 The National Institute of Neurological Disorders and Stroke rtPA Stroke Study Group (1995) Tissue plasminogen activator for acute ischemic stroke. *New England Journal of Medicine*, **333**, 1581–7.

25 Hill MD & Hachinski V (1998) Stroke treatment: time is brain. *Lancet*, **352** Suppl 3, SIII10–SIII144.

26 Warach S, Boska M & Welch KMA (1997) Pitfalls and potential of clinical diffusion-weighted MR imaging in acute stroke. *Stroke*, **28**, 481–2.

27 Albers GW (1999) Expanding the window for thrombolytic therapy in acute stroke. The potential role of acute MRI for patient selection. *Stroke*, **30**, 2230–7.

28 Warach S, for the GAIN Americas and GAIN International MRI Investigators (1999) Recruitment in diffusion and perfusion MRI-based stroke drug trials: the GAIN MRI sub-study. *Annual Meeting of the American Society of Neuroradiology*, Atlanta, 2–8 April, 2000 (Abstract).

29 Sacco RL, DeRosa JT, Haley EC, Levin B, Ordonneau P, Phillips SJ, Rundek T, Snipes RG & Thompson JLP, for the GAIN Americas Investigators (2001) Glycine antagonist in neuroprotection for patients with acute stroke. GAIN Americas: a randomized controlled trial. *JAMA*, **285**, 1719–28.

30 Intravenous Magnesium Efficacy in Stroke Trial Study Group (1999) Intravenous magnesium efficacy in stroke trial (IMAGES). *Stroke*, **30**, 2259 (Abstract).

31 Bradford A, for the IMAGES Study Group (2000) Intravenous magnesium efficacy in stroke trial and MRI substudy (IMAGES & MR IMAGES). *Cerebrovascular Diseases*, **10**, 80 (Abstract).

32 Seelig JM, Wei EP, Kontos HA, Choi SC & Becker DP (1983) Effect of changes in magnesium ion concentration on cat cerebral arterioles. *American Journal of Physiology*, **245**, H22–H26.

33 Adams JH & Mitchell JR (1979) The effect of agents which modify platelet behaviour and of magnesium ions on thrombus formation in vivo. *Thrombosis & Haemostasis*, **42**, 603–10.

34 Marinov MB, Harbaugh KS, Hoopes PJ, Pikus HJ & Harbaugh R (1996) Neuroprotective effects of preischemia intraarterial magnesium sulfate in reversible focal cerebral ischemia. *Journal of Neurosurgery*, **85**, 117–24.

35 Smith DH, Okiyama K, Gennarelli TA & McIntosh TK (1993) Magnesium and ketamine attenuate cognitive dysfunction following experimental brain injury. *Neuroscience Letters*, **157**, 211–14.

36 McIntosh TK, Vink R, Yamakami I & Faden AI (1989) Magnesium protects against neurological deficit after brain injury. *Brain Research*, **482**, 252–60.

37 Blair JL, Warner DS & Todd MM (1989) Effects of elevated plasma magnesium vs. calcium on cerebral ischemic injury in rats. *Stroke*, **20**, 507–12.

38 Kass IS, Cottrell JE & Chambers G (1988) Magnesium and cobalt, not nimodipine, protect neurons against anoxic damage in the rat hippocampal slice. *Anesthesiology*, **69**, 710–15.

39 Thordstein M, Bagenholm R, Thiringer K & Kjellmer I (1993) Scavengers of free oxygen radicals in combination with magnesium ameliorate perinatal hypoxic–ischemic brain damage in the rat. *Pediatric Research*, **34**, 23–6.

40 Hallak M, Berman RF, Irtenkauf SM, Evans MI & Cotton DB (1992) Peripheral magnesium sulfate enters the brain and increases the threshold for hippocampal seizures in rats. *American Journal of Obstetrics & Gynecology*, **167**, 1605–10.

41 Ram Z, Sadeh M, Shacked I, Sahar A & Hadani M (1991) Magnesium sulfate reverses experimental delayed cerebral vasospasm after subarachnoid hemorrhage in rats. *Stroke*, **22**, 922–7.

42 Cox JA, Lysko PG & Henneberry RC (1989) Excitatory amino acid neurotoxicity at the N-methyl-D-aspartate receptor in cultured neurons: role of the voltage-dependent magnesium block. *Brain Research*, **499**, 267–72.

43 Favaron M & Bernardi P (1985) Tissue-specific modulation of the mitochondrial calcium uniporter by magnesium ions. *FEBS Letters*, **183**, 260–4.

44 Davies J & Watkins JC (1977) Effect of magnesium ions on the responses of spinal neurones to excitatory amino acids and acetylcholine. *Brain Research*, **130**, 364–8.

45 Thurnau GR, Kemp DB & Jarvis A (1987) Cerebrospinal fluid levels of magnesium in patients with preeclampsia after treatment with intravenous magnesium sulfate: a preliminary report. *American Journal of Obstetrics & Gynecology*, **157**, 1435–8.

46 ISIS-4 (Fourth International Study of Infarct Survival) Collaborative Group (1995) ISIS-4: a randomised factorial trial assessing early oral captopril, oral mononitrate, and intravenous magnesium sulphate in 58,050 patients with suspected acute myocardial infarction. *Lancet*, **345**, 669–85.

47 Muir KW & Lees KR (1995) A randomized, double-blind, placebo-controlled pilot trial of intravenous magnesium sulfate in acute stroke. *Stroke*, **26**, 1183–8.

48 Lees KR, Lavelle JF, Cunha L, Diener HC, Sanders EACM, Tack P, Wester P for the GAIN Phase II European Study Group (2001) Glycine antagonist (GV150526) in acute stroke: a double-blind placebo-controlled phase II trial. *Cerebrovascular Diseases*, **11**, 20–29.

49 Diener HC, Hacke W, Hennerici M, Rådberg J, Hantson L & De Keyser J, for the Lubeluzole International Study Group (1996) Lubeluzole in acute ischemic stroke. A double-blind, placebo-controlled phase II trial. *Stroke*, **27**, 76–81.

50 Lees KR, Haley EC, Warach S & Dyker AG (1999) GV150526: an overview of phase II studies in stroke patients. *Stroke*, **30**, 265 (Abstract).

51 Weir CJ & Lees KR (1998) Value of minimisation for treatment allocation in acute stroke trials. *Cerebrovascular Diseases*, **8**, 32 (Abstract).

52 Weir CJ & Lees KR (1999) Power of treatment allocation by adaptive stratification in an acute stroke trial. *Cerebrovascular Diseases*, **9**, 114 (Abstract).

53 Yatsu FM & Zivin J (1985) Hypertension in acute ischemic strokes. Not to treat. *Archives of Neurology*, **42**, 999–1000.

54 Rordorf G, Cramer SC, Efird JT, Schwamm LH, Buonanno F & Koroshetz WJ (1997) Pharmacological elevation of blood pressure in acute stroke. Clinical effects and safety. *Stroke*, **28**, 2133–8.

55 Brott T, Lu M, Kothari R, Fagan SC, Frankel M, Grotta JC, Broderick J, Kwiatkowski T, Lewandowski C, Haley EC Jr, Marler JR & Tilley BC, for the NINDS rtPA Stroke Study Group

(1998) Hypertension and its treatment in the NINDS rtPA stroke trial. *Stroke*, **29**, 1504–9.

56 Potter JF (1999) What should we do about blood pressure and stroke? *Quarterly Journal of Medicine*, **92**, 63–6.

57 Saxena R, Wijnhoud AD, Koudstaal PJ & van den Meiracker AH, on behalf of the DCLHb in Acute Stroke Study (2000) Induced elevation of blood pressure in the acute phase of ischemic stroke in humans. *Stroke*, **31**, 546–8 (Letter).

58 Weir CJ, Murray GD, Dyker AG & Lees KR (1997) Is hyperglycaemia an independent predictor of poor outcome after acute stroke? Results of a long term follow up study. *British Medical Journal*, **314**, 1303–6.

59 Kiers L, Davis SM, Larkins R, Hopper J, Tress B, Rossiter SC, Carlin J & Ratnaike S (1992) Stroke topography and outcome in relation to hyperglycaemia and diabetes. *Journal of Neurology, Neurosurgery & Psychiatry*, **55**, 263–70.

60 Castillo J, Martinez F, Leira R, Prieto JM, Lema M & Noya M (1994) Mortality and morbidity of acute cerebral infarction related to temperature and basal analytic parameters. *Cerebrovascular Diseases*, **4**, 66–71.

61 Reith J, Jorgensen HS, Pedersen PM, Nakayama H, Raaschou HO, Jeppesen LL & Olsen TS (1996) Body temperature in acute stroke: relation to stroke severity, infarct size, mortality, and outcome. *Lancet*, **347**, 422–5.

62 The RANTTAS Investigators (1996) A randomized trial of tirilazad mesylate in patients with acute stroke (RANTTAS). *Stroke*, **27**, 1453–8.

63 Lees KR, Sharma AK, Barer D, Ford GA, Kostulas V & Chen Y-F and for the SA-NXY-003 Investigators (2001) Tolerability and pharmacokinetics of the nitrone NXY-059 in patients with acute stroke. *Stroke*, **32**, 675–680.

64 Jiang N, Moyle M, Soule HR, Rote WE & Chopp M (1995) Neutrophil inhibitory factor is neuroprotective after focal ischemia in rats. *Annals of Neurology*, **38**, 935–42.

36

Basic research and stroke therapeutics: what have we learned?

Justin A. Zivin

Department of Neurosciences, University of California, San Diego, CA

Although there now is a generally accepted method for acute stroke therapy in patients, we have encountered many problems in developing additional ones in the last few years. Only one treatment has been unequivocally proven to be beneficial; thrombolytic therapy with tissue plasminogen activator (tPA) is effective in reducing neurological damage with adequate safety. Two other clinical trials have also produced positive results. These were studies of prourokinase, which is also a thrombolytic, and ancrod, which reduces fibrinogen levels and may have some thrombolytic properties. Neither of these treatments has yet been approved by regulatory agencies for treatment of stroke victims.

At the time of writing, all clinical trials of neuroprotective agents have failed to provide clear evidence of reduction in neurological injury. Table 36.1 provides a list of many of these drugs. There are probably a number of reasons for the difficulties that were encountered. Examination of the successful trials, as contrasted with the failures, may give us some insight into how to better design future studies. The National Institutes of Health (NIH) tPA trial [1] was the only unambiguously successful trial. There was approximately a 50% relative risk improvement in neurological function recovery when the scales were dichotomized to unimpaired vs. impaired, and there was not an increase in adverse outcomes (including death). A critical feature of the NIH tPA trial was that all of the patients were treated within 180 minutes after onset of systems, and half of the subjects were treated within 90 minutes.

Three studies exploring longer time windows for tPA therapy were conducted. In the European Cooperative Acute Stroke Study I (ECASS I) [2], the patients were treated within 6 hours after symptom onset, but less than 20% of the patients were treated during the first 3 hours. In that study, there was no overall improvement in neurological function. There were, however, a large number of protocol violations, predominantly caused by difficulties that the investigators had in recognizing early signs of large infarcts on the initial computed tomography scans (absence of, or

Table 36.1. Recent failed drug development programs

Fibroblast growth factor II
CDP-choline
Heparinoid
Glutamate antagonists
Fosphenytoin
Intracellular adhesion molecule antibody
Lubeluzole
Nalmefene
Tirilazad

Notes:
CDP, cytosine diphosphate.

only small, lesions were a required entry criterion). When these patients were removed as part of a secondary analysis, the results favored benefit with tPA therapy. Also, if the NIH trial criteria for improvement had been employed in the ECASS I trial, the results also might have been positive [3]. However, these are retrospective analyses and inadequate to provide proof of benefit. Subsequently, a second ECASS trial (ECASS II) was conducted [4]. Several changes were made in the protocol from the ECASS I trial. The most important were that the patients with large early infarct signs were not eligible for entry into the trial and the investigators were better trained to recognize them. This procedure decreased the average degree of stroke severity sustained by the patients who were enrolled in this trial. Again, although the treatment window was 0 to 6 hours, over 80% of the patients were treated 3 to 6 hours after symptom onset. The results of ECASS II did not demonstrate efficacy of tPA when treatment was administered more than 3 hours after stroke onset. Conversely, there was no evidence that the patients were harmed by the tPA treatment. The fraction of patients who developed symptomatic intra-cerebral hemorrhages increased in the tPA-treated cohort, but it appears that this was simply a conversion of severe ischemic strokes into hemorrhages, since there was no overall increase in poor outcomes or mortality. A second possible reason for the failure of thrombolytic therapy efficacy in ECASS II was that the patients had, on the average, less severe strokes, so the placebo group had a much higher rate of spontaneous recovery than had been observed in previous studies. Thus any benefit that tPA may have provided was probably obscured by this ceiling effect.

The third trial, the Alteplase Thrombolysis for Acute Noninterventional Therapy in Ischemic Stroke (ATLANTIS) study, was conducted in the United States and Canada [5]. Inclusion and exclusion criteria virtually identical to those of the

ECASS II trial were used and the time window was 3 to 5 hours after symptom onset. No significant benefit was shown. However, as in the ECASS studies, patients who were treated beyond the 3 hour window were not harmed, despite the increased symptomatic intracerebral hemorrhage rate. Again, the hemorrhages were counterbalanced by a decrease in the rate of infarctions so that there was no net increase in poor outcomes.

The Prolyse in Acute Cerebral Thromboembolism (PROACT) study was the first in which thrombolytic therapy was administered intra-arterially to stroke victims [6]. The time window for this study was 0 to 6 hours after symptom onset and nearly all of the patients were treated beyond the 3 hour time period. The results showed an improvement in neurological outcome in these patients, although the degree of improvement was not as large as in the intravenous tPA trial. The patients did sustain increased intracerebral hemorrhages, but again, not at the expense of increased poor outcomes. Large numbers of patients were screened in order to obtain the sample examined in this trial and only 180 patients were ultimately randomized. As a consequence, when the results were presented to the Food and Drug Administration, the agency requested a confirmatory study. One possible reason that this trial showed positive results was that the thrombolytic agent was administered intra-arterially. A relatively high dose of the drug was concentrated at the site of the vascular occlusion and this substantially accelerated the rate of clot lysis. Therefore the time of vessel reopening may not have differed appreciably from that produced by intravenous drug studies. In other words, the increased speed of clot lysis compensated for the time lost in conducting the intra-arterial procedure.

The other drug that was found to be effective in reducing neurological damage is ancrod, which is Malaysian pit viper venom. Recently published results show a 16% relative risk improvement in neurological function outcome [7]. The rate of intracranial hemorrhages increased 2.5 times, but the death rate did not change. Therefore, it is possible that the drug produces less symptomatic intracranial hemorrhages than tPA. An important aspect of this trial was that, aside from the NIH tPA trial, it was the only one that was placebo controlled and required treatment initiation within 3 hours after symptom onset. This again supports the need for rapid commencement of therapy. It is important to note that all of the neuroprotective studies used treatment windows that exceeded 3 hours in duration.

There are a number of lessons that can be drawn from the development programs that have been completed. In nearly all instances, the treatments that ultimately were tested in clinical trials showed positive results in preclinical animal studies. Therefore, the question arises as to how valid animal models are for predicting the outcomes of human trials for acute stroke. Re-examination of the preclinical literature shows that there were important differences between the preclinical studies and the subsequent clinical trials in most cases. In many instances, preclinical data were inadequate. Some animal models were used that do not simulate the human problem. Treatment was administered either before the onset of ischemia or within a few minutes after vascular occlusion. This is not possible in stroke patients. Doses of drugs used in animal models often markedly differed from those administered to the stroke patients. In some investigations, the drug doses that were given to the animals were substantially higher than those that were ultimately used in the human trials. In these cases the patients were unable to tolerate high doses due to side effects that did not produce excessive difficulties in the animal models. For example, N-methyl-D-aspartate-type glutamate antagonists cause psychiatric side effects in patients, so in all of the human trials, the doses were lowered to levels that did not cause severe reactions. As a consequence, the blood levels attained in many human trials were approximately an order of magnitude less than efficacious levels in the animal models. In other instances, it is entirely possible that the drug doses that were administered to the patients were either too high or continued for too long. In all of the animal studies, treatments were administered for relatively brief periods of time, whereas in some clinical trials, patients received a drug for days or even weeks. For example, this was true of the intracellular adhesion molecule antibody program. The discrepancies between the clinical trials and the preclinical model studies may well explain some of the differences in the ultimate results.

The issue of the time window for therapy appears to be crucial. There are, at present, no unequivocal data from human studies as to the maximum duration of ischemia that the human brain can withstand. The reason is that current technology does not make it possible to identify when cerebral circulation is restored. No methods exist to continuously monitor the status of most occluded vessels; we cannot therefore establish the precise relationship between duration of ischemia and extent of neurological injury. Figure 36.1 provides the only available primate data relevant to this question. Jones et al. [8] published a study that appeared in 1981 in which the effects of ischemia on cerebral damage was evaluated in macaque monkeys. The animals were anesthetized and an externally accessible occlusion devise was implanted around the middle cerebral artery. The animals were permitted to recover from the surgery and then the vessels were occluded for prespecified periods from 15 minutes to 3 hours or permanently. The neurological function was rated and measurements of regional cerebral blood flow and histopathology were performed. I recalculated the results to attempt to quantify the critical periods of ischemia associated with various degrees of neurological dysfunction. Using the histological end-points, the data analysis revealed that greater than 95% recovery occurred when there was an average of 19.5 minutes of ischemia. There was a greater than 95% chance of no recovery when blood flow was restored after 398 minutes. The average duration of ischemia that produced damage in 50% of the

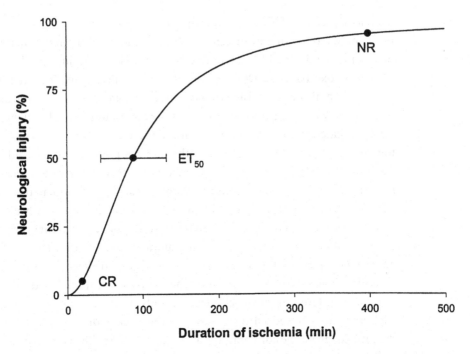

Figure 36.1   The neuropathological data from the paper by Jones et al. [8] was used to generate this figure. In this instance, the neurological damage is the percentage of monkeys exhibiting infarcts of any size. CR is the maximum duration of ischemia compatible with complete recovery. NR is the minimum time for no recovery. ET_{50} represents the duration of ischemia that results in half-maximal damage. The error bar is the standard error at ET_{50}. (From ref. 10.)

animals (ET_{50}) was 88.2 ± 43.2 minutes ($\pm$ standard error). These are reasonable results. A good deal of clinical literature obtained from asphyxia or drowning accidents suggests that irreversible brain damage occurs in people who are subjected to less than 20 minutes of loss of oxygen in the brain. The idea that there may be something to salvage up to 6 hours after symptom onset is suggested by this data analysis and is in accord with a fair number of other animal model studies. Also, as shown in the curve, approximately 75% of maximum damage occurs by 200 minutes after vessel occlusion. This suggests that it would be very difficult to show restoration of function produced by thrombolysis in patients who have suffered vascular occlusion that lasts for more than approximately 3 hours. This is in concordance with the results of the clinical trials mentioned previously. Another clear implication of this data analysis is that the optimal time for studying potential therapeutic agents is treatment at approximately 90 minutes after symptom onset. This is approximately the ET_{50} and this point has the lowest variance on the curve. Studies that average treatment at this duration of ischemia will require the smallest number of patients, since shorter durations of ischemia will increase the number of patients that spontaneously recover, and longer durations of ischemia increase the likelihood that the patients will suffer irreversible damage.

It is now reasonable to attempt to synthesize these lessons and design future studies that are likely to increase the chances of success. Thrombolytic therapy has been shown to be effective and there are ways to improve the efficacy of clot lysis. If drugs can be identified that increase the rate of thrombolysis, they are likely to improve efficacy. Vessel reopening can be facilitated by (i) drugs that dissolve clots more rapidly than currently available agents, (ii) implementation of intra-arterial techniques that increase the concentration of thrombolytic agents at the clot site, or (iii) injecting the substance using mechanical devices that permit increased penetration of the drug into the clot. Techniques that reopen the vessel by a variety of mechanical means such as ultrasound probes or stents may provide alternative methods for reopening vessels that cannot be adequately treated with intravenous therapies. Of course, intra-arterial techniques delay the time from vascular occlusion to vessel reopening because the occlusion site has to be identified and the device inserted into the appropriate location. Another problem is that intra-arterial therapy will markedly increase the cost due to the requirement for specialized equipment and the presence of appropriately trained therapists. Furthermore, the duration of time that the brain can tolerate ischemia will continue to be an important limitation and such therapies will necessarily have to be initiated within 6 hours after vascular occlusion.

A second technique that may improve the outcome of clinical trials is better patient selection. The tPA trials were unable to define additional exclusion criteria that might determine a subset of patients who would be harmed by therapy. Conversely, aside from the 3 hour time limit, no subset was found that was especially likely to benefit from tPA treatment. It is, however, quite probable that there are important differences amongst patients regarding the degree of benefit that can be derived from thrombolytic therapy. We have been unable to find clinical factors that specify such patients, but it is possible that various types of imaging technique will be useful. Identification of patients who are more likely to benefit may also reduce the risk of complications. However, at the present time, imaging techniques have not been shown to be useful in patient trials. The studies required to prove the validity of these new methods will be time consuming because it is necessary to show that the imaging technique is effective and better than the currently available clinical methods.

A third new approach to stroke therapy would be to find treatments that reduce the consequences of intracerebral hemorrhaging. Such hemorrhages are the principle complication of thrombolytic therapies and, at the present time, we have no treatment for primary intracerebral hemorrhages. It is possible that neuroprotective therapies can reduce the ischemic damage that is associated with rupture of intra-cerebral vessels and some treatments may decrease the size or frequency of hemor-rhages [9].

Finally, since thrombolytic therapy already has been proven to be effective, future studies will be required to include combination therapy designs. It is possible that thrombolysis plus neuroprotective agents will increase the efficacy of the combina-tion because thrombolysis will provide improved access of the neuroprotective agent to the threatened tissue. Alternatively, neuroprotectives may increase the time window for administration of thrombolysis. However, combined therapy studies increase the complexities of trial designs.

In summary, acute stroke therapy has finally arrived. Unfortunately, we have had many more trial failures than successes and thrombolysis with tPA remains the only treatment approved by the Food and Drug Administration. The short time window and perceived dangers of this type of treatment have limited the number of patients who have received it. Conclusions can be drawn from the studies that have failed to show improved neurological outcome and our successes are reasonably consistent with our understanding of the disease process. It is now time to utilize this infor-mation to guide our preclinical studies to better predict clinical circumstances and to suggest new methodologies for the next generation of clinical trials.

REFERENCES

1 The National Institute of Neurological Disorders; Stroke rtPA Stroke Study Group (1995) Tissue plasminogen activator for acute ischemic stroke. *New England Journal of Medicine*, 333, 1581–7.

2 Hacke W, Kaste M, Fieschi C, Toni D, Lesaffre E, von Kummer R, Boysen G, Bluhmki E, Hoxter G, Mahagne M-H & Hennerici M (1995) Intravenous thrombolysis with recombinant tissue plasminogen activator for acute hemispheric stroke. The European Cooperative Acute Stroke Study (ECASS). *Journal of the American Medical Association*, 274, 1017–25.

3 Hacke W, Bluhmki E, Steiner T, Tatlisumak T, Mahagne M-H, Sacchetti ML & Meier D (1998) Dichotomized efficacy end points and global end-point analysis applied to the ECASS inten-tion-to-treat data set. Post hoc analysis of ECASS I. *Stroke*, 29, 2073–5.

4 Hacke W, Kaste M, Fieschi C, von Kummer R, Davalos A, Meier D, Larrue V, Bluhmki E, Davis S, Donnan G, Schneider D, Diez-Tejedor E & Trouillas P (1998) Randomised double-blind placebo-controlled trial of thrombolytic therapy with intravenous alteplase in acute ischaemic stroke (ECASS II). *Lancet*, 352, 1245–51.

5 Clark WM, Wissman S, Albers GW, Jhamandas JH, Madden KP & Hamilton S (1999) Recombinant tissue-type plasminogen activator (Alteplase) for ischemic stroke 3 to 5 hours after symptom onset: The ATLANTIS Study: a randomized controlled trial. *Journal of the American Medical Association*, 282, 2019–26.

6 Furlan A, Higashida R, Wechsler L, Gent M, Rowley H, Kase C, Pessin M, Ahuja A, Callahan F, Clark WM, Silver F, Rivera F, for the PROACT Investigators (1999) Intra-arterial prourokinase for acute ischemic stroke: the PROACT II study: A randomized controlled trial. *Journal of the American Medical Association*, **282**, 2003–11.

7 Sherman DG, Atkinson RP, Chippendale T, Levin KA, Ng K, Futrell N, Hsu CY & Levy DE (2000) Intravenous ancrod for treatment of acute ischemic stroke: the STAT study: a randomized controlled trial. *Journal of the American Medical Association*, **283**, 2395–403.

8 Jones TH, Morawetz RB, Crowell RM, Marcoux FW, FitzGibbon SJ, DeGirolami U & Ojemann RG (1981) Thresholds of focal cerebral ischemia in awake monkeys. *Journal of Neurosurgery*, **54**, 773–82.

9 Hu B, Liu C & Zivin JA (1999) Reduction of intracerebral hemorrhaging in a rabbit embolic stroke model. *Neurology*, **53**, 2140–5.

10 Zivin JA (1998) Factors determining the therapeutic window for Stroke. *Neurology*, **50**, 599–603.

Index

Numbers in *italics* indicate *tables* or *figures*; 'p' indicates a plate.